Researches
in
SEPARATION
ANXIETY

Henry G. Hansburg, PhD is former (1955–1976) senior psychological consultant, psychotherapist, and research associate of the Jewish Child Care Association in New York City. From 1949 to 1955, he was professor of psychology and chief psychologist of the Education Clinic at Brooklyn College. From 1935–1943, he was a psychologist in the Bureau of Child Guidance in New York City and, from 1943 to 1949, chief psychologist for the Borough of Brooklyn in that agency. From 1932 to 1935, he was a psychological consultant in a probationary school for boys.

As a consultant to many centers in the 1940s, Dr. Hansburg made special contributions to the Child Study Association of America and to the Brooklyn Association for Mental Hygiene. He was one of the organizers of the Brooklyn Psychological Association, served two years on the Executive Board of the Clinical Division of the New York State Psychological Association, and, from 1963 to 1965, was actively involved on the New York City Mental Health Planning Commission. During World War II, he served as examiner of draftees, and, in 1945–1946, he created the German Attitude Scale for a special commission of the U.S. State Department, headed by Dr. Margaret Mead.

Dr. Hansburg has authored numerous articles in educational and psychological journals and is best known for his creation of the Separation Anxiety Test, publishing two previous volumes on this subject. He received the Distinguished Service Award from the Brooklyn Psychological Association and in recent years has been a Visiting Professor at the California School of Professional Psychology in Los Angeles.

RESEARCHES
IN
SEPARATION
ANXIETY

A Third Volume on the Separation Anxiety Test

Henry G. Hansburg

ROBERT E. KRIEGER PUBLISHING COMPANY

Original Edition 1986

Published by
ROBERT E. KRIEGER PUBLISHING COMPANY, INC.
KRIEGER DRIVE
MALABAR, FLORIDA 32950

Printed in the United States of America

Library of Congress Cataloging-in-Publication Data
(Revised for vol. 3)

Hansburg, Henry G., 1910-
    Adolescent separation anxiety.

    Vol. 1 was first published in 1972 under title: Adolescent separation anxie-
ty; a method for the study of adolescent separation problems.
    Vol. 3: "Separation anxiety test."
    Bibliography: v. 1, p. 141-146; v. 2, p. [191]-193.
    Includes indexes.
    Contents: v. 1. A method for the study of adolescent separation problems.
— v. 2. Separation disorders. — v. 3. Researches in separation anxiety.
        1. Separation anxiety in children—Collected works.
        2. Separation (Psychology)—Collected works
        3. Separation Anxiety Test—Collected works.
        4. Adolescent psychology—Collected works.
        I. Title. II. Title: Separation anxiety test.
BF724.3.S38H35   1980   616.8'522   79-21798
ISBN 0-89874-042-8 (Vol. 1)
ISBN 0-89874-043-6 (Vol. 2)
ISBN 0-89874-973-5 (Vol. 3)

10 9 8 7 6 5 4 3 2

This volume is dedicated to the students and faculty of the California School of Professional Psychology, whose ceaseless interest in researching the areas of attachment, separation, and loss has won my sincere appreciation, admiration, and respect.

CONTENTS

FOREWORD

In the last ten years growing interest and widening investigation into those human behaviors coming under such designations as bonding, separation, reunion, loss, etc., whether viewed from perspectives of object relations or Bowlby's attachment theory, have made evident the need for a method of appraising subjects' current personality vulnerability to separation and loss. In the last five or six years indications have appeared that the potential of Henry Hansburg's method, known as the Separation Anxiety Test, to fill that need is being realized and is certainly being put to the test. This volume will better enable those interested to determine how well and in what ways the Separation Anxiety Test is indeed capable of filling that need.

On a note more of acknowledgment and appreciation, since 1978, when Dr. Pauline DeLozier put me in touch with his work, Dr. Hansburg has proven of inestimable value and unflagging assistance to graduate students and faculty at many graduate training settings in psychology, CSPP-LA among them.

Over these years Dr. Hansburg has conducted workshops and conferences at many academic and clinical centers, including CSPP, on the Separation Anxiety Test's design and development, the theories underlying it, the evidence it rests upon, and potential contributions to clinical diagnosis and research endeavors. Studies completed at CSPP-LA alone, including the Separation Anxiety Test as a measure, have investigated a wide variety of interrelated clinical and social problems, such as the origins of child abuse, the structure of marital relationships, the effects of divorce on children, patients exploited by their psychotherapists, sources of fear of death in college students, father-son relationships, battered women, schizophrenic young adults, fears of children and mothers in the hospital, personality factors predisposing children to prostitution, and the mother's role in father-daughter incest. In a large number of these studies, inclusion of the Separation Anxiety Test as a predictive measure has contributed in major and insightful ways to the studies' outcomes.

For his warm friendship, for his scientific achievement, for his

ready availability and thoughtful responsiveness in consultation with
graduate students or faculty, whether in person, by mail, or by long-
distance telephone, for his sharing in a common affinity, for his asking
of rare questions that probe beyond common and popular answers, we
will always be in his debt.

KARL E. POTTHARST
February 1985

PREFACE

The current volume is a follow-up to two previous volumes entitled *Adolescent Separation Anxiety*. Its purpose is to provide a compendium of researches with the Separation Anxiety Test which were not reported in either of the previous volumes, and to carry the scope of the research into preadolescent childhood and stages of adulthood.

Researches using the test method of studying human reactions to separation have burgeoned. This volume is only representative of them and cannot possibly encompass them all. I have tried to indicate the use of the method at various stages of the life cycle and in the understanding of varying human problems. The research has addressed many aspects of the effect of separations on human character, feelings, thoughts, and behavior and is, of course, never-ending. I have included an introduction which I hope will prove to be of some use in interpreting and understanding what follows. I have also presented a Summary of what the researches have contributed to our understanding.

This volume was first planned in 1980 and is now long overdue. It was originally meant for university graduate students who were searching for additional literature and research to assist them in the formulation of their hypotheses with regard to human separation problems. While much of this literature is listed in various abstracts, the original works have not been available to them. By bringing the material together, I hope that the book will serve a real purpose to both university students and their graduate professors.

Nearly all of the graduate research papers are summaries which I have written myself with the permission of the researchers. I have done this to relieve them of the burden and also to be able to highlight certain factors in the research. The special section on adaptations of the Separation Anxiety Test has been provided to demonstrate how it is possible to adapt the method for varied ages and problem situations. And for purposes of completeness I do not wish to ignore the several attempts to provide foreign-language translations of the test. The first was in Hebrew, made at the author's request in 1972 by a rabbi specializing in psychology. An attempt was made to arrange for a study to make comparisons of adolescents raised in the Israeli kibbutzim with those raised in their own homes. Unfortunately, numerous priorities of the Department of Education in Israel prevented the attempt at investigation. A more successful result attended the efforts of Marjorie C. Mitchell at a translation into Spanish. This was used in a study of maternal child abuse in the Mexican-American community in Los Angeles and is included in this volume in the Appendix. Finally, of my own papers, which are presented in full, three have not been published previously.

HENRY G. HANSBURG
January 1985

ACKNOWLEDGMENTS

The cooperation of many psychologists has made this volume possible. First and foremost, my sincere gratitude goes to Professor Karl E. Pottharst, coordinator of graduate programs in the field of attachment theory at the Los Angeles branch of the California School of Professional Psychology. He organized seminars at the school and invited me to present current data of a clinical and research nature. He continuously informed me of all new studies in the graduate program and encouraged students to undertake studies of various aspects of separation and attachment with a view to learning more about the Separation Anxiety Test as well. His constant willingness to pursue any meaningful approach to the problems discussed in this volume has earned my sincere respect. I know that he is writing a book that will include all of the researches in attachment, separation, and loss which have been conducted at the school, and I wish him well in this undertaking.

I would like to thank all of the psychologists who made it possible for me to obtain the dissertations which are included in this book. I am especially indebted to Dr. Pauline DeLozier, whose initial work with the Separation Anxiety Test sparked many other researches and who gave so much of her time and effort to other psychologists who undertook work in this area. I also thank those psychologists who devised new methods of presentation, scoring, and interpretation of the Separation Anxiety Test. These include Dr. Christine Duplak, Dr. Lynn M. Varela, Dr. Marjorie Mitchell, Dr. Nancy Brody, and Dr. Donald Burger. My further thanks go to Dr. Joyce Miller, Dr. Thomas Kaleita, Dr. Anne-Marie Kelly, Dr. Michael Sherry, Dr. Ellen Levitz, Dr. Pauline Schwartz, Dr. Arlene Noble, Dr. Peter C. Fisk, and Dr. Hugh Black for their willingness to participate in this project. I am greatly indebted to Dr. Black for his study of the reliability of the Separation Anxiety Test and his subsequent recommendations. The affiliations of these and other researchers important to the work reflected in this volume are listed on pages xvii-xviii.

My thanks go to a group of social workers at the Jewish Child Care

Association prior to 1975 who aided the author in working with the case records of the families involved. By this date, most of these workers have either retired or gone to other agencies. Considerable assistance was provided by clerks in the case library, as well as the librarians of the Psychiatric Clinic.

I am especially grateful to Mrs. Hazel Schnurr, a graduate student, for her collection of data in the study of the elderly in a number of the institutions discussed in the chapter dealing with that subject. Dr. George Train, psychiatrist and psychoanalytic psychotherapist, was instrumental in assisting her in working at the Maimonides Hospital Geriatric Center. I am indebted to Dr. Stephanie Warshall, who did the examination and studies of the elderly patients at the Kingsbrook Medical Center. With the kind assistance of my wife, Rose Hansburg, who was engaged in occupational art therapy with the elderly, I was able to study the elderly men and women at the Ocean Parkway Jewish Center in Brooklyn.

I am further indebted to Christine Duplak for her assistance in the examination of youngsters in the Psychiatric Clinic at the Jewish Child Care Association.

Thanks also go to Dr. Arye Rohn, principal of the East Midwood Day School, who made it possible to examine the mothers of the five-year-olds in the kindergarten. I also wish to express my gratitude to the mothers who willingly submitted to interviews and testing at the school.

I thank the *British Journal of Projective Psychology and Personality Study* for permission to reprint the paper by Klagsbrun and Bowlby. I also thank Dr. Duplak, Dr. Varela, Dr. Brody, Dr. Burger and Dr. Mitchell for permission to reprint their techniques. Further thanks go to Dr. D.V. Siva Sankar and PJD Publications Limited, Westbury, N.Y., for permission to reprint one of my own papers published in *Mental Health in Childhood*, Volume III, in 1976.

I am continually mindful of the encouragement that I received from Dr. John Bowlby to continue the explorations represented by the studies in this volume. His work has always been an inspiration to me, and I shall be progressively mindful of his theoretical formulations. Wherever possible, I have made an effort to expand on his concepts and to develop them further in an effort to locate new truths in hidden corners.

H.G.H.

PARTICIPATING RESEARCHERS

Black, Hugh (Ph.D.). Clinical Director of Intermountain Deaconess Home for Children, a treatment center for disturbed children, Helena, Montana.

Bowlby, John (M.D., F.R.C.P., F.R.C. Psych.). Emeritus Chairman, Staff Committee, School of Family Psychiatry and Community Mental Health, Tavistock Institute of Human Relations, London. Honorary Consultant Psychiatrist, Tavistock Clinic, London.

Brody, Nancy (Ph.D.). Former instructor in Educational Psychology at Loyola University, Chicago; formerly instructor in Child Development, De Paul University, Chicago.

Burger, Donald (Ph.D.). Clinical Psychologist, private practice, San Diego.

DeLozier, Pauline P. (Ph.D.). Clinical Psychologist, Ross Loos Medical Group, Dept. of Mental Health, West Covina, Calif.; Research Associate, Child and Family Development Program, Children's Institute, Los Angeles.

Duplak, Christine (Ph.D.). Psychologist, Reading Laboratory, Cedarhurst, N.Y.; Psychologist, Reading Laboratory, Great Neck, N.Y.

Fisk, Peter C. (Ph.D.). Psychologist, La Puente Valley Community Mental Health Center, La Puente, Calif.

Kaleita, Thomas (Ph.D.). Assistant Clinical Professor of Pediatrics, Division of Pediatric Neurology, University of California at Los Angeles Medical Center.

Kelly, Anne-Marie C. (Ph.D.). Senior Staff Psychologist, St. John's Hospital and Health Center, Child Study Center, Santa Monica, Calif.; Clinical Assistant Professor, Fuller Graduate School of Psychology, Pasadena, Calif.

Klagsbrun, Michelle (M.A.). Graduate of Tavistock Institute, London. Current address unknown.

Levitz-Jones, Ellen (Ph.D.). Graduate of University of Missouri, St. Louis. Psychological Consultant, Head Start Program, St. Louis (Webster Groves), Missouri.

Miller, Joyce B. (Ph.D.). Assistant Clinical Professor, University of California at Los Angeles School of Nursing, Community Mental Health; private practice, Westwood Village, Calif.

Mitchell, Marjorie C. (Ph.D.) Former Supervisor in Children's Services, Los Angeles County Dept. of Mental Health; private practice, Long Beach, Calif.

Noble, Arlene S. Psychologist, Mt. Zion Hospital, San Francisco Crisis Clinic; private practice, El Cerrito Counseling Associates, El Cerrito, Calif.

Schwartz, Pauline K. (Ph.D.). Assistant Professor, Dept. of Psychology, California State University, Northbridge; Co-director, Omega Center for Mental Health, Woodland Hills, Calif; Psychologist lecturer, Sirkin Institute, Encino, Calif.

Sherry, Michael (Ph.D.). Psychologist, McClean Hospital; Instructor, Harvard Medical School; private practice, Holyoke, Mass.; Director of Psychology Training, McClean/Northhampton Program.

Varela, Lynn M. (Ph.D.). Private practice in Clinical Psychology, Woodland Hills, Calif. Former predoctoral intern in Pediatric Psychology, School of Medicine, University of California, Los Angeles.

INTRODUCTION

Research begins with the need for an answer to a problem. The need may be derived from either social pressure, crisis, scientific curiosity, intellectual exercise, or perhaps some idiosyncratic creative impulse. Whatever it may be, the researcher regards what is being done as a search for truth. But truth has many aspects and, if pursued, may become highly elusive. The dictionary defines truth as "fact or facts; matter or circumstance as it really is—a fixed or established principle, law, etc; proven doctrine; verified hypothesis; a basic scientific truth." However, as Thomas Huxley said, "It is the customary fate of new truths to begin as heresies and to end as superstitions"; and, as Bernard Shaw said, "All great truths begin as blasphemies."

Truth depends upon the observation of the viewer, the circumstances of viewing, and the viewing tools. Its variability is enormous and almost infinite in its possibilities. To be a valid observation, it must be verifiable and capable of replication by others. Thus, if a consensus is formed about an observation by various viewers under similar viewing circumstances and with similar viewing tools, it is established as valid; it becomes a truth.

But it may be that, for some reason, it does not have this established validity; nevertheless, it may have some truth under circumstances that are further limited and very difficult to determine. Truth is so complicated that often only minor aspects of truth are uncovered and major truths remain hidden. In the basic sciences, such as chemistry or physics, there are laws governing the various reactions which occur under different degrees of temperature and pressure.

However, psychology as a science is far more complicated than the basic sciences. Therefore, the combinations of viewer, viewing circumstances, and viewing tools are extraordinarily varied, more subject to error, and more difficult to validate because of the problems involved in all of the aspects of viewing. Even when a degree of validation is obtained, the problem of replication and, therefore, reliability is more complicated because variations occur in viewer observations, circumstances, and tools during any given experiment at any other point in time. For these reasons human behavioral patterns may, to some degree, be unpredictable from one set of conditions to another, even when the tools, the viewer, and the major circumstances are apparently held constant. Very few individuals or populations are exactly the same, and no matter how strict the viewer, variations in results are bound to occur. Furthermore, even the same individual varies in reactions to similar circumstances at different times and places and under different physical states.

This problem becomes even more difficult when we consider the variations in the manner of usage of any given psychological tool by the same viewer at different times and by different viewers. Viewing often becomes so highly personalized that it is almost impossible to control the behavior of the viewer, much less control the reporting of what is being viewed. Imagine, then, what must occur when changes are made in the instruments of viewing while efforts are made to control the viewing circumstances and the viewers.

Nevertheless, the only method by which truths are established in the various sciences is for different viewers using the same or similar tools under varied circumstances to study their subjects and to vary the vantage points from which their studies are conducted. In this way the obtained truths will be gradually enriched and broadened. With the above considerations in mind, the current series of studies, conducted by various investigators with different subjects in varied milieus and with the use of varied tools in addition to the Separation Anxiety Test (S.A.T.), has been collected to shed greater light not only on the validity and reliability of the latter instrument but also on how separation experiences affect personality and behavior at various periods of the life cycle.

In presenting this series a major effort has been made to explore the use of the S.A.T. not only at varied age levels but also in varied kinds of situations and problems, and thereby not only contribute to knowledge but also increase our understanding of the test and its various ramifications. From these studies it has become possible to broaden the norms of the test and to make certain changes in the currently used norms. Although these norms are not concisely presented anywhere in this volume, there are implications spread throughout these studies of what they may well be. (The new norms have been patiently gathered for a large population by Dr. Karl Pottharst and will be published in the near future.)

Because of the ever-present concern with the problems of the disruptions in family life by death, separation, divorce, and major social cataclysms, a number of studies in these areas are included. Several studies have been incorporated here which deal with the distress of children subsequent to separation and/or divorce (Miller with 9- to 12-year-olds and Brody with 8-year-olds). Further, one study deals with its effect upon the male spouse (Burger). In some of these studies a new form of the test was developed to adapt to the problem of testing adults.

Studies of mothers were begun by me in 1974, at which time whole families were examined (see Chapter 16). Subsequently, DeLozier did a study of abusive mothers in which the same test was used without any revisions except for directions. Mitchell followed this with a study of Mexican-American mothers in which she translated the test into Spanish and was also concerned with the mothers' abuse of children. I did a study of mothers of 5-year olds from the point of view of the relationship to closeness of the extended family (see Section Three). Bennett, who was interested in father-daughter incestuous relations, made a study of the mothers of such daughters (see references in the Summary). Lesser used the test to study battered women and their return to their own mothers after a shelter program (see references in the Summary). Problems of using and interpreting the test with adults were minimal in those studies, and the workers reported considerable satisfaction with the test.

Studies of early and late adolescence were continued. I did a study of suicidal trends in young adolescents (see Section Three), while Sherry did an interesting evaluation of college freshmen and their separation problems in relation to presence or absence of the father from the home during their childhood. Kaleita studied a group of abused adolescents and, in a way, paralleled the work of DeLozier with abusive mothers. Marquart examined the families of schizophrenic adolescents with a view to some further understanding of their separation problems and characteristics (see references in the Summary). Lewis, who has used the test extensively with adolescents in institutions, has described interesting results with the tests in the Youth Development Center, New Castle, Pa., and the State Regional Rehabilitation Center, Mercer, Pa. (no reference in this volume).

Some miscellaneous studies of various problems were conducted. Among these was a study by Stone (1980) of the relationship between attachment and separation problems and sexual involvement of women patients with their therapists (no reference in this volume). Another study by Schwartz concerned the fear of death as related to separation problems. Both of these studies represented further work with adults.

With the same S.A.T., several studies were done with the elderly. These, of course, represented a far greater deviation from the adolescent than the other studies on adults. My study (see Chapter 18) of the elderly, written in 1979, ranged over five areas of elderly living styles, while Fisk (1979) was concerned with the effect of loss of meaning on the physical and mental well-being of the elderly.

Further attempts to use the S.A.T. in children ranging from ages 4 through 8 were undertaken by revising the test to accommodate the desired age. Klagsbrun (1976), working under Bowlby and gearing her revision much more closely to Bowlby's theoretical formulation, developed a test for 4- and 5-year-olds. Varela (1982), exploiting the latter development, compared the results of this test for young hospitalized children with the results of the S.A.T. for the mothers of these children. She developed her own form of the test. Duplak, working with reading disabilities in latency-age children and using her own adaptations of the test, studied separation problems of such children.

The most recent effort to check on the reliability and consistency of the S.A.T. was undertaken by Black in a study of pairs of adolescents and their mothers. This study is reported here at length. Further, through the efforts of Dr. Karl Pottharst, it has been possible to establish norms for adults which should be quite useful in further research studies.

Studies in various universities and mental health agencies using the S.A.T. are in progress and are too numerous to mention here. Through such studies we shall be able to establish various techniques for the research use of the instrument and also be able to suggest further approaches to the problems of separation as they relate to various aspects of development and of personality.

At this point I would like to discuss the reasons why I consider researches on separation problems of significance in understanding human personality and, further, why I consider a psychological instrument of importance in studying separation problems. While I discussed these issues in Volume I of *Adolescent Separation Anxiety*, I believe that these current research studies require some replication of these reasons.

Since separation from close and significant persons in our lives occurs daily in various minor and, occasionally, major forms, various theories of attachment agree that the phenomenon of person (object) permanence within the structure of psychic life is a significant ingredient of personality development. The degree to which this intrapsychic configuration becomes intact and relatively secure provides us with some indication of developmental personality health and environmental adjustment. Minor and major separation experiences, or what is referred to by Ainsworth as "strange situations," represent tentative threats to this personality ingredient and to other aspects of the personality and its consequent human behavior. The establishment of this internalized secure image (Mahler) or model (Bowlby) of an attachment figure is highly complicated, and while evidence points to some genetic factors, it is largely the parental handling of critical life moments or stages in early infancy and childhood which produces an internally secure base by which the person is guided during separations of varied intensity and frequency. Much of this appears from various studies to hinge on the ability of the maternal attachment figure to remain sensitive to significant signals during development as well as at critical stages. This ability, in turn, appears to depend upon the maternal strength to withstand the threats to her own protective role.

Further, the evidence suggests that once an attachment between the mother and the child has developed, any threat to this attachment which is signaled to the child and is experienced as such produces stress with its concomitant anxiety. It may well be a formidable task to determine the extent to which an individual experiences anxiety when the degree of separation and the nature and significance of the separation vary. Anxiety manifests itself in such considerable and idiosyncratic patterns that, in a developing or mature person, it must no longer be considered as pure anxiety. For this reason reactions to varied separation experiences must be examined by studying as many features of the personality as may be necessary to arrive at a more comprehensive evaluation of the effects of separation experiences. Therefore, the S.A.T. was developed to measure not simply a psychological entity known as "separation anxiety" but rather the whole gamut of the patterns by which an individual reacts to and handles separation experiences of varied quality and intensity (see Volume II of *Adolescent Separation Anxiety*).

It is not enough to develop a method by which one may detect these patterns since it must be tested and retested on varied populations of varied ages, circumstances of life, sex, levels of mental development, sociocultural-economic status, and the like. Further, whatever patterns of response are demonstrated by a particular youngster or adult at any given time require further study to determine the degree to which these patterns are fairly stable and the degree to which they change with circumstances, developmental stages of life, and social pressures. In addition, the meanings and significance of the various patterns and categories must be checked and rechecked against other known criteria in order to continually improve the diagnostic and predictive character of the method.

Without a reasonably good method of studying human reactions to separation, we will certainly find it more difficult to understand human personality and behavior. I believe very strongly that the phenomenon of attachment and its corollaries, separation and loss, are of such significance in the formation of personality and are of such importance throughout the life cycle that, if we neglect methods of studying these developmental characteristics, we will have less success in our theoretical formulations, our clinical diagnosis and treatment, and our psychological researches.

Using the S.A.T. in research has occasioned many and varied designs, different statistical stratagems, varied adaptations of the test itself, and emphases on different responses, patterns, and categories. In design many have used a variety of test materials with which to correlate the S.A.T., hoping thereby either to validate concepts derived from the S.A.T. or to verify certain hypotheses with regard to a specific area of investigation. Thus, both Sherry and Black used the Spielberger State and Trait Anxiety Scales with the S.A.T.; the former studied background separation in relation to current separation from family in college freshmen, while the latter was seriously concerned with testing the reliability and stability of the S.A.T. Schwartz explored the relationship between the fear of death and various aspects of separation anxiety and used two other scales besides the S.A.T.—Templer's Death Anxiety Scale and Feifel and Branscomb's Word Association Test—as well as an Attachment Separation History Questionnaire of her own adaptation.

Many of the current researches gave a good deal of attention to the use of questionnaires, generally involving the history of relationships in the past, the family of the parents, separation experiences, etc. For example, DeLozier revised Wallace's Questionnaire, which she then utilized for her study of the attachment history experiences of abusive mothers. This provided a lengthy and detailed study of the mother's background relationship experiences, attachments and separations, experiences of abuse, etc., which might possibly be related to current reactions to separation experiences. Miller then revised the same questionnaire in studying the effects of divorce on children and then created a similar questionnaire for use with children. Comparisons between the mother's and children's questionnaires were then obtained. A number of studies used short questionnaires to establish for each subject an information index of their family experiences, such as the one used by Bergenstal in a study of father availability and separation anxiety, referred to in the Summary.

Bennett, in studying the mothers of daughters involved in an incestuous relationship with the father, used several other types of scales to relate to the S.A.T.: the Tennessee Self-Concept Scale and an Anger Direction Questionnaire. He was concerned about the self-esteem level of these mothers because of the possibility that low levels of self-esteem would be responsible for their continued tolerance of the sexual relationship between father and daughter. The Anger Direction Questionnaire was used to determine whether the mothers tended to turn anger inward. The combination of low self-esteem and inwardization of anger would be considered a significant factor in their personalities. Bennett's study sought to determine whether pathological separation patterns existed in these mothers (see references in the Summary).

Mitchell was concerned with studying abusive mothers of Mexican background. Therefore, in addition to using an attachment questionnaire of the type used by DeLozier, she introduced the Olmedo Acculturation Scale to study the effect of cultural factors on separation reactions. This was done in addition to interviews.

The populations used in these various studies were largely composed of persons dwelling in cities or suburban communities. Rarely do we find individuals who have lived their lives in rural areas, mainly because the studies are initiated by graduate students in large universities or professional schools or by college professionals who find it simpler to draw their subjects from the surrounding urban centers. Thus, the studies become limited by cultural factors. The class levels of many of the individuals examined varied considerably and ranged from the poor to the fairly affluent. In addition, there were blacks, Mexicans, Chinese, Jews, Catholics, and Protestants, as well as other groups. This

mixture of classes, races, nationalities, and religions has broadened the
scope of these researches.

A number of these studies have used the S.A.T. with adults, including mothers of young children, mothers of adolescents, young unmarried women, divorced young men, and elderly persons. The test
was not designed for adults, and its use with adults posed certain
problems. Since the persons in the pictures who are the central characters are youngsters, older persons are required to identify with these
children. The question of how successful an adult can be in trying to
identify with a youngster becomes important because there may
readily be a tendency to intellectualize rather than to experience. On
the other hand, a youngster might readily do the same. Yet we assume
that there is a degree of projection and that unconsciously an adult
selects those responses which satisfy a feeling with regard to the picture. It will be seen from the researches presented in this book that
interesting and worthwhile knowledge concerning the separation patterns of adults has been obtained with the present form of the S.A.T.

Many of these studies have not been truly experimental but have
depended largely on studying groups of individuals who have shown
certain known characteristics. The effort has been to relate separation
reactions of these persons with known behaviors or personality constructs and thus to determine whether there is any causal relationship
between the two or any noteworthy parallelisms. For example,
DeLozier, in her effort to study the application of attachment theory to
maternal abuse of children, used the S.A.T. to compare patterns of
separation reactions in abusive mothers with those in mothers who
were known not to be abusive. The results clearly demonstrated
pathological separation disorders in the abusive mothers. She referred
to these as "high levels of attachment disorder." Brody compared 8-
year-old children of divorced parents with children of intact families
by using an adaptation of the S.A.T. for that age level. Her major finding was that the former group showed higher levels of denial, self-
esteem, preoccupation, and individuation, suggesting their awareness
of the greater need for independent action and denial of stress from
separation. This was corroborated by Miller in her study of children of
divorce aged 9 to 12. These are some examples of efforts to compare
groups in separation reactions who show a particular variable in
behavior, personality, or social condition.

One study of the reliability and stability of the S.A.T. was done by

Black, who introduced an experimental element. Sixty-nine families (a mother and an adolescent between 13 and 16) were tested and retested six months after initial testing with the S.A.T. to determine not only internal consistency but also reliability and stability. This experimental use resulted in both high levels of internal consistency and generally good stability for the test.

A number of researchers have had problems in dealing statistically with the S.A.T. The reason lies largely in the effort to relate specific responses of the test to the variables with which the researcher may be concerned. Each test item, such as anger or loneliness or anxiety, is correlated with the various variables to determine whether there is any statistical relationship. Hypotheses are created around the variables and the test response, as though the test response itself were a very significant or meaningful life reaction. Failure to achieve satisfaction with these hypotheses leaves the researcher with consternation and disappointment. Similar problems have arisen surrounding the various eight patterns of responses, which are more meaningful than single responses. The correlation of each of the patterns with the hypothecated variables has also frequently resulted in unsatisfactory findings which do not correlate with what appear to be rational assumptions.

The fact is that the S.A.T. presents us with a clinical picture of how an individual tends to react to separation experiences of varying levels of intensity. The picture obtained shows the interaction of various forces within the individual and which of these forces tend to dominate the reactions. The clinical picture presents us with these interplays, which are of more significance than any given response or any pattern of reaction. For example, there is evidence that when the attachment and pain patterns are dominated by the individuation and hostility patterns in any given test protocol, the individual who produced this protocol reacts to separation experiences with a relative self-sufficiency and annoyance or a degree of detachment in contrast to individuals who suffer attachment needfulness and strong anxiety-pain-fear syndrome. Representing this statistically can be done by utilizing nonparametric methods in which the so-called normal distribution is not postulated.

Thus, to follow up the latter tactic statistically, a comparison may be made between one group which contains the constant factor a researcher may be studying—such as a group in which there has been the death of a parent at an early age—and another matched group for most meaningful factors. The groups are compared by taking the per-

xxviii   RESEARCHES IN SEPARATION ANXIETY

centage of individuals who, for example, show an excess of individuation and hostility over attachment and pain. The significance of the difference between these two percentages may then be determined by appropriate statistical calculations. Many of the most meaningful characteristics of the S.A.T. may be studied in this manner. An example of this tactic may be found in DeLozier's study in which a group of abusive mothers were compared to a control group with regard to anxious attachment and hostile detachment. Nonparametric techniques have been found to be especially useful in medical research and in many types of population studies.

Parametric methods may be found useful in handling some of the data in which normal distributions are noted. For example, if we were to subtract the following combinations: (the attachment index plus the pain index) minus (the individuation index plus the hostility index), the resulting percentage score would approach the normal curve. This score would then respond readily to statistical calculations, such as median, mean, range, middle 50%, standard deviation of the difference, probable error, and Pearson Product Moment method of correlation. This same method could apply to a number of the mathematical calculations for the scores of the S.A.T. My own predilection is to employ nonparametric techniques.

Another statistical problem relates to the use of the norms provided for the test. The norms shown in the appendixes of both Volumes I and II of *Adolescent Separation Anxiety* were derived from the studies of adolescence. The second set of somewhat more precise norms shown in Volume II have been those utilized more widely. However, subsequent research indicates that the test norms were not quite satisfactory for adults. It was noted, for example, that the norms for identity stress reactions in adolescents were much higher than for adults. Adults approximate on the average about 4% of their responses in this area, while 11- to 12-year-olds show 8% and 13- to 14-year-olds show approximately 12%. It appeared that as children grow into adolescence, the identity stress response becomes more emphatic but tends to gradually dissipate with increasing maturity. Attachment and pain reactions are higher, percentagewise, among adults than among children and adolescents, while avoidance (or defensive maneuvers) occur more strongly in adolescents. These variations in norms do suggest caution in the proper use of the norm charts for making clinical appraisals, as well as for the interpretation of results in research studies. The norms for adults have been incorporated in statistical calculations by Dr. Karl E. Pottharst of the California School of Professional Psychology, but at this writing they are not available.

Some research difficulties arise when the researcher attempts to correlate, either through Spearman Rank method, Pearson Product Moment method, or χ^2, scores or patterns from other tests, questionnaires, or interviews with the varied characteristics of the S.A.T. Self-reporting questionnaires depend to such a degree on memory for past events, the manner of reacting to them, and an awareness of current situations in the subject's life that whether their statements are accurate and unbiased must be called into question. Comparisons of these reports with the S.A.T. are, therefore, often tricky and difficult to interpret. It follows, further, that correlations of this type are likely to vary from one population to another, from one type of interview or questionnaire to another, from one researcher to another, and from one period of time to another. The reasons often lie in the meanings of questions to varied populations and to the same population at different times. At various periods of time one's memory for past events may be focused differently. The net result of all of these variations is to create distortions which are often difficult to explain.

Why, then, do researchers use these instruments to correlate with the S.A.T. if they are aware of all these pitfalls? Obviously, there are some advantages to this method, such as ease of scoring, lack of subtlety (and, therefore, ease of interpretation), and relative ease of statistical analysis. Further, if sufficient studies and experiments are conducted on large populations and if sufficient care is taken that significant variables are held constant and the same or similar instruments are utilized, the results may well cancel out many of the errors which accumulate from smaller and more isolated studies. This suggests why more studies of the same problems with the same instruments and at different times with varied populations are necessary. Gradually, some consensus is likely to arise which will provide the truths with regard to human separation problems.

It is not planned to present the complete studies in each of the chapters included in this volume. The effort will be made to concentrate on the manner in which the S.A.T. was used by the researcher, what problems were being studied, how the test was analyzed, and what comparative statistical data were used to understand the problems involved.

SECTION ONE

The fourteen chapters in this section are devoted to summaries of various dissertations utilizing the Separation Anxiety Test. These are divided into studies pertaining to child abuse, mothers and children, college students, and, finally, the elderly. They demonstrate the utility of the test for a variety of human problems and represent different experimental designs and various statistical approaches.

The considerable interest that has been generated concerning child abuse and divorce, the development of Bowlby's attachment theory, and the simultaneous concern with measurement in the areas of attachment, separation, and loss—these have prompted the use of the S.A.T. Furthermore, applying it to the many experiences of childhood, including the problematic areas of children hospitalized and away from their mothers, hyperactivity, and learning disability, the studies provide insights into attachment and separation in the lives of children and their mothers.

Extending the studies to college students, four summarized papers are presented dealing with a variety of problems, including the fear of death and attraction to cultist groups. The extension of the use of the S.A.T. to college students has proven to be very revealing with regard to attachment, separation, and loss in the lives and personalities of late adolescents and young adults.

The final study in this group is an interesting examination of how the S.A.T. was utilized in evaluating the reactions of elderly persons. This study deals with a deeply significant element in the lives of elderly people—the loss of life meaning.

STUDIES OF CHILD ABUSE

1

DeLozier's Application of Attachment Theory to Abusive Mothers

Several studies have used the S.A.T. to study mothers who abused their children and adolescents who were abused and neglected. One such study was conducted by Dr. Pauline P. DeLozier of Hacienda Heights, California, and was completed for her doctorate at the California School of Professional Psychology at Los Angeles in 1979. The study made comparisons between eighteen abusive and eighteen nonabusive mothers in their reactions to the S.A.T. and to the Wallace Attachment Questionnaire. It was entitled "An Application of Attachment Theory to the Study of Child Abuse."

In this study the S.A.T. was employed to determine differential reactions of eighteen known abusive mothers as compared with eighteen mothers who were considered to be nonabusive. The theoretical basis for this study lay in Bowlby's attachment theory (1969), which suggested that pathology of maternal behavior grows out of the disruption of early attachment bonds in the mother's own childhood experience.

DeLozier's explanations of attachment theory suggested that it draws heavily upon psychoanalytic and object relations theories but differs from the analytic view in several crucial areas. She proposed the general hypothesis that the attachment process is dysfunctional in child-abusing families. Patterns of attachment difficulty seem to be evident along generational lines. Further, she noted that child-abusing parents are known to be isolated, demanding, unable to maintain close relationships, and expectant of care-taking from their children (Helfer and Kempe, 1974, 1976; Steele and Pollack, 1968). The role-reversing aspect of mother-child relationships was considered by DeLozier—following Bowlby's concept—to be a central issue in child abuse. She quoted extensively from Bowlby (1973) but also from Kempe (1976) and Martin (1976).

Another significant factor is that alarming events, including the unavailability of the mother, considerably reduce exploratory behavior. Attachment theory postulates this interplay of attachment behavior and exploratory behavior throughout an individual's lifetime. Early attachment difficulties or early misparenting could significantly diminish later capacity to master the environment. Such a pattern seems reflected in the description of the abusing parent as dependent, passive, and immature. The fact that alarm increases attachment behavior (proximity seeking) at the expense of exploratory behavior seems evident in abused children.

DeLozier presented a very extensive and intensive review of the literature dealing with attachment theory, especially Bowlby (1969, 1973) and Ainsworth (1970, 1971, 1972, 1973). Her literature extended into child abuse, with material from Fontana (1968), Justice and Justice (1976), Klaus and Kennell (1976), Klein and Stern (1971), Stern (1973), Steele and Pollack (1968), and Steele (1975). Significant was the conclusion from the literature that abusive parents were abused as children and forced into parental roles.

DeLozier used her own revision of the Wallace Attachment History Questionnaire (1973) and the Hansburg S.A.T. (1972) as her main instruments of investigation. The self-reported background in the attachment area was considered to be highly important to this study because DeLozier wished to discover the nature of the differences in the attachment and separation experiences of abusive mothers. It was hoped that the Wallace questionnaire would reveal such data.

In order to use the S.A.T. with adults, she altered the instructions somewhat so that the mothers could identify with the child in the pictures. Since several studies made by me (reported in this volume) had already been made with adults without any serious problems, DeLozier felt on solid ground in using the test.

DeLozier defined an abusive mother according to the following criteria: (a) being reported to the Department of Public Social Service, Child Protective Services (Los Angeles); (b) being judged by the Director and Program Director of a hospital day treatment program; (c) being judged by other professionals (social worker, physician, therapist, etc.); or (d) being self-referred to an agency or clinic as having abused her children. The most recent abuse had occurred within the last two years prior to the study, and the child was a preadolescent. Typical mothers for a control group were selected with the aid of the school system parent-teacher organization and were from a comparable socioeconomic level. All mothers in both groups were Caucasian. The interviewers who administered the instruments were clinically trained social workers who received training sessions with DeLozier.

DeLozier hypothesized that since, in general, in child-abusing families there is inadequate or faulty development of attachment, it would show in the mothers' responses to their own attachment history as well as on the S.A.T. She developed four major hypotheses:

1. Abusive mothers would report experiencing a greater number of disruptions or threats of disruptions in early attachments. She divided this hypothesis into four subhypotheses referrable to her attachment history questionnaire.
2. They would also report markedly fewer significant others perceived to be available as support figures. She divided this hypothesis into two sections.
3. At the time surrounding the birth of the identified abused child, abusive mothers would report a greater number of stressful incidents, including many factors, such as separation from spouse, financial problems, illnesses, etc. She divided this hypothesis into four sections, each of which had many subtitles. Included also were many other elements.
4. Abusive mothers would demonstrate more serious problems of attachment on the S.A.T. both in an individual clinical analysis of the test patterning and in statistical evaluation of the various items and patterns. She divided this hypothesis into two sections, of which the second section had nine subtitles.

The control group was selected from volunteer mothers of elementary school children, since the age of children of the abusive mothers was largely in the range of 6 to 14 with a mean of 9 years. While the main source of difficulty was related to the availability of Caucasian mothers in a sufficiently low-income bracket, it was not a problem to obtain volunteers from some elementary schools and other private sources who would fit the criteria. A statistical analysis of the demographic data showed the two groups to be similar, with no significant differences in major cultural and socioeconomic conditions, as well as age and sex levels of the children and ages of the mothers.

It is not the intention of this summary to present in detail the results that were obtained with the revision of the Wallace Questionnaire, except to make brief mention of the findings. It is my intention to provide a detailed summary of the S.A.T. results.

During the course of this study, DeLozier sent the protocols to me for analysis of six factors dealing with anxious attachment, as was originally outlined in a paper published in 1976. Further, I examined the protocols for those with detachment patterns and for those with good core strength. Following this clinical analysis, the Mann-Whitney nonparametric test was utilized to test whether two independent groups came from the same population. Further, the Glass rank biserial correlation for the strength of association with the Mann-Whitney was obtained for significant findings.

DeLozier began her analysis of the S.A.T. by first presenting the data with regard to the presence or absence of severe dysfunctional attachment in each group. When the data were examined for severe cases of anxious attachment, it was found that twelve (66.7%) mothers of the eighteen in the abusive group were so diagnosed as compared with two (11%) of the control group. A large number of milder cases were found in the control group (ten, or 55.5%), while only a small number (three, or 17%) were found among the abusive mothers. When severe anxious attachment cases were combined with detachment cases, the data appeared as follows:

Table 1.1

FREQUENCY OF PATHOLOGICAL ATTACHMENT S.A.T. PROTOCOLS

Group	Severe Anxious Attachment or Detachment	Neither
Abusive	84% (15)	16% (3)
Typical	34% (6)	66% (12)

$\chi^2 = 51.67$; $df = 1$; p (1) = $<$ .0005.

These data provided such a clear indication of pathological attachment patterns among the abusive mothers in comparison with typical mothers as to leave little doubt of its significance. Further, the core strength levels (defined as high levels of both attachment capacity and individuation, or self-reliance) were generally quite low among the abusive mothers (only 6% in the high group), while a much higher percentage of mothers with good core strength was noted in the typical group (33%) ($p < .05$). Hostility reactions were far more prevalent in the abusive group (67%) than in the control group (39%) ($p < .05$).

The abusive mothers were studied further for the depressive syndrome, and 83% showed self-love loss greater than or equal to self-esteem preoccupation, while only 40% of the typical mothers fell into this category with a $p < .01$. Reality avoidance reactions (defensive maneuvers) above the norms were found in 76.5% of the abusive mothers as compared with 41% of the typical mothers with a $p < .02$. Table 1.2 provides a χ^2 analysis of the data described above.

Table 1.2

χ^2 ANALYSIS OF FREQUENCY AND PERCENTAGE OF S.A.T. PROTOCOLS WITH FACTORS INDICATING ANXIOUS ATTACHMENT FOR ABUSIVE VERSUS TYPICAL MOTHERS

(Based on Clinical Interpretation)

Group	n	None (0 Factors)	Mild (1 2)	Strong (3 4)	Severe (5 6)
Abusives	18	0	17% (3)	17% (3)	66.67% (12)
Typical	18	5.5% (1)	55.5% (10)	28% (5)	11% (2)

The results of this analysis further supported the first section of DeLozier's fourth hypothesis, with findings of lower core strength, higher percentages of rejection and self-blame responses, and higher levels of anger and separation avoidance responses in the protocols of the abusive mothers.

DeLozier presented samples of clinical analysis of the protocols and then stated:

Although occasionally differing from attachment theory concepts in the use of terminology such as "symbiosis," "individuation," etc., whereas attachment theory utilizes the concepts of "attachment" and "self-reliance," the clinical analysis of the Separation Anxiety Test protocols strongly supports the predicted hypothesis of inadequate attachment, primarily, [severe] anxious attachment in the child abusing group (of mothers). This finding in conjunction with the findings regarding the early attachment experience of the child abusing mothers and their reported expectations of significant others, clearly supports the prediction of both childhood and adult attachment disorders in the child abusing mothers studied.

DeLozier proceeded to do a statistical analysis of many of the response items of the S.A.T. for both the abusive and typical mother groups. Higher attachment responses and lower self-reliance responses on mild pictures were the rule for abusive mothers. This indicated a heightened sensitivity to separation. (See Mitchell's study on abusive mothers in the Mexican-American community for similar results.) Comparable results were found in an examination of responses to the hostility pattern in that they were significantly higher for abusive mothers, especially because of their reactions to the strong separation pictures. Further, anxiety reactions were found to be stronger on the mild pictures. Thus, there was verification of the results for adolescent disturbance (Hansburg, 1972, pp. 79–80), indicating that abusive mothers tended to shift reactions from anxiety to hostility when they moved from mild to strong separation stimuli. DeLozier concluded that "while overall the total 'inner turmoil' responses remain significantly higher for the abusing group, a different emphasis is found as the degree of intensity of stimulus varies" (p. 255).

It was further noted that avoidance responses were stronger for the abusive group on the mild pictures, but as the intensity of the stimulus increased, avoidance responses became less prominent for the abusive mothers and more prominent for the typical mothers. It is obvious that more severe avoidance to a mild stimulus, such as was found with the abusive mothers, is more pathological than if avoidance were greater on the strong stimulus.

The self-love loss pattern was significantly higher for the abusive mothers on mild, strong, and total pictures. This is a depressive phenomenon. It was also noticed that an increase in the strength of the separation stimulus caused a shift from feelings of rejection to self-blame in comparison with the patterns of the typical mothers. The significance of these data should not be overlooked and should be compared to that of the data on the depressive syndrome. While depressive reactions to separation are common in the general population, they appear on the Hansburg S.A.T. to be extremely prevalent among abusive mothers (83% as compared with 40%). (The 40% figure for the depressive syndrome in the control population of DeLozier's study compares exactly with the same figure obtained by me with the group of thirty-one mothers studied at the East Midwood Day School in Brooklyn, N.Y., and reported in Chapter 19.) The fact that the strong stimuli produced a significantly greater shift from feelings of rejection to self-blame in the abusive mothers than in the more typical mothers was interpreted by DeLozier to mean that abusive mothers tend to feel a greater sense of responsibility for strong family separations (and therefore a greater sense of personal guilt). She remarked, "This is also consistent with the childhood information which indicates that the mothers felt anxiously concerned for the well-being of their caretakers (role reversal)."

Of further interest was the excessive number of absurd or inappropriate responses to the various pictures, whether mild or strong. The statistics were quite startling, as shown by the Mann-Whitney analysis of the S.A.T. On the mild pictures the rankings were M(abusive) = 21.53, M(typical) = 15.47, Z = 7.893, $p < .05$. On the strong pictures M(abusive) = 23.17, M(typical) = 13.83, Z = -2.668, $p < .005$, Total M(abusive) = 22.94, M(typical) = 14.06, Z = -2.541, $p < .01$. These data strongly suggested that abusive mothers tend to have poorer reality testing than typical mothers and, therefore, some impairment of judgment.

Results of that portion of the study using the S.A.T. may be summarized as follows. They indicated:

. . . clear patterns of severe attachment disorder in the abusive mothers as compared with the typical mothers, with a probable origin related to threatened disruptions of attachments and caretaking, as well as severe discipline in childhood. Present manifestations of attachment difficulties in the abusing group . . . included significantly more frequent indicators of anxious attachment (and detachment) in both blind clinical interpretations of protocols and statistical analyses of protocol data by Mann-Whitney non-parametric tests. Indicators of anxious attachment (severe) obtained significantly more frequently for the abusing group included high percentages of attachment responses, especially in response to mild separation pictures; low percentages of self-reliant responses; higher percentages of anger and anxiety responses and higher percentages of rejection and self-blame responses. In addition the abusive mothers showed significantly more inappropriate responses than typical mothers.

DeLozier discussed her findings as they relate to attachment theory. I now quote at length from her section entitled "Convergence of Findings" (pp. 344–346):

All of the results about earlier difficulties (obtained from the Wallace Attachment History Questionnaire) were found to be consistent with the present manifestations of attachment difficulties as assessed by the Separation Anxiety Test. The abusing mothers indicated on this test a high present level of attachment disorder, primarily anxious attachment (severe) but with some degree of tendency toward detachment as well. They responded with overall high levels of attachment response, although a crucial shift was noted in the high attachment response to mild separations and a slight decrease in attachment response to strong situations, higher levels of both anger and anxiety responses, overall low levels of self-reliance, and high levels of rejection and self-blame. Thus, the abusing mothers in this study demonstrated their overall sensitivity to separation, especially mild separation.

It should be noted that DeLozier strongly suggested that abusive mothers are so sensitive to small daily separation experiences that they can become very disturbed by the slightest suspicion of an insignificant separation. This excessive reaction makes these women extremely vulnerable to normal experiences of aloneness.

DeLozier continued:

These findings suggest the prediction that the abusive mothers in this study have experienced difficulty in their childhood attachments and in the development of internal representations of significant others as accessible and reliable, resulting in consequent adult attachment difficulties as well as in possible difficulties in the development of caretaking behavior. . . .

On the basis of the present findings it is clear that the protective functioning of the attachment system is not adequately operating in the abusing family, at least to the extent measured in this study. The result is that individuals in the abusing family appear to live in a more or less constant state of arousal or alertness to signals of danger, especially separation from significant others. The maintenance of proximity to the discriminate caretaker appears to be constantly in jeopardy. Therefore, the sensitivity to separation and the increased attachment behavior at the slightest signal of potential danger would appear to serve a survival function in abusing families.

From this perspective the dependency, depression, anxiety, hostility and distrustfulness frequently noted in abusing families is reinterpreted as indicators of anxious attachment (severe), a state reflecting uncertainty regarding the availability of caretakers in childhood and the resulting anger, anxiety and lack of ability to rely on others and self. The inappropriate anger expressed toward the child is seen as the anger engendered by anxious attachment by a parent toward an inappropriate "attachment figure." The frozen watchfulness noted in abused children and proposed as characterizing abusing parents also, is seen as *adaptive behavior resorted to when (a) retreating from danger and (b) increasing proximity to an accessible significant other, are in conflict.*

Furthermore, when the accessibility of a dependable attachment figure or significant other is uncertain, attention must be paid to any signals warning of danger. Thus, the hypersensitivity and danger orientation of both the abused child and the abusing parent is interpreted as a continuing alertness to the environment, as alertness necessary for survival in what is experienced as an unpredictable and unreliable environment. The experience of the individual in the abusing family has *not* involved, as it has for individuals in typical families, learning that the natural clues warning of increased risk of danger are *not* necessarily associated with increased actual danger.

From the attachment theory perspective the generational pattern of abuse, including the deficit in adequate parenting, can be seen then, as the transmission of attachment disorders through diversions in the development of the attachment and caretaker behavioral systems. The pattern of findings in the present study strongly supports such a formulation.

REFERENCES

Ainsworth, M. D. S., and Bell, S. "Attachment, Exploration and Separation: Illustrated by the Behavior of One-Year-Olds in a Strange Situation." *Child Development*, 1970, *41*, 49–67.

Ainsworth, M. D. S., Bell, S. M., and Stayton, D. J. "Individual Differences in Strange Situation Behavior in One-Year-Olds," in H. R. Shaffer (ed.), *The Origin of Human Social Relations.* New York: Academic Press, 1971.

Ainsworth, M. D. S. "Attachment and Dependency: A Comparison," in J. L. Gewirtz (ed.), *Attachment and Dependency.* New York: John Wiley and Sons, 1972.

Ainsworth, M. D. S. "The Development of Infant-Mother Attachment," in B. M. Caldwell and H. N. Ricciuti (eds.), *Review of Child Development Research*, Vol. III, Chicago: University of Chicago Press, 1973.

Bowlby, J. *Attachment and Loss*, Vol. I. New York: Basic Books, 1969.

Bowlby, J. *Attachment and Loss*, Vol. II. New York: Basic Books, 1973.

DeLozier, P. P. *An Application of Attachment Theory to the Study of Child Abuse.* Unpublished doctoral dissertation, California School of Professional Psychology, Los Angeles, 1979.

Fontana, V. J. "Further Reflections on Maltreatment of Children." *New York Journal of Medicine*, 1968, *68*, 2214–2215.

Hansburg, H. G. "Separation Problems of Displaced Children," in R. S. Parker (ed.), *The Emotional Stress of War, Violence and Peace.* Stanwyx House, 1972.

Hansburg, H. G. *Adolescent Separation Anxiety*, Vol. I, Springfield, Ill.: C. C. Thomas, 1972. Reprinted, Huntington, N.Y.: R. E. Krieger, 1980.

Hansburg, H. G. "Adolescent Separation Hostility: A Prelude to Violence." *Abstract Guide of the Congress of International Psychology*, Tokyo, 1972.

Hansburg, H. G. *Adolescent Separation Anxiety*, Vol. II. Huntington, N.Y.: R. E. Krieger, 1980.

Hansburg, H. G. "The Use of the Separation Anxiety Test in the Detection of Self-Destructive Tendencies in Early Adolescence," in D. V. S. Sankar (ed.), *Mental Health in Children*, Vol. III. Westbury, N.Y.: P. J. D. Publications, 1976.

Helfer, R. E., and Kempe, C. H. (eds.). *The Battered Child* (2nd ed.). Chicago: University of Chicago Press, 1974.

Helfer, R. E., and Kempe, C. H. *Child Abuse and Neglect: The Family and the Community*. Cambridge: Ballinger Publishing, 1976.

Justice, B., and Justice, R. *The Abusing Family*. New York: Human Sciences Press, 1976.

Klaus, M. H., and Kennell, J. H. *Maternal Infant Bonding—The Impact of Early Separation or Loss on Family Development*. St. Louis: Mosby, 1976.

Klein, M., and Stern, L. "Low Birth Weight and the Battered Child Syndrome." *American Journal of Diseases of Children*, 1971, *122*, 15–18.

Martin, H. P. (ed.). *The Abused Child: A Multidisciplinary Approach to Developmental Issues and Treatment*. Cambridge: Ballinger Publishing, 1976.

Steele, B. F. *Working with Abusive Parents from the Psychiatric Point of View*. U.S. Department of Health, Education and Welfare Publication No. (OHD) 75-70. Washington, D.C.: U.S. Government Printing Office, 1975.

Steele, B. F., and Pollack, C. B. "A Psychiatric Study of Parents Who Abuse Infants and Small Children," in R. E. Helfer and C. H. Kempe (eds.), *The Battered Child* (2nd ed.). Chicago: University of Chicago Press, 1968.

Stern, L. "Prematurity as a Factor in Child Abuse." *Hospital Practices*, 1973, 8, 117–123.

Wallace, A. *An Application of Attachment Theory to the Study of Divorced People*. Unpublished doctoral dissertation, California School of Professional Psychology, Los Angeles, 1977.

2

Mitchell's Application of Attachment Theory to Mexican-American Abusive Mothers

Dr. Marjorie C. Mitchell of Long Beach, California, did a study of child abuse for her doctorate at the California School of Professional Psychology at Los Angeles, which she completed in 1981. It was entitled "An Application of Attachment Theory to a Socio-Cultural Perspective of Physical Child Abuse in the Mexican-American Community." This study made an analysis of abusive and nonabusive mothers (thirty mothers in each group) in a Mexican-American population. Methods utilized included the Olmedo Acculturation Scale, The Attachment and Support Systems Questionnaire, and a Spanish translation of the Hansburg S.A.T.

This research was an intensive study of a group of thirty abusive mothers with a group of thirty nonabusive mothers as a control from the Mexican-American community in California. Mitchell translated the S.A.T. into Spanish and gave it to all sixty of these mothers. In addition, she made a careful study of sociocultural factors which utilized the Olmedo Acculturation Scale to differentiate levels of abusive mothers in this area. Further, along the lines of DeLozier's study of abusive mothers, she used a revision of Wallace's Attachment History Questionnaire. Since this chapter deals mainly with the use and interpretation of results of the S.A.T., there will be very little discussion of how Mitchell utilized the other material of her study.

Mitchell's review of the literature dealing with the Mexican-American community was extensive. In addition, she reviewed the

studies of the serious effects of poverty on the abusive behavior of
parental figures. The failure of the use of support systems emerged
from these studies as a significant factor in the lives of these people. In
addition, she referred to studies of the effect of an unemployed father
on many abusive families. The relatively low level of formal education
was also found to be a significant sociocultural factor.

Mitchell quoted from important studies of the farm families of
Mexican background, indicating that while the Mexican-Americans
were traditionally, as a group, living with extended families, abusive
families had a weaker kinship network. Yet her evidence indicated that
Mexican-American farm workers are a minority of their culture, with
the majority (83%) living in urban areas. Mitchell suggested that any
or all of these factors, while significant, do not fully explain the
phenomenon of child abuse and that it was necessary to look elsewhere
for fundamental causes. Mitchell stated, "Although the poverty groups
have been over-represented in the literature, this has not explained
why not all indigent people abuse their children." She posited the importance of attachment theory in explaining this form of behavior. She
proceeded to discuss the theoretical formulations of Bowlby, Ainsworth, Harlow, Hansburg, et al. There was considerable explication of
the concepts of separation anxiety as a factor in attachment theory.

Mitchell provided a long chapter dealing with the family system
present in the farm families, as well as the urban families, of the
Mexican-American community. Gradually, the compadrazo system of
the extended family has become more akin to that of the Anglo-
American group, and the younger generation has adopted another
cultural setting. This has resulted in greater isolation and less security.

Mitchell formulated a hypothesis that the S.A.T. would show
pathological functioning of the attachment system in abusive Mexican-
American families. This pathological dysfunction would be represented by severe anxious attachment and hostile detachment. She
hypothesized that hostility would be predominant in the protocols of
the abusing mother group.

Although it is not my intention to present here other parts of the
study, nevertheless it might be worthwhile to present some of the
results obtained by using the revised Wallace Attachment History
Questionnaire in order to throw some light on significant elements of
the background of the abusive mothers. They were found to make less
use of supportive figures. As predicted, the abusive group had more

and longer separations from attachment figures than the nonabusive mothers, with more deaths of attachment figures in childhood. Fewer years were lived with the nuclear family, and longer years were lived with alternate living arrangements. More threats of abandonment were experienced by the abusive mothers—often threats of suicide—as well as threats of divorce and of punishment. In addition, the various support systems, including their number, appeared to be more questionable among the histories of the abusive mothers. These included immediate relatives and friends. The above data leave no doubt of the extreme insecurity, instability, and threatened or actual abuse suffered by the abusive mother group in childhood—a finding similar to that of DeLozier. Keeping these data in mind, we can understand the results that were obtained from the S.A.T.

I quote from Mitchell (p. 252):

The Hansburg Separation Anxiety Test measures the current level of attachment and individuation as well as the pathological levels of inadequate attachment and self-reliance. This hypothesis predicted that on five measures of the test there would be significant differences between the two groups, with the abusing group showing more evidence of pathology. These five included (a) responses to both mild and strong stimuli, as well as total responses, (b) total responses to each of the twelve stimulus cards, (c) attachment and individuation subscales, (d) indices of pathological attachment, and (e) specific response patterns. . . .

Significant differences were found in the total responses to all of the stimuli on this instrument (Ab mean 100, N − Ab mean 67.1, p_2 = .001). The child abusive mothers responded . . . with significantly greater frequency than the non-abusing mothers. Further more alarm was elicited from the abusing mothers in response to the mild stimuli compared to the non-abusing mothers (Ab mean = 45.27, N − Ab mean 29.23, p_2 = .002).

Following this pattern, the abusing mother also made significantly greater numbers of responses to the strong stimuli than the non-abusing mother (Ab mean = 54.73, N − Ab mean = 37.87, p_2 = 0.001). Abusing mothers responded significantly to all levels of separation stimuli with higher numbers of responses when compared to the non-abusing mothers. . . .

The abusing mothers differed significantly from the nonabusing mothers in a characteristic pattern of acknowledging far greater responses to the hypothetical experiences represented by the pictures. Consistently, the abusing mothers found every card, mild and strong, to be *anxiety-inducing*, with resultant higher numbers of answers.

Mitchell divided the balances of attachment and individuation into five subscales, which include (a) attachment, (b) individuation,

(c) mild separation response, (d) strong separation response, and (e) attachment versus individuation.

The significant areas on the subscales showed up in an interesting way. Since mild separation experiences should not occasion *higher* levels of attachment, the nonabusing mothers, as expected, had significantly greater differences between the mild levels of individuation and the mild attachment responses, indicating a healthier response to mild separation (Ab mean dif $= -.733$, $N -$ Ab mean dif $= 6.93$, $p_2 = 0.0001$).

The reverse of this result was expected and obtained when Mitchell compared the differences between self-reliance and attachment need on the strong pictures. The child-abusing mothers showed a definitely larger difference between attachment and individuation responses on the strong pictures, indicating the strong attachment needs that are stimulated in abusing mothers in more severe separation situations (Ab mean $= 8.0$, $N -$ Ab mean $= 3.7$, $p_2 = .025$).

When the total individuation responses were subtracted from the total attachment responses for both groups, the differences were quite significant (Ab mean dif $= 8.77$, $N -$ Ab mean dif $= -3.17$, $p_2 = .005$), suggesting a lower level of independent functioning under separation in the abusive mothers.

Mitchell then analyzed each of the seventeen responses to the S.A.T. for both groups, and the differences were significant in twelve of these. The following items were responded to more significantly among the abusive than the nonabusive mothers: rejection, phobic feelings, anxiety, loneliness, withdrawal, somatic complaints, anger, projection, empathy, evasion, intrapunitive feelings, and fantasy.

Doing a pattern analysis, Mitchell found that the abusing mothers gave statistically significant more responses than the nonabusing mothers on the *attachment pattern* (Ab mean $= 22.82$, $N -$ Ab mean 18.37, $p_2 = .008$). The individuation pattern was significantly higher for the nonabusing mothers (Ab mean $= 13.79$, $N -$ Ab mean $= 21.66$, $p_2 = .001$), suggesting that they maintained greater self-reliance during separation experiences in contrast to the abusing group.

While there was a trend toward a higher percentage of patterned hostility responses in the abusive mothers, it was not statistically significant. There was no significant difference in the painful tension response pattern, although the trend showed a higher mean for the abusive group. Defensive patterning showed no trends between the abusive and nonabusive groups.

It was of considerable importance that the self-love loss pattern (rejection and intrapunitiveness) was greater in the abusive mothers, but the difference was not statistically significant. The reverse was true in the area of concentration impairment. My further analysis of Mitchell's data showed that when a comparison was made between the means of the self-love loss pattern and the means of the self-esteem preoccupation pattern, a more reliable measure of depressive tendency was found. The abusive mothers showed a self-love loss mean of 12.4 and a self-esteem preoccupation pattern mean of 9.1. The nonabusive mothers showed a reverse but more typical pattern difference, with self-esteem preoccupation pattern at 12.13 and a self-love loss pattern of 10.06. Regardless of whether there is a statistical significance here, the fact that the reversal of the typical trend by the abusive mothers is shown demonstrates a definitely increased depressive tone in the abusive mothers. I pointed out (in *Adolescent Separation Anxiety*, Vol. II) that the depressive syndrome is an important aspect of the pathology of the attachment system, and it is quite probable that abusive mothers more often suffer from feelings of isolation and depression.

Reality testing problems were more often seen in the abusive group. They compared to the nonabusive group on absurd (inappropriate) responses as follows: Ab mean = 4.23, N − Ab mean = 2.1, p_2 = .21. Mitchell stated:

Examples of such absurd responses to the separation pictures were on picture IV (school) "sorry for the mother" and "somebody else is causing all this trouble"; a response on picture VII "that if the child had behaved better, her brother wouldn't have left her to go to sea" and a response on picture XI, "the child feels like reading a book or watching TV (death of the mother picture)."

In interpreting the above results, Mitchell stated that the abusive mothers showed more pathological responses to the separation stimuli when compared to the nonabusive mothers. Of nine response patterns, the abusive mothers differed significantly on five, with higher indices of problems with separation. Three other response patterns were not significantly different but were in the anticipated direction.

Unfortunately, Mitchell did not do a clinical analysis of the patterns of each of the sixty mothers in the study with a view to determining the presence or absence of varying degrees of anxious attachment or detachment. Instead, she evaluated the statistical results on the various six factors derived from the material referred to in *Adolescent Separation Anxiety*, Vol. II and previously noted here. She determined that three of the six factors were more prevalent in the abusive mother group. She referred to the higher levels of attachment and the lower levels of individuation (mean below the norm), with the difference greater in the abusive group and, therefore, less self-reliance. Further, she noted again the larger number of attachment responses on the mild pictures among abusive mothers and finally indicated that self-love loss was significantly stronger among abusive mothers. She concluded from this that separation reactions among abusive mothers fell more often into moderate anxious attachment than those of the nonabusive mothers. She stated, "On a continuum of mild to severe levels of anxious attachment, the child abusing mothers had moderate levels of anxious attachment when compared to the nonabusing mothers" (p. 267).

It would be of value to present here Table 2.1, in which the significant factors of anxious attachment appear.

It should be noted that at least five of the original factors are stronger for the abusive group than for the nonabusive group, even though only three are statistically significant. Thus, it could be suspected that a clinical analysis would have shown a considerable number of abusive mothers with severe anxious attachment patterns. It is also probable that more cases of pathological detachment would have occurred, as was found in DeLozier's study (1979).

Mitchell made an effort to compare various levels of acculturation (from the Olmedo Scale) to reports of loneliness on the Hansburg S.A.T.; she said:

There were no significant differences when the low and high levels of acculturation abusive mothers were compared on the number of loneliness responses (Ab "low" mean 8.2, Ab "high" mean 8.33 with p_1 not significant). . . . However, differences were discovered when the more recent immigrant abusive mothers were compared to both levels of acculturation in the nonabusive group. The "low" level of acculturation abusive mothers reported significantly higher indices of loneliness on the S.A.T. when compared to her counterpart in the "low" level of acculturation of the non-abusive mothers (Ab "low" 8.2, N – Ab "low" 3.73, p_1 .0001).

In an ex post facto statistical analysis, Mitchell reported eighteen factors in her study which were "the best predictors of physical child

Table 2.1

t-TEST ANALYSIS OF THE SIX FACTORS ASSOCIATED WITH ANXIOUS

ATTACHMENT, AS MEASURED BY THE HANSBURG S.A.T. FOR ABUSING

MOTHERS COMPARED TO NONABUSING MOTHERS

	N	Mean	S.D.	t	df	p level (two tailed)
Factor 1						
Attach.						
vs.						
Indiv.						
Abusing	30	8.767	9.526			
Nonabusing	30	-3.167	13.115	3.091	58	.005
Levels of						
Self-rel.						
Abusing	30	13.786	5.788			
Nonabusing	30	21.663	9.209	3.97	58	.0001
Factor 2						
% Responses						
to mild						
stimulus						
Abusing	30	45.267	18.525			
Nonabusing	30	29.233	16.001	-3.25	58	.002
Factor 3						
Hostility						
Response						
Pattern						
Abusing	30	18.057	4.607			
Nonabusing	30	16.422	4.551	-1.38	58	.172
Painful						
Tension						
Abusing	30	20.063	4.589			
Nonabusing	30	18.415	6.597	-1.12	58	.266
Factor 4						
Separation						
Avoid.						
Abusing	30	14.767	4.206			
Nonabusing	30	13.173	5.508	-1.26	58	.213
Factor 5						
Self-L.L./						
Self-E.P.						
Abusing	30	3.333	5.504			
Nonabusing	30	-2.300	8.404	3.019	58	.005
Factor 6						
Identity						
Stress						
Abusing	30	5.061	2.573			
Nonabusing	30	6.025	3.992	1.11	58	.271

abuse in the Mexican-American community." Many of these were items obtained from the S.A.T. These were:

1) total percent of mild responses, 2) total percent of strong responses, 3) total responses to all separation stimuli, 4) total percent of the attachment response pattern, 5) total percent of individuation (self-reliance) response pattern and 6) total percent of self-love loss response pattern.

To put this statement in better perspective, it would imply that child abuse by mothers in the Mexican-American community could be best predicted on the S.A.T. by higher percentages of responses to mild and to strong separation pictures, a greater number of responses to all the pictures, a larger percentage of responses included in the attachment response pattern, a lower percentage of response to the individuation pattern, and a higher percentage of self-love loss responses. She reported that the three strongest predictors of physical child abuse among Mexican-American mothers were the frequency of physical punishment during the mother's childhood, the number of separations from attachment figures during childhood, and the low individuation percentage on the S.A.T.

Later, Mitchell noted that the combination of the total individuation responses to the mild pictures and the total individuation responses were found to be significant. She stated further:

. . . of these 16 variables only the response pattern to mild stimuli on the Hansburg Separation Anxiety Test and the individuation (self-reliance) response pattern from the same instrument were found to contribute significant variance to the total multiple regression when combined with the remaining variables.

In summary, Mitchell suggested that abusive mothers react with greater alarm to all separation stimuli with little differentiation in regard to the severity of the separation scene. Abusing mothers reacted to the separation pictures "as if they were real," with emotionally charged acknowledgments that the child must feel terrible.

Many of the abusive mothers lost distance from the stimulus card and consistently added addendums of "this happened to me and I know how this child must feel." Affective responses such as crying and sighing were noted consistently more with the abusing group of mothers and there was no difference based on level of acculturation. One of the diagnostic features of this test is the correlation between the intensity of the separation stimulus and the resulting

frequency and intensity of the reactions. . . . Attachment should increase and self-reliance should decrease when faced with a strong
separation stimulus with the reverse order for mild separations.

There is no doubt that abusive mothers in comparison to nonabusive
mothers were much more readily alarmed by separation experiences
and showed greater preference for attachment responses and less
preference for self-reliance responses *on the mild pictures.* The
nonabusive mothers were by far much more attracted to attachment
responses on the strong separation pictures, suggesting a healthier
response to separation. Yet they also maintained their self-reliance and
autonomy far better than the abusive mothers on the mild separation
pictures. Further, the abusive mothers were inclined to give more inappropriate reactions to the test, which Mitchell explained as follows:

With the numerous separations during childhood, it appears that mothers who
abuse their children have never been sure of the reasons for the rejections [they
experienced] and [therefore] must attempt to justify their disruptions in attachment by any explanation even if it is not logical.

Referring to the depressive problem, Mitchell stated:

As a result of the earlier disruptions in attachment, the abusing mothers self-
evaluation has been profoundly affected. . . . [They] have been exposed to
negative evaluations by their caretakers during childhood with a resultant self-
love loss. [They] are filled with self-blame and feelings of rejection. Whenever
faced with separation, . . . they feel unwanted and responsible for the perceived rejection. Regardless of the strength of the impending separation . . .
[they] feel more responsibility for the rejection than non-abusive mothers.

This conclusion was based on the much stronger response to the pattern
of self-love loss on the S.A.T., which included rejection and intrapunitiveness.

There were some indications that identity stress responses to the
strong pictures were more prevalent among the abusive mothers but
were not similarly so for the mild pictures. Although Mitchell did not
indicate anything with regard to this, experience with S.A.T.s has
shown that poor differentiation here heightens the level of anxious attachment.

In conclusion, Mitchell stated (p. 365):

The results of this study showed a clear correlation between the histories of
inadequate attachment during childhood for the abusing mothers and anxious

attachment during adulthood. [In my terms, read "anxious attachment" as
strong-to-severe anxious attachment.] . . . As the abused children developed
into adulthood, they continued to manifest separation disorders as assessed by
the Hansburg Separation Anxiety Test. . . . Compared to non-abusing mothers
significantly more pathological responses to the separation stimulus were noted
in the protocols of the abusing mothers. . . . They were unable to differentiate
the degree of separation stimulus, reacting to (both) mild and strong stimuli
with heightened attachment responses. . . . (Their) level of self-reliance was
markedly decreased with resultant feelings of depression. . . .

In addition to the data on the S.A.T., Mitchell pointed out that
her study definitely disproved the notion that the socioeconomic and
cultural levels are cardinal factors in the abuse of children by their
mothers. Experiential and psychological factors explainable by attachment theory are shown to be of greater significance. Abusive
mothers demonstrated significantly less desire to talk to their own
mothers, fathers, stepparents, and spouses, indicating a difficulty in
dealing with and communicating with close family members. The
presence of numerous close relatives and support systems does not ob-
viate a potential for child abuse, but it changes the use made of
closeness, which is more primary.

REFERENCES

(Since Mitchell includes twenty pages of references for her study, I
have taken the liberty of reducing this list to those I consider most pertinent to this summary. Those who wish the complete list should refer
to the original dissertation.)

Ainsworth, M., and Bell, S. M. "Attachment, Exploration and Separations:
    Illustrated by the Behavior of One-Year-Olds in a Strange Situation."
    Child Development, 1970, *41*, 49–69.
Ainsworth, M. D., Bell, S. M., and Stayton, D. J. "Infant-Mother Attachment
    and Social Development," in M. Richards (ed.), *The Integration of a
    Child into a Social World*. London: Cambridge University Press, 1974.
Alvarez, R. "The Psycho-Historical and Socio-Economic Development of the
    Chicano Community in the United States." *Social Science Quarterly*,
    1973, *53*, 921–949.
Alvy, K. "Preventing Child Abuse." *American Psychologist*, 1975, *30*,
    921–928.

Arling, G., and Harlow, H. "Effects of a Social Deprivation on Maternal Behavior of Rhesus Monkeys." *Journal of Comparative and Physiological Psychology*, 1967, *64*, 371–377.

Avery, N. "Viewing Child Abuse and Neglect as Symptoms of Family Dysfunctioning," in N. Eberling and D. Hill (eds.), *Child Abuse*. Acton, Mass.: Publishers Sciences Group, 1975.

Blumberg, M. "Psychopathology of the Abusing Parent." *American Journal of Psychotherapy*, 1974, *28*, 21–29.

Bowlby, J. *Loss, Detachment and Defence*. London: Tavistock Child Development Research Unit, 1962.

Bowlby, J. *Attachment and Loss*, Vol. II: *Separation: Anxiety and Anger*. New York: Basic Books, 1973.

Buriel, R., Loya, P., Gonda, T., and Klessen, K. "Child Abuse and Neglect Referral Patterns of Anglo and Mexican-Americans." *Hispanic Journal of Behavioral Sciences*, 1979, *1*, 215–227.

Clarke, A., and Menzel, R. *Child Abuse in Pierce County's Non-Community: A Study of Perceptions and Attitudes*. Unpublished paper, sponsored by Panel for Family Living, Tacoma, Wash. (Grant 90-0-77, DHEW), May 1976.

Cohen, J., and Cohen, P. *Applied Multiple Regression/Correlation and Analysis for the Behavioral Sciences*. Hillsdale, N.J.: Lawrence Erlbaum Associates, 1975.

DeLozier, P. P. *Application of Attachment Theory to the Study of Child Abuse*. Unpublished doctoral dissertation, California School of Professional Psychology, Los Angeles, 1979.

Fontana, V. J. *Somewhere a Child Is Crying: Maltreatment, Causes and Prevention*. New York: Macmillan, 1973.

Garbarino, J. "A Preliminary Study of Some Ecological Correlates of Child Abuse: The Impact of Sociological Stress on Mothers." *Child Development*, 1976, *47*, 178–185.

Gelles, R. J. "Child Abuse as Psychopathology: A Sociological Critique and Reformulation." *American Journal of Orthopsychiatry*, 1973, *43*, 611–621.

Gil, D. G. *Violence Against Children: Physical Child Abuse in the United States*. Boston: Harvard University Press, 1970.

Giavanonni, J. M. "Parental Mistreatment: Perpetrators and Victims." *Journal of Marriage and the Family*, 1971, *33*, 649–657.

Grebler, L., Moore, J., and Guzman, R. *The Mexican-American People: The Nation's Second Largest Minority*. New York: Free Press, 1970.

Griswold, B., and Billingsley, A. *Personality and Social Characteristics of Low-Income Mothers Who Neglect or Abuse Their Children.* Unpublished manuscript, University of California at Los Angeles, 1967.

Guerrero-Pavich, E. *Study of the Cultural Differences Among Mexican-Americans and Mexican Nationals Regarding Consensus of Opinion of the Relative Seriousness of Sexual Child Abuse.* Unpublished master's thesis, University of California at Los Angeles, 1978.

Hansburg, H. G. *Adolescent Separation Anxiety.* Springfield, Ill.: Charles C. Thomas, 1972. Reprinted, Melbourne, Fla.: R. E. Krieger, 1980.

Hansburg, H. G. *Some Conceptualizations in Regard to Studies of Families with the Separation Anxiety Test.* Unpublished paper, available from the author, 1975.

Hansburg, H. G. *Separation Disorders: A Manual for the Interpretation of Emotional Disorders Manifested on the Separation Anxiety Test.* Melbourne, Fla.: R. E. Krieger, 1980.

Hansburg, H. G. Personal communication, May 1979.

Harlow, H. F., Harlow, M. K., and Hansen, J. "The Maternal Affectional System," in H. Rinegold (ed.), *Maternal Behavior in Mammals.* New York: John Wiley and Sons, 1963.

Justice, B., and Justice, R. *The Abusing Family.* New York: Human Sciences Press, 1976.

Keefe, S. E., Padilla, A. M., and Carlos, M. L. "The Mexican-American Extended Family as an Emotional Support System." *Human Organization*, 1979, *38*, 144–152.

Maden, M., and Wrench, D. "Significant Findings in Child Abuse Research." *Victimology: An International Journal*, 1977, *2*, 196–224.

Mirande, A. "The Chicano Family: A Reanalysis of Conflicting Views." *Journal of Marriage and the Family*, 1977, *39*, 747–756.

Mitchell, M. C. *An Application of Attachment Theory to a Socio-Cultural Perspective of Physical Child Abuse in the Mexican-American Community.* Unpublished doctoral dissertation, California School of Professional Psychology, Los Angeles, 1980.

Navarro, J., and Swinger, H. "Child Abuse and the Chicano Family," in *Child Abuse, Neglect and the Family within a Cultural Context*, DHEW Publication No. (OHDS) 78-30135, Washington, D.C.: U.S. Govt. Printing Office, 1978.

Olmedo, E., and Padilla, A. "Empirical and Construct Validation of a Measure of Acculturation for Mexican-Americans" *Journal of Social Psychology*, 1978, *105*, 179–187.

Paulson, M. "A Discriminant Function Procedure for Identifying Abusing Parents." *Suicide*, 1975, *5*, 104–114.

Spinetta, J. "Parental Personality Factors in Child Abuse." *Journal of Consulting and Clinical Psychology*, 1978, *4*, 1408–1414.

Spinetta, J., and Rigler, D. "The Child Abusing Parent." *Psychological Bulletin*, 1972, *77*, 296–304.

Steele, B. F., and Pollock, C. B. "A Psychiatric Study of Parents Who Abuse Infants and Small Children," in R. Helfer and C. Kempe (eds.), *Battered Child*. Chicago: University of Chicago Press, 1968.

Uhlenberg, P. "Marital Instability among Mexican-Americans: Is It Following the Pattern of the Blacks?" *Social Problems*, 1972, *20*, 49–56.

U.S. Department of Health, Education and Welfare. "Americans of Spanish Origin," in *A Study of Selected Socio-Economic Characteristics of Ethnic Minorities*, Vol. I. Washington, D.C.: U.S. Govt. Printing Office, 1974.

Wallace, A. *An Application of Attachment Theory to the Study of Divorced People*. Unpublished doctoral dissertation, California School of Professional Psychology, Los Angeles, 1977.

3

Kaleita's Study of Attachment and Separation Anxiety in Abused and Neglected Adolescents

A study of child abuse by Dr. Thomas A. Kaleita was completed for a doctorate at the California School of Professional Psychology at Los Angeles in 1980. It was entitled "The Expression of Attachment and Separation Anxiety in Abused and Neglected Adolescents." This study used the Roberts Apperception Test and the Hansburg S.A.T. on adolescent boys from 12 to 15 years of age. In addition, the Conners Rating Scale was given to social workers and counselors at residential institutions and to teachers at each school to rate each boy's behavior.

The principal goal of this study was to investigate the effects of abusive and neglectful environments on attachment and separation patterns of male adolescents. After a review of the literature, the author spent some time in defining both abuse and neglect, quoting from the works of Lourie (1976, 1977, 1979), Martin (1972, 1974, 1976), Helfer and Kempe (1972), Green (1968), Friedrich and Boriskin (1976), and Gregg and Elmer (1969), but neglecting the significant studies of DeLozier (1979) and Mitchell (1980) dealing with abusive mothers. He discussed the phenomenal growth of attention to child abuse in general and the institution of law and legal methods for the reporting and handling of child abuse cases in particular. In his efforts to develop the theoretical aspects of the problem, he presented a discussion of Bowlby, Ainsworth, Harlow, and Mahler's theories of attachment, to which he gave weight in his study.

27

The author's main hypothesis was that unpredictable attachment relationships in the past result in dysfunctional attempts by adolescents to resolve their developmental tasks. The S.A.T. came into use in this effort in the hope that variables in this test would differentiate between those who had been abused and those from an apparently healthier family environment. Other tests which were extremely helpful were the Roberts Apperception Test, an instrument designed to elicit a variety of emotional reactions to supportive and conflictive relationships, and the Conners Behavior Rating Scale-Teachers Form, a measure of behavior and symptoms as observed by teachers.

Kaleita used three groups of adolescents: (a) physically abused, (b) emotionally neglected, and (c) relatively normal, and he was largely interested in differential facts between them on these tests. In this presentation the emphasis will be largely on how he used the S.A.T. to determine such differentiation. Additionally, since he considered Bowlby's theory of attachment as significant in studying child abuse, he felt that the test would evaluate aspects of attachment disorders in such youngsters. Because ethnic factors seemed important to him, he divided his subjects into Caucasian, black, and Latino.

The subjects in this study consisted of ninety-six adolescent males, aged 12 through 15, evenly divided between Caucasian, black, and Latino ethnic backgrounds. The mean age for all these ethnic groups was approximately 14½, but the Caucasian group showed a generally higher economic status. The "normal" group was selected from four parochial schools, while the abused and emotionally neglected adolescents were obtained from five residential placement facilities in Los Angeles County. The physically abused group of thirty-one adolescents placed in this group had been defined as such by their history of injury by parents or other care-taking adults and validated by a court, agency, or institutional reports. There was a considerable range of periods of stay in institutions for these boys, from weeks to several years. Most had been declared delinquent, and the reasons were often quite varied.

The group of thirty-two adolescents who were defined in the study as emotionally neglected had been in residential institutions as well, but nowhere in their histories was there evidence of physical abuse. Kaleita suggested that all had experienced dramatic parental failure to provide nurturance, protection, or supervision. All had been placed because of repeated delinquent behavior. Similarly to the abused group, all had been in residence from weeks to several years. The thirty-three "normal" adolescents showed no evidence in their histories of emotional neglect, significant behavior problems, emotional disorder, or academic underachievement.

Kaleita hypothesized that the physically abused group would report a significantly higher number of responses on the following response patterns than the "normal" group: hostility, reality avoidance, self-love loss, separation pain, attachment, individuation, and identity stress. Apparently, he felt that the group of separation patterns would be affected by physical abuse—a highly unlikely set of reactions. No explanation for this hypothesis was offered. Further, he reasoned that emotionally neglected adolescents would report a significantly higher number of responses in the same areas as the physically abused. Again, he offered no explanation for this theorizing.

The study utilized a two-factor approach between subjects, an experimental design to facilitate comparison of the similarities and differences between the three groups. The two factors were abuse level and ethnic background, and each factor had three categories, thus yielding nine combinations. Two major statistical analyses were conducted, using the Statistical Analysis System package of the S.A.S. Institute Inc. of Raleigh, North Carolina. In addition, analyses of variance were performed to examine differences in age and socioeconomic class among the nine subgroups. Age and socioeconomic class were then covaried to eliminate the effects of these variables from the dependent measures.

A two-way analysis of variance was first performed to examine the main effects and interactions of abuse level and ethnicity. The dependent variables were examined for significant differences, and this was followed by tests of simple main effects to clarify the location of these differences.

The second major statistical analysis involved a two-way multivariate analysis of variance. This procedure utilized the combination of all dependent variables to examine the main effects and interactions of the three levels of the two factors. In the interest of brevity, the analysis of variance for the age variable and for the socioeconomic variable will not be presented. Nor will the data on the Roberts Apperception Test or the Conners Rating Scale be presented. We shall confine the test results to the Separation Anxiety Test.

Here the two-way analyses of variance indicated significant differences with respect to abuse level ($p < .008$) and interactions of abuse level and ethnicity ($p < .04$) on the *individuation response pattern*. Interaction effects of abuse level and ethnicity also produced significant findings ($p < .006$) on the *reality avoidance response pattern* (defensive processes). The summaries of the analyses of these two variables are located in Tables 3.1, 3.2, 3.3, and 3.4.

The results of this study with the S.A.T. corroborated other studies suggesting that delinquent boys tend to show excessive self-

Table 3.1

TWO-WAY ANALYSIS OF VARIANCE OF INDIVIDUATION RESPONSE

PATTERN SCORES ON THE HANSBURG S.A.T.

Source of Variation	df	Sum of Squares	Mean Squares	F Ratio	p Level
Ethnicity	2	1.55	.78	.04	.97
Abuse Level	2	222.29	111.15	5.05	.008
Ethnicity & Abuse Level	4	229.36	57.34	2.60	.04
Error	87	1916.10	22.02		
Total	95	2377.49			

Table 3.2

TWO-WAY ANALYSIS OF VARIANCE OF REALITY AVOIDANCE RESPONSE

(DEFENSIVE PROCESSES) SCORES ON THE HANSBURG S.A.T.

Source of Variation	df	Sum of Squares	Mean Squares	F Ratio	p Level
Ethnicity	2	70.29	35.15	1.41	.25
Abuse Level	2	76.03	38.02	1.53	.22
Ethnicity & Abuse Level	4	386.49	96.02	3.89	.006
Error	87	2161.85	24.85		
Total	95	2707.33			

sufficiency syndromes and often show high defense levels. It should be noted that emotionally neglected blacks showed similar levels to Caucasians and Latinos in the individuation area. Emotionally neglected blacks also showed high levels of reality avoidance, but the physically abused Latinos were the most defensive of all the groups. Nevertheless, all the physically abused and emotionally neglected were derived from delinquent institutions and generally showed excessive self-sufficiency patterns and defensive reactions. In the original research with the S.A.T., it was found that the most dominant defensive pattern was evasion, a common characteristic of acting out youngsters (see Hansburg 1972, 1980). There was no analysis by Kaleita of the three responses making up the pattern referred to as reality avoidance.

Referring to his results, Kaleita stated that they demonstrated an excessive dependency on self and a trend toward creating emotional distance from others because of previously unsatisfied needs. "Hans-

Table 3.3

MEANS ACCORDING TO ABUSE LEVEL AND ETHNICITY ON THE

INDIVIDUATION RESPONSE PATTERN OF THE HANSBURG S.A.T.

	Physically Abused	Emotionally Neglected	Normal
Black	8.10	12.36	8.36
White	12.20	8.82	6.91
Latino	12.55	8.80	6.82

Table 3.4

MEANS ACCORDING TO ABUSE LEVEL AND ETHNICITY ON THE

REALITY AVOIDANCE RESPONSE PATTERN OF THE HANSBURG S.A.T.

	Physically Abused	Emotionally Neglected	Normal
Black	5.30	9.45	7.18
White	7.20	7.82	6.18
Latino	13.73	6.80	6.45

burg (1972) had suggested that adolescents with high scores on this response pattern are likely to act out in various ways depending on other psychological characteristics." Adolescents who experienced neither abuse nor emotional neglect showed lower frequencies of individuation responses on the test. The author further indicated that physical abuse and emotional neglect result in inadequate attachments.

Each subject in the two mistreatment groups had documented histories of rejection, abandonment or separation of some sort by a parental figure. . . . It is suggested that the expression of "pseudo-independence" is centered around increasing uncertainty about the availability of attachment figures as well as cognitive representations developed from past experience. Moreover, there is substantial evidence that a natural course of changing attachment-separation patterns is a general characteristic of this age. It would appear that intense anxiety from past and present separation experiences combined with the developmental tasks of this stage would combine to establish cyclical patterns of pathological conflict. An adolescent in these circumstances may, therefore, be compelled to adapt by becoming "pseudo-mature" and self-protective through avoidance of contact with others who would normally provide this function.

Kaleita continued to discuss the results on the reality avoidance response pattern, which he thought complicated understanding of these defensive processes. He raised the issue of defensive styles of various ethnic groups. Because of the considerable variability demonstrated in the study, he urged further research to clarify the issue.

In his summary Kaleita included, among others, the conclusion that physical abuse and emotional neglect result in a deficit in the ability to perceive available attachment figures in the environment. "Furthermore, because of the unavailability of attachment figures, they demonstrate an excessive self-dependency for satisfaction of their needs, supporting the description of the abused child as 'pseudo-mature' or 'pseudo-independent.' "

An enhancement of this study in regard to the use of the S.A.T. might have been achieved if the clinical evaluation of each protocol had been carefully appraised. By examining the clinical aspects of the S.A.T. patterns and determining to what extent different patterns existed in the three groups of adolescents, perhaps another dimension of understanding might have been obtained. Further, an additional index in which individuation-hostility (consisting of six items) was subtracted from the attachment-pain pattern (consisting of another six items) might have been very useful. (See Chapter 17 for a discussion of this index.)

Various forms of detachment have been fairly consistently noted in children exposed to abuse, neglect, or other traumatic forms of either abandonment or threats of separation. The similarity of these results in Kaleita's study to those of children of divorce in Brody (1981) and Miller (1980), although in the latter two studies the children were younger, is noteworthy. However, in adults the patterns on the S.A.T. tend to move in the directions of severe anxious attachment (DeLozier (1979) and Mitchell (1981)) and detachment. It was surprising that Kaleita did not find differentiating hostility and hostile detachment among delinquents, especially those who have been in residential care and treatment (see Hansburg, "Separation Hostility: A Prelude to Violence," International Congress of Psychology, Tokyo, 1972).

In a significant discussion of his subjects, Kaleita indicated some of the problems which might well have mitigated against a truer determination of the truth or error of many of his hypotheses. These included accessibility, identification, parenting and residential variables, and ethnicity. I quote from some of this discussion:

The problem of identification is a critical issue from a number of perspectives. The subjects in this study were from predominantly lower and lower middle class socio-economic backgrounds, a bias consistent with recent literature which connects low income and low occupational status with child abuse and neglect (e.g., Gelles, 1979; Pelton, 1978). The existing literature also contains evidence that there are significant differences in child rearing patterns between families from various socio-economic classes (Miller and Swanson, 1966). Nonetheless, it seems reasonable to argue that children from higher socio-economic classes have also been abused and neglected, yet their presence in residential care systems is virtually nil. [Kaleita is probably referring here to public institutions rather than private or private agency facilities.] The reasons for this phenomenon and the effects of abuse on child development independent of socio-economic class have been elaborated by Kent (1976), who believes that upper class families have greater ability to contain maladaptive familial interactions. Thus, it remains a possibility that the institutional population studied may represent a predetermined bias if residential placement is considered a more likely consequence for adolescents from lower socio-economic backgrounds.

Kaleita was also impressed with the considerable variations in parenting contacts and similar variations in the nature and degree of treatment while in the residence; he stated:

The resultant effect of these differences in familial contact and treatment time no doubt accounted for variations in responses to the measures employed. Despite these differences . . . these adolescents did demonstrate profound deficits (especially in attachment reactions).

The division of subjects along ethnic dimensions was implemented as an initial investigation into possible cultural differences in the expression of attachment and separation anxiety. . . . The present study did not yield essential differences between ethnic groups on the measures employed. The fact that all Caucasian groups were from significantly higher socio-economic backgrounds is consistent with the generally accepted view of socio-economic stratification in our culture.

Despite Kaleita's efforts here to introduce differences in child rearing in various cultures as a limiting factor, it may well be that his results demonstrated that abuse and neglect have very similar effects on children even in different settings; witness the similarity of results of Mitchell (1981) and DeLozier (1979) on abusive mothers.

REFERENCES

Bowlby, J. "The Nature of the Child's Tie to His Mother." *International Journal of Psychoanalysis*, 1958, *39*, 350–373.

Bowlby, J. *Attachment and Loss*, Vol. I: *Attachment*. New York: Basic Books, 1969.

Bowlby, J. *Attachment and Loss*, Vol. II: *Separation: Anxiety and Anger*. New York: Basic Books, 1973.

Brody, Nancy P. *An Investigation of the Effects of Parental Divorce on Third Graders, etc.* Unpublished doctoral dissertation, Loyola University, Chicago, 1981.

Conners, C. "A Teacher Rating Scale for Use in Drug Studies in Children." *American Journal of Psychiatry*, 1969, *126*, 884–888.

DeLozier, P. P. *An Application of Attachment Theory to the Study of Child Abuse*. Unpublished doctoral dissertation, California School of Professional Psychology, Los Angeles, 1979.

Fontana, V. J. *Somewhere a Child Is Crying: Maltreatment, Causes and Prevention*. New York: Macmillan, 1968.

Freedman, S., and Morse, C. "Child Abuse: A Five Year Follow-up Study of Early Case Findings in the Emergency Dept." *Pediatrics*, 1974, *54*, 404–410.

Friedrich, W., and Boriskin, J. "The Role of the Child in Abuse: A Review of the Literature." *American Journal of Orthopsychiatry*, 1976, *46*, 580–590.

Galdston, R. "Violence Begins at Home: The Parents' Center Project for the Study and Prevention of Child Abuse." *American Academy of Child Psychiatry Journal*, 1971, *10*, 336–350.

Gelles, R. "Violence toward Children in the United States." *American Journal of Orthopsychiatry*, 1978, *48*, 580–592.

Gil, D. G. *Violence Against Children: Physical Child Abuse in the United States*. Cambridge, Mass.: Harvard University Press, 1970.

Green, A. "Self Destruction in Physically Abused Schizophrenic Children: Report of Cases." *Archives of General Psychiatry*, 1968, *19*, 171–197.

Gregg, G., and Elmer, E. "Infant Injuries, Accident or Abuse?" *Pediatrics*, 1969, *44*, 434–439.

Hansburg, H. G. *Adolescent Separation Anxiety*, Springfield, Ill.: Charles C. Thomas, 1972. Reprinted, Melbourne, Fla.: R. E. Krieger, 1980.

Hansburg, H. G. "The Use of the Separation Anxiety Test in the Detection of Self-Destructive Tendencies in Early Adolescence," in D. V. Siva Sankar (ed.), *Mental Health in Children*, Vol. III. Westbury, N.Y.: P. J. D. Publications, 1976, 161–199.

Helfer, R., and Kempe, H. (eds.). *Helping the Battered Child and His Family*. Chicago: University of Chicago Press, 1972.

Kagan, J. "The Stability of TAT Fantasy and Stimulus Ambiguity." *Journal of Consulting and Clinical Psychology*, 1959, *23*, 266–271.

Kaleita, T. A. *The Expression of Attachment and Separation Anxiety in Abused and Neglected Adolescents*. Unpublished doctoral dissertation, California School of Professional Psychology, Los Angeles, 1980.

Lourie, I. "The Phenomenon of the Abused Adolescent: A Clinical Study." *Victimology*, 1977, *2*, 268–274.

Lourie, I. *Family Dynamics and the Abuse of Adolescents: A Case for a Developmental Phase Specific Model of Child Abuse*. Unpublished paper, 1979.

Lourie, I., and Cohen, A. "Abuse and Neglect of Adolescents." *Child Abuse Reports*, 1976, *1*, 6.

Lynch, M. "Risk Factors in the Child: A Study of Abused Children and Their Siblings," in H. Martin (ed.), *The Abused Child: A Multidisciplinary Approach to Developmental Issues and Treatment*. Cambridge, Mass.: Ballinger, 1976.

Martin, H., Beezley, P., Conway, E., and Kempe, H. "The Development of Abused Children," in I. Schuman (ed.), *Advances in Pediatrics*. Chicago: Yearbook Medical Publishers, 1974.

McArthur, D., and Robert, G. *Manual for Roberts Apperception Test*. Los Angeles: Western Psychological Services, 1980.

Miller, J. B. *The Effects of Separation on Latency Age Children as a Consequence of Separation-Divorce*. Unpublished doctoral dissertation, California School of Professional Psychology, Los Angeles, 1980.

Mitchell, M. C. *An Application of Attachment Theory to a Sociocultural Perspective of Physical Child Abuse to the Mexican-American Community*. Unpublished doctoral dissertation, California School of Professional Psychology, Los Angeles, 1980.

Morris, M., and Gould, R. "Role Reversal: A Concept in Dealing with the Neglected/Battered Child Syndrome," in *The Neglected-Battered Child Syndrome*. New York: Child Welfare League of America, 1963.

Pelton, L. "Child Abuse and Neglect: The Myth of Classlessness." *American Journal of Orthopsychiatry*, 1978, *48*, 608–617.

Steirlin, H. *Separating Parents and Adolescents*. New York: Quadrangle Books, 1974.

Wick, E. *A Study of the Development of Self-Concept in Physically Abused Children*. Unpublished doctoral dissertation, California School of Professional Psychology, Los Angeles, 1978.

STUDIES OF DIVORCE

4

Miller's Study of the Effects of Separation and/or Divorce on Latency-Age Children

Several studies of divorce and its effect on children, adolescents, and adults were done with the S.A.T. as one of the instruments of research. The first of these studies was undertaken by Dr. Joyce B. Miller at the California School of Professional Psychology in Los Angeles. This study, entitled "The Effects of Separation on Latency Age Children as a Consequence of Separation-Divorce," was completed in 1980. The subjects were children ages 9 through 12 in two comparable groups, one group of thirty from separated-divorced families and the other group of thirty from intact families. Comparisons were made between both groups with regard to maternal backgrounds and the history of separation reactions in mothers and children. Differential studies were made comparing both groups' reactions to the S.A.T.

In this study, Miller hypothesized that the S.A.T. would uncover characteristic reactions of children from separated/divorced families. These included the following: (a) greater overall sensitivity to separation as measured by the attachment subscale, (b) less self-reliance as measured by the individuation scale, (c) more anxious attachment, (d) a greater number of attachment responses, (e) more depressive factors, (f) a higher percentage of separation hostility, (g) greater painful tension, and (h) the highest score on separation hostility for those with attachment dysfunction. It was further hypothesized that, regardless of marital status, the mother who, in the analysis of their attachment history, (a) disclosed significant disruptions of early attachment bonds, or (b) disclosed significant threats of separation, parental suicide, and disciplinary threats, or (c) reported with significant frequency anxious concern for their parents, or (d) had significantly fewer numbers of significant others whom they could turn to in childhood, as well as less assurance or perception of accessibility and help, would have children who exhibited attachment dysfunction.

Similarly to the preceding, theories with regard to the children's attachment history in relation to the four indicated factors and their resultant attachment dysfunction were to be examined and compared without regard to the parents' marital status. Finally, two more hypotheses were to determine whether or not children from separated and divorced families who had significantly less access to their mothers as a result of the separation or divorce would exhibit attachment dysfunction.

In her review of the literature, Miller was impressed with the minimal number of research studies in this field which were of acceptable quality; she stated:

Except for a few prospective studies (Wallerstein & Kelly, 1976; Hetherington, Cox, & Cox, 1977; Jacobson, 1977) all research is retrospective. Also, although longitudinal studies seem a most appropriate way of assessing factors of importance regarding children and divorce, only two studies to date employed this design (the first two listed above). There is much to be learned concerning separation/divorce and the ways in which separations, as well as threats of separation, may affect a child's development. Although research has been sparse, those variables which have been identified as important in the study of the effects of parental separation include: 1) the age and developmental stage of the child at the time of separation, 2) sex of the child, 3) sex of the non-custodial parent, 4) the length and frequency of the separation, 5) the quality of the parent/child relationships, both pre- and post-divorce, and 6) time lost with both parents post-divorce. Most children are unhappy about their parents' divorce but emotional and behavioral responses vary. Children are often depressed, angry, and anxious when their parents separate. As the literature also states, children who are raised in unhappy, never-divorced households may also exhibit disturbed behaviors, depression, anxiety and anger. This study also examines children from never-divorced families in the hope of obtaining data which will either support or refute this thesis.

Attachment theory will be used as a theoretical base for this study and it is assumed that in order to explain and understand the ways in which a child is affected by separation experiences, one must have knowledge not only of the child's attachment history but also that of the child's primary caretaker. It is further assumed that in order for a child to have a healthy balance between attachment and self-reliance, he or she must have had and have a secure base.

Separation and threats of separation early in life as well as later on may be responsible for a child's increased sensitivity to any separation experience. Further, significant disruptions of early attachment bonds, as well as the lack of available support systems, can lead to different forms of attachment dysfunction, namely anxious attachment and detachment.

Miller selected sixty children from ages 9 to 12 and their mothers as her subjects for study. Thirty of these were from never-divorced families, and thirty were from separated or divorced families. The criteria for inclusion in the separated or divorced group included the following: (a) the parents had been separated between one month and two years, (b) the mother was the custodial parent, and (c) neither parent had remarried. The study included fifteen girls and fifteen boys in the control group and eighteen girls and twelve boys in the experimental group. All subjects for the study were voluntary. Subjects for the never-divorced group were obtained from the following sources: friendship networks of the researcher (eight subjects), a local community synagogue (eight subjects), and a PTA leader of a Los Angeles school district (fourteen subjects). Subjects from the separated and divorced group were obtained from the following sources: friendship networks of the researcher (three subjects), alumni resources from previous schools the researcher attended (nineteen subjects), clients at the Center for Legal Psychiatry, Post-Divorce Clinic (six subjects), and the PTA (two subjects).

When the two groups were compared with respect to demographic characteristics, there were no significant differences in the distribution of the children's age, sex, birth order, or religion. Results showed that the separated/divorced group was more likely to have had psychotherapy than the children from never-divorced families (separated/divorced = 20.0, $p > .05$).

The mean age of mothers at time of marriage was 21.86 for the mothers in the never-divorced group and 21.83 for those in the separated/divorced group. There were no differences in the socioeconomic status between the mothers of both groups preseparation. There was a significant drop in income, however, in the separated/divorced group postseparation. The never-divorced mothers' mean monthly income was about $4,260.00, while the separated/divorced mothers' mean monthly income was $2,295.00 ($t = 3.87$, $p > .05$). Mothers from separated/divorced families showed significantly higher levels of education than never-divorced mothers (never-divorced group:

H.S. = 44.8, A.A. = 10.3; separated/divorced group: B.A. = 46.7, M.A. = 30.0, $p > .05$). At the time of the study, separated/divorced mothers also, like their children, participated in counseling and psychotherapy with significantly greater frequency than the never-divorced mothers (never-divorced mothers' group mean = 10.08, t = 3.22, $p > .05$).

The children were given the S.A.T. and a revised form of the Wallace Attachment History Questionnaire, while the mothers were administered the appropriate Attachment History Questionnaire and a Marital Adjustment Scale which had been incorporated as part of the questionnaire. Aside from the tests, an additional dependent variable was introduced, the time spent with parents and extended family, both prior and subsequent to parental separation.

The areas for statistical analysis of the data were as follows: (a) patterns of attachment and individuation (self-reliance), (b) group differences on various subscales of the S.A.T., (c) the relationship between attachment dysfunction and affective measures of the S.A.T., (d) the relation of a mother's attachment history to her child's attachment dysfunction (as measured by the S.A.T.), (e) the relation of a child's early attachment history to his or her attachment dysfunction, and (f) the relation of a child's attachment dysfunction to his or her accessibility to parents. Basic analysis was performed by independent t tests. However, multiple regression/correlation analysis was performed on all hypotheses to determine the relationship of a variety of demographic characteristics, as well as group membership, to the dependent variable. These characteristics included the subject's birth order, sex, and religion, the length of the parent's separation, whether the child or the mother was currently in psychotherapy, and whether the child was from a never-divorced or separated/divorced family.

RESULTS

The first hypothesis (Subject A) tested the overall sensitivity to separation by subtracting the attachment responses on the mild pictures from those on the strong pictures. The mean sensitivity score for the separated/divorced group was 9.63 (S.D. = 6.10), and the mean score for the never-divorced group was 11.4 (S.D. = 5.63) (+ score of 1.16 N.S.). (This score, as a measure of overall sensitivity to separation, is highly doubtful. More to the point is the index of attachment-pain minus individuation hostility, to be discussed later.) The first hypothesis (Subject A) was not confirmed by this particular method of expressing overall sensitivity to separation.

The first hypothesis (Subject B) tested the ability to be self-reliant, theorizing that separated/divorced children would show less self-reliance. This was done by subtracting individuation responses under the strong stimulus from the individuation responses under the mild stimulus. While this hypothesis was not confirmed, *there was a strong tendency in the opposite direction to that which was predicted*. The mean score for the separated/divorced group was 6.26 (S.D. = 4.33), and the mean score for the never-divorced group was 3.06 (S.D. = 9.34) ($t = -1.70$ N.S.).

The first hypothesis (Subject C) tested anxious attachment by subtracting the total percentage of attachment responses on the mild separation situations frog the percentage of individuation responses on the mild separation situations. (Unfortunately, Miller here used only one of the six factors of anxious attachment described in the study of early adolescents to make the comparison. The fuller evaluation is noted later). These data did not confirm the hypothesis. The mean score for the separated/divorced group was 8.56 (S.D. = 9.39), and the mean score for the never-divorced group was 5.73 (S.D. = 11.38) ($t = -1.05$ N.S.).

The first hypothesis (Subject D) tested whether children from separated/divorced families would exhibit significantly greater attachment responses to separation when compared with children from never-divorced families. This was done by subtracting the strong individuation responses from the strong attachment responses. This method of studying this hypothesis proved abortive and was not confirmed, and there was a strong trend in the opposite direction to that which was predicted. The mean score for the separated/divorced group was 7.33 (S.D. = 8.45), and the mean score for the never-divorced group was 11.4 (S.D. = 8.47) ($t = 1.86$ N.S.).

With regard to the first hypothesis (Subject D), subsequent analysis revealed that those children who had had therapy (or counseling) and the children of mothers who were currently in counseling or therapy tended to have more attachment responses than the others. This finding was more true of the males than of the females.

The first hypothesis (Subject E) examined the degree to which children from separated/divorced families would exhibit an overall higher level of attachment responses, combined with an overall lower level of self-reliance responses, as compared with children from intact families. This was determined by subtracting the total individuation percentage from the total attachment percentage. Although this hypothesis was not confirmed, there was a definite trend in the predicted direction. The mean score for the separated/divorced group was -2.13 (S.D. $= 19.38$), and the mean score for the intact family group was 5.43 (S.D. $= 16.10$) ($t = 1.64$ N.S.).

The second hypothesis predicted that children from separated and divorced families, regardless of length of separation, would show more depressive factors when compared with those from intact families. Depressive factors were measured by scores on the self-love loss subscale of the S.A.T. (Unfortunately, the better measure of depressive reaction, which consisted of a higher self-love loss percentage than self-preoccupation percentage, was not used in this study.) This hypothesis was not confirmed. The mean score for the separated/divorced group was 8.63 (S.D. $= 5.20$), and the mean score for the intact group was 8.36 (S.D. $= 4.52$) ($t = -.21$ N.S.).

Further analysis of the latter hypothesis indicated that only children tended to exhibit fewer depressive factors than children of any other birth order, children whose mothers had previously been in therapy tended to have fewer depressive factors than children whose mothers had not, and children who were currently in therapy tended to have a greater number of depressive factors than children who were not currently in therapy.

The third hypothesis predicted that children from separated/divorced families would exhibit a total percentage of separation hostility on the S.A.T. which would be significantly higher than those scores of children from intact families. This was measured by the sum of anger, projection, and intrapunitive responses. The hypothesis was not confirmed. The mean score for the separated/divorced group was 14.93 (S.D. $= 6.04$), and the mean score for the intact group was 14.13 (S.D. $= 6.65$) ($t = -.49$ N.S.).

The fourth hypothesis stated that children from separated/divorced families would exhibit a total percentage of separation pain which would be a significantly higher percentage than that for the children from intact families. Separation pain was measured by the total of anxiety, phobic, and somatic responses. This hypothesis was not confirmed. The mean score for the separated/divorced group was 19.03 (S.D. = 6.92), and the mean score for the intact group was 18.43 (S.D. = 7.80) (t = − .32 N.S.).

The fifth hypothesis (Subject A) took the third and fourth hypotheses together and was not confirmed. The mean score for the separated/divorced group was 23.56 (S.D. = 9.96), and the mean score for the intact group was 22.50 (S.D. = 9.67) (t = − .42 N.S.). There was, however, a significant relationship between birth order, mother's current therapy, and the child's current therapy and the sum of hostility and pain. Only children tended to lower scores on the combined subscales of hostility and pain, but children and mothers in current therapy tended to higher scores on these scales.

A number of hypotheses were posited with regard to the relationship between attachment dysfunction and various other factors of the S.A.T., as well as factors of the mother's and the child's history. Attachment dysfunction (anxious attachment) was determined by six factors in the S.A.T.: (a) high attachment with low self-reliance, (b) strong attachment reaction to mild stimulus, (c) high levels of separation hostility and anxiety, (d) high separation avoidance, (e) loss of self-love exceeding self-esteem preoccupation, and (f) unusual levels of identity stress. Attachment dysfunction (detachment) was measured by (a) attachment subscale percentage below 20% and (b) percentage of separation avoidance responses above 13%. Both factors had to be present for a detachment diagnosis (p. 73). Children without attachment dysfunction (anxious attachment) showed a mean of 15.65 (S.D. = 7.31) on the painful tension subscale, and children with anxious attachment showed a mean of 21.08 (S.D. = 6.48) with a t ratio of − 3.04 ($p < .05$), clearly significant in the predicted direction. However, when all attachment dysfunction (detachment) children were compared on painful tension with nondetached children, the differences were not significant.

When similar comparisons were made on the separation-hostility scale, those with no attachment dysfunction were significantly lower in hostility than those with attachment dysfunction. However, when the attachment dysfunction (detachment) group was studied for the hostility measurement, there was no significant difference among high and low scores for the separated/divorced group.

Analysis of the mother's attachment history did not reveal any relationship between early attachment bond disruptions of the mother's and the child's attachment dysfunction (either anxious attachment or detachment). However, there was evidence that mothers who had anxious concern for their parents had children who showed less attachment dysfunction. Mothers who had a smaller number of significant others to appeal to for guidance did not necessarily have children with attachment dysfunction.

Interesting findings were that the mother's religion, the mother's current therapy, and the child's current therapy had significant effects on the number of attachment dysfunctions. Jewish children tended to have a greater number of attachment dysfunctions than any of the other children. Further, children of mothers in therapy showed a greater number of attachment dysfunctions. Accessibility to parents (measured by selected questions on the Child's Attachment History Questionnaire) among the separated/divorced families did not show a relationship to attachment dysfunction. With regard to therapy, there was a definite positive correlation which indicated that the mother's therapy was related to the child's lessened sensitivity to separation. Thus, on the S.A.T. the children of mothers in therapy gave fewer responses to the mild pictures and more responses to the strong pictures.

An important finding (using chi-square analysis) showed that, although not quite statistically significant, many children of separated/divorced parents tended to show an increasing self-sufficiency, coupled with detachment of a hostile character. (See confirmatory evidence in Brody's study of 8-year-olds of divorced parents.) Further, chi-square analysis was also performed, using the Yates correction for discontinuity, to determine if the occurrence of excessively self-sufficient children significantly differed from chance occurrence in the never-divorced and the separated/divorced groups. Results indicated a significant chi-square of 4.3439. While only nine of the thirty never-divorced respondents exhibited excessive self-sufficiency, seventeen of the thirty in the separated/divorced group demonstrated the existence of excessive self-sufficiency.

Another index that appeared to have interesting implications for separated/divorced children was derived from the relationship of attachment-pain index (six items) and individuation-hostility index (six items). It was assumed that attachment and emotionally painful reactions should be normally higher under painful separation experience than self-assertion and hostility. The closer these two indices came to each other, the greater was the likelihood that the personality would be influenced to direct itself toward acting out and toward feelings of greater self-sufficiency. A study was made of the closeness of these two indices to each other in both groups. The mean difference for the intact group was 9.73 (S.D. = 18.09), and for the separated/divorced group, 3.03 (S.D. = 20.22). While not statistically significant, it was fairly clear that there was a definitely increased chance that the children of divorce would be under greater impetus to assert opposition to separation experiences, to be more exploratory of the environment, and to be more hostile. It would also appear that in some cases hostility would dominate and in others the assertion of individuality would be the most characteristic. In intact families it appears that separation would occasion more dominance from either attachment need or the fear-anxiety pain complex. Usually, a more homeostatic balance between attachment and pain levels ensures increasingly better insights into the self, relations with others, and reduced acting out. This changes when the balance moves into the detachment direction.

Individual blind clinical analyses of the S.A.T. protocols (performed by DeLozier) revealed meaningful differences between the two groups of children. When looking at attachment percentages of individual protocols, fourteen of the children of intact families showed attachment percentages greater than 25%, whereas only six of the separated/divorced group were in this category. I indicated (Vol. II,) that mild anxious attachment is a common phenomenon in the general population. (See Chapter 19 for a study of thirty-one mothers.) This reduction of anxious attachment in children of separated/divorced families is consonant with the other statistical findings of this study. While the statistical data show that hostility levels were high for both groups, it is noteworthy that fourteen of the children from the intact families had hostility levels below 12%, but only seven of the children from the separated/divorced group were in this category. This indicated a greater variation in separation hostility level, as well as a more pervasive anger within the children of the separated/divorced families.

Both groups demonstrated high fear-anxiety-pain levels, with nineteen of the control group and twenty-one of the experimental group scoring over 17% of the total number of responses to the test in separation pain. (Miller ascribed this result to the presence of high levels of threats of separation in both groups of children and quoted

Bowlby, 1973, p. 226: "Threats by parents that, if a child is not good, they will not love him any more have frequently been referred to as playing a part in the genesis of anxiety." Miller's own data—see Hypothesis 9-B, p. 81—did not support this conclusion, although there appeared to be some minor trends to greater threats in the separated/divorced group.)

DISCUSSION

This study raised many questions with regard to the validity of overall conclusions about the serious psychological effects of parental separation and/or divorce on children. It also indicated how approaching the results statistically from varying perspectives may lead to varying conclusions. However, there are certain facets of this study which appear to be solidly backed by the data and which may be emphasized in this discussion. The first of these deals with the increased demands made on children of divorce for self-sufficiency.

There is no doubt from these data that children of divorce show a definite increase in individuation and assertion. This is compatible with Wallerstein and Kelly's (1976) finding of pseudo-adolescent behavior in latency-age children. While the latter did not have a control group, the present study, utilizing one, strengthened Wallerstein and Kelly's conclusion. Children's conscious anger, specifically directed at divorcing parents, was evident in both studies. Hetherington, Cox, and Cox (1977) also observed that, after two years postdivorce, parents demanded more mature and independent behavior for their children than they had previously expected, which is compatible with findings in our study. Weiss (1978) described the need for latency-age children and adolescents from single-parent families to assume more adult behavior and responsibilities as a result of either direct demands from mothers or situational factors which place the children in a position where they feel they must behave as adults.

This research study showed no significant differences on affective or cognitive measures (S.A.T. scores) for children who lost time spent with the father after separation, in contrast to Jacobson's study (1977), which showed a significant inverse association in children of ages 7–13 between adjustment to parental separation and amount of time lost with the noncustodial father. The explanation for this differential finding may be multifaceted. Jacobson found a positive correlation between adjustment to parental separation and the child's experience of interparental turbulence. It is possible that the children's attachment to the primary care-giver may have been weakened or threatened as the remaining parent attended to marital conflict. It is difficult to imagine that any care-giver can be sufficiently available to a child during this stressful period. Miller's study relied on self-report from children for this finding, and, in many cases, children reported not only that fathers were more accessible postseparation, but also that the quality of time spent with father was improved. In contrast, the Jacobson study relied on the custodial mother's report of the child's responses to the father's absence. It is highly likely that the mother's impression and the child's experience do not necessarily coincide.

The discrepancies between the findings of these two studies suggest that time lost with father postseparation does not necessarily, in all cases, have a detrimental effect on children. It also suggests that what children are responding to may not be the time lost with the non-custodial parent but the decreased availability of the custodial parent.

Despert (1962) deals with the importance of the marital relationship when assessing a child's well-being. She believes unhappy intact marital stress to be more harmful to children than divorce but presents no systematic evidence to support her belief. Although almost one-quarter of the married mothers identified themselves as unhappily married in the current study, there was no evidence that these particular children were necessarily affected by this factor. There is some evidence that, in compiling data for this study, there were some mothers in the never-divorced group whose children experienced their parents as unhappy and argumentative, although these mothers did not report themselves as such. Therefore, it is difficult to make a definitive statement in regard to the "unhappily-happily married" issue. This is undoubtedly one of the limitations of information based solely on self-report and subjective evaluation. This may also be an example of what Bowlby refers to as suppression of family context (Bowlby, 1973), in which he describes the inclination that parents have to either omit, suppress, or falsify the role that their behavior or feelings may be playing in their children's emotional problems.

The results of the statistical analysis of the S.A.T. protocols (group means of separate scores) revealed a trend in the predicted direction for the separated and divorced group to give more responses to separation

stimuli, although the difference between the groups was not significant. The children of separated and divorced parents tended to be
less sensitive to separation stimuli, more self-reliant, and less anxiously
attached, and to have fewer responses to separation.

Analysis of differences in a measure of depressive factors revealed
that, although there were no significant differences in depression scores
between children from separated and divorced parents and children
from never-divorced parents, birth order had a significant effect on the
subject's depression score. Only-children tended to exhibit fewer
depressive factors than children with siblings. This may be accounted
for by the fact that only children do not have to share their parents
with other siblings. Thus, even if their parents are less available, they
do not sustain as great a loss of parental time as children who must
share their divorced or never-divorced parents with other siblings. (As
previously noted, the measure of the depressive factor in this study was
obtained by the use of the self-love loss percentage—a combination of
feelings of rejection and intrapunitiveness. Actually, it might have
shown a different result if the depressive factor had been obtained by
checking out those children who show a higher self-love loss than self-
esteem preoccupation percentage. A comparison of the number of such
children in each group would have been more definitive.)

Contrary to expectation, there were no significant differences in
separation hostility between the control and experimental groups.
However, both groups had an unusually high percentage of hostility
level compared with the S.A.T. test norms, which consider 12% to
14% of the responses to be within the normal range. This will be
discussed further in the clinical analysis of the S.A.T.

There were no significant differences on the painful tension scale
between the two groups. However, according to the multiple
regression correlational analysis, there is a significant relationship between birth order and the separation hostility and painful tension subscales. Again, it is plausible that only children experience less stress as
they need not be concerned with sibling rivalries. Also, their parents
may be less stressed as they only have one child to give care to.

Exploration of the relationship between how happily married the
mothers were and the amount of the children's separation hostility and
painful tension on the S.A.T. yielded no significant finding. This did
not corroborate findings of other studies reporting some negative effects for children reared in unhappy intact homes (Despert, 1962). As

mentioned earlier, there may be unhappily married families who participated in the study but did not identify themselves as unhappily married, even though their children sometimes perceived them as unhappily married.

In supplementary analysis of my revised indices, children classified as hostile-detached were found to be more prevalent among the separated/divorced children. In addition, the percentage of excessive self-sufficient children was statistically significant, supporting the finding that there were twice as many detached children in the experimental group than in the control group. There is strong indication here that many children of separated or divorced parents developed an increasing self-sufficiency in addition to detachment of a hostile character.

Findings on the Attachment-Pain Index score minus the Individuation-Hostility Index score revealed a trend for the individuation-hostility pattern to be in far greater control of the personality for the children in the separated/divorced group than in the children from never-divorced couples. Theoretically, the healthy power of attachment and pain levels, if properly balanced, is commonly associated with better insights into the self, enhanced relations with others, and reduced acting out. Such effects, however, are considerably reduced in the experimental group by the increased hostility and self-sufficiency. It appears likely that children from separated/divorced families are apt to exhibit detachment as the more dominant form of attachment dysfunction in response to their exposure to parental separation.

When the relation of individual children's attachment dysfunction, as measured by the number of anxious attachment and detachment indices present in individual test protocols, was examined, the results were in the predicted direction. That is, all children with attachment dysfunction, regardless of group membership, scored significantly higher on painful tension than children without attachment dysfunction. The prediction that children with detachment would not score significantly higher on painful tension was also confirmed. The outcome of these hypotheses simply contributed toward internal validation of what the S.A.T. purports to measure.

A significant predicted result was found in the relation between attachment dysfunction and separation hostility in children from separated and divorced families. Children with anxious attachment scored the highest percentage of all divorced children on the separation hostility subscale. Children with detachment did not score significantly higher percentages. Again, this validated the significance of S.A.T. measures.

The analysis of the data on the Child's Attachment History Questionnaire pertaining to early childhood separation experiences revealed no significant differences between the children from separated and divorced families on any variables. It appears that none of the children in the study had significant disruptions of early attachment bonds, other than the experience of parental separation and divorce in the experimental group. An additional finding, revealed by the multiple regression correlational analysis, was that, regardless of group membership, Jewish children tend to have a greater number of attachment dysfunctions. Also, more Jewish children are in therapy than any other religious group. The study revealed that those individuals currently in therapy had more attachment dysfunctions than those not currently in therapy. This study had a large group of Jewish subjects, which may help to account for this finding. Also, Jewish parents may possibly be more predisposed to involve themselves and their children in the therapeutic experience. It also appears likely that those individuals with attachment dysfunction would be in more pain than individuals without attachment dysfunction and, therefore, more likely to seek professional help with their emotional difficulties.

The mother's attachment history in this study was not predictive of attachment dysfunction in the children, except for the item of anxious concern for parents, which was statistically significant, but in the opposite direction to which it was predicted. It was not possible to obtain a meaningful result on this item.

Therapy appeared to have had an impact throughout this study. Regression analysis revealed that children who had previously been in therapy, as well as those whose mothers were currently in therapy, regardless of group membership, gave more attachment responses than those who had not. Mothers and children currently in therapy tended to be less depressed, anxious, and hostile than those subjects who were not currently in therapy across groups of both divorced and never-divorced. Therapy is considered by many to be a mitigating factor in helping people work through and resolve distressing situational factors surrounding the experience of separation and divorce. This therapeutic effect may also be responsible for diminishing the appearance of differences between groups, as well as for the large standard deviations.

The lack of significant differences between the control and experimental group on depression, anxiety, and hostility variables in this study is an important issue which warrants further discussion. Statistically speaking, there is a large within-group variance for both groups which diminishes the possibility of achieving between-group differences. It appears to be of importance to explore the possible causes of this large within-group variance. One possible explanation is that there is something inherent in the divorce experience for children which produces a wide variability in response to that phenomenon.

When we consider the finding that children from separated and divorced families tend to be excessively self-sufficient, more likely to be detached, and less likely to be anxiously attached than children from never-divorced families, it is further interesting to speculate on whether these again are the children who were willing to participate because they were less uncomfortable with their situation. Since one of the requirements for participation in the study was willingness on the part of the child as well as the mother, it is conceivable that those eligible subjects who were approached to be subjects but refused to participate may have had more pain and discomfort with the separation experience. This is something that ought to be seriously thought about by future researchers in the area, and perhaps some way of trying to deal with this problem and adequately meet it methodologically needs to be developed. It does become increasingly clear that there exist some serious limitations in the use of self-selected samples in this kind of research. A clinic population could provide individuals who were in too much pain to ignore it. These people are likely to be anxiously attached and to have sought therapy for help in separating. By using a clinic population, it may be possible to reach some of those people who, in a self-selected population, would refuse to participate.

The individual blind clinical analyses of the S.A.T. protocols, as performed by Dr. DeLozier, revealed meaningful differences between the two groups of children. When we look at attachment percentages of individual protocols, we find that fourteen of the never-divorced group had an attachment percentage greater than 25%, whereas six of the separated/divorced group had an attachment percentage greater than 25%, indicating a large group of anxiously attached children in the never-divorced group. (Bowlby stated, " . . . anxious attachment develops because his experiences have led him to build a model of an attachment figure who is likely to be inaccessible and/or unresponsive to him when he desires her. The more discontinuous and unpredictable the regime, the more anxious his attachment" (1973, p. 225). There is nothing in the attachment history scores of either the mothers or the anxiously attached children to account for this finding.)

Hostility levels were high for both groups. However, it is of interest to note that fourteen of the children from the never-divorced group had hostility levels below 12% compared to only seven of the children from the separated/divorced group, indicating a greater variation in hostility level in the divorced group, as well as a more pervasive anger within the separated/divorced children's group.

In addition to high hostility percentages, both groups had extremely high separation pain levels, with nineteen of the control group and twenty-one of the experimental group scoring over 17% of the total protocol on separation anxiety. This nonpredicted finding may be supportive of Bowlby's view on the effects of parental threats to children. Bowlby (1973, p. 226) stated, "Threats by parents that, if a child is not good, they will not love him any more have frequently been referred to as playing a part in the genesis of anxiety."

In a further attempt to understand and explain the unexpected findings of high levels of anxiety, hostility, and anxious attachment evidenced in the children from never-divorced families in this study, Miller suggested the importance of viewing this Southern California subject population in its cultural and environmental context, as well as its psychological context. The following statement appeared in a report to the President at the White House Conference on Children (1971):

In today's world, parents find themselves at the mercy of a society which imposes pressures and priorities that allow neither time nor place for meaningful activities and relations between children and adults, which downgrade the role of parents and the functions of parenthood, and which prevent the parent from doing things he wants to do as a guide, friend, and companion to his children.

Women and children are not highly valued in our society. Economically speaking, children have been considered inconsequential from the time they were no longer part of the work force. Since the role of motherhood is currently without status, women who choose to be housewives and mothers in our contemporary society often suffer from low self-esteem. As the burden of parenting falls predominantly on women, it is the mother who has a major influence on the child's development.

It is Miller's opinion that mothers in this middle- to upper-middle-class Southern California community are, in all probability, unduly stressed and experiencing diminished status and self-esteem. They are an upwardly mobile group whose husbands are in pursuit of successful careers and acquiring material possessions. Historically speaking, the economic crisis of inflation is eating away at their income, making it difficult for them to achieve economic goals. Socially, these women are expected to be supportive of their husbands' careers, whatever that might entail, and, at the same time, be intellectually, socially, and sexually stimulating. When we consider the role of the working mother, of which there were a number in the current study, the problems are compounded. Since parenting is a difficult, time-consuming, and often exhausting job, it is nearly impossible to be a good parent if one works, maintains a household, has adult social relationships, and attends to at least one child, unless one receives a great deal of support (Bronfenbrenner, 1979). When we consider such realities, it seems plausible that those individuals who are married and have available an extended family and network of friends will be most capable of being available and accessible to their children.

Geographically speaking, it is probable that, in this specific subject population, children are physically isolated from other people. Factors contributing to this condition include full-time working mothers (60%), little or no public transportation, little or no extended family, frequent lack of neighborhood relationships, children socializing mostly within their own age groups, and parenting often delegated to housekeepers, baby sitters, or the television (Bronfenbrenner, 1970, p. xviii). One, or several, of these prevailing conditions may contribute to the development of anxious attachment in some of these children, since they are far more physically dependent upon their primary care-givers for contact with other people.

REFERENCES

Bowlby, J. *Attachment and Loss*, Vol. II: *Separation*. New York: Basic Books, 1973.

Bronfenbrenner, U. *Report to the President: White House Conference on Children*. Washington, D.C.: U.S. Govt. Printing Office, 1971.

Despert, L. *Children of Divorce*. Garden City, N.Y.: Doubleday, 1962.

DeLozier, P. P. *An Application of Attachment Theory to the Study of Child Abuse.* Unpublished doctoral dissertation, California School of Professional Psychology, Los Angeles, 1979.

Hansburg, H. G. *Adolescent Separation Anxiety*, Vol. I. Springfield, Ill.: C. C. Thomas, 1972. Reprinted, Melbourne, Fla.: R. E. Krieger, 1980.

Hansburg, H. G. *Adolescent Separation Anxiety:* Vol. II. *Separation Disorders.* Melbourne, Fla.: R. E. Krieger, 1980.

Hetherington, E. M., Cox, M., and Cox, R. "The Aftermath of Divorce," in J. H. Stevens, Jr., and M. Mathews (eds.), *Mother-Child–Father-Child Relations.* Washington, D.C.: NAEYC, 1977.

Jacobson, D. "The Impact of Marital Separation/Divorce on Children." *Journal of Divorce*, 1977, *1*(4).

Klagsbrun, M., and Bowlby, J. "Responses to Separation from Parents: A Clinical Test for Young Children." *British Journal of Projective Psychology*, 1976, *21*, 7–27.

Locke, H. J., and Wallace, K. M. "Short Marital Adjustment and Prediction Tests: Their Reliability and Validity." *Marriage and Family Living*, 1959, *21*, 251–255.

Miller, J. B. *The Effects of Separation on Latency Age Children as a Consequence of Separation/Divorce.* Unpublished doctoral dissertation, California School of Professional Psychology, Los Angeles, 1980.

U.S. National Center for Health Statistics. *Summary Report: Final Divorce Statistics, 1973* (Monthly Vital Statistics Report, Vol. 24, No. 4). Washington, D.C.: U.S. Govt. Printing Office, 1975.

Wallace, A. *An Application of Attachment Theory to the Study of a Population of Court Referred Divorced People.* Unpublished doctoral dissertation, California School of Professional Psychology, Los Angeles, 1977.

Wallerstein, J., and Kelly, J. "The Effects of Parental Divorce: Experiences of the Child in Later Latency," *American Journal of Orthopsychiatry*, 1976, *46*, 256–269.

Weiss, R. *Marital Separation.* New York: Basic Books, 1975.

Weiss, R. "Single Parent Households as Settings for Growing Up," paper presented at the National Institute of Mental Health Conference on Divorce, February 1978.

5

Brody's Study of the Effects of Divorce on Third-Grade Children

Another study of divorce was done by Dr. Nancy P. Brody of Paradise Valley, Arizona. Entitled "An Investigation of the Effects of Parental Divorce on Third Graders, etc.," it was completed for her doctorate in 1981 at Loyola University in Chicago. The study involved 120 third-grade children averaging 8 years of age from four Catholic schools in the Phoenix, Arizona, area. The S.A.T. was adapted to 8-year-olds by the use of a tape recording to avoid the problem of reading, and special interpretation was given to some vocabulary words which in the original test were not adequately understood by this age group. Comparisons were made of the test results between children of divorce and those from intact families.

In 1977, when her children were ages 5 and 8, Dr. Brody moved to Paradise Valley in Arizona, where they soon discovered that many children whom they met and played with were from divorced families. They began asking questions about divorce which Dr. Brody could not answer despite her background as a teacher of educational psychology at Loyola University and child development at De Paul University in Chicago. She took an interest in the problems of children from divorced families, noting that all children have questions and anxieties about divorce regardless of their parents' marital status. She determined to find out more about how elementary-school-age children in the 7-, 8-, and 9-year-old age group react to or have reacted to divorce in their families.

She was impressed with the great variety of results that had been

obtained in various studies of children of divorce. Studies including children seeking psychiatric help (Kalter, 1977; McDermott,
1970) yielded different results from studies of children judged to be free
of psychological disturbance. Comparisons of children whose parents
were divorced with children whose parents were still married (Glueck
and Glueck, 1950; McDermott, 1970; Morrison, 1974) yielded different results than when children whose parents were divorced were
compared with children whose parents were still married but unhappily married (Bane, 1976; Gettleman and Markowitz, 1974; Krantzler,
1974; Landis, 1960; Magrab, 1978; Nye, 1957). She stated, "Although
there is not one specific reaction to parental divorce, children faced
with this kind of family disruption do seem to be susceptible to
psychological problems (Anthony, 1974; Kapit, 1972; Kelly and
Wallerstein, 1977; Mahler and Rabinovitch, 1956)." Brody conceded
that there was also a difference in studying long- and short-term effects
of divorce and referred to Rorlich, Ranier, Berg-Cross, and Berg-Cross
(1977) for documentation.

Brody engaged in some theoretical discussion with regard to the
stages of reaction to divorce which have been deduced from various observations. She referred to stages devised by Elizabeth Kubler-Ross in
studying death and translated by Froiland and Hoznan (1977) to
children of divorce—denial, anger, bargaining, depression, and,
finally, acceptance. She compared these to both Freud's (1926) and
Bowlby's (1973) conceptualizations, with emphasis on the latter's now
quite familiar three stages of protest, despair, and detachment. Brody
did not work with these formulations in her actual study but confined
herself to theorizing about them.

Brody's main emphasis in this study was the school-age child's
reactions to divorce, whether or not the child was living in a divorced
family, and the degree of knowledge and intellectual understanding
the child had about this problem. Since school played such a large part
in the lives of children, she was concerned with the role of that institution in helping children to adjust to divorce and educating them
about the problems. She documented this assertion with the researchers of this problem (including Black, 1979; Boyer, 1979; Gardner, 1976; Hammond, 1979; Kelly and Wallerstein, 1977; Parks, 1977;
Ricci, 1979; Rubin and Price, 1979; and Wilkenson and Bleck, 1977).
She stated, "The teacher often takes on added importance because,
with one parent leaving the home and the other usually unable to func-

tion well as a parent at the time of great emotional turmoil, the teacher may take on the role of parent surrogate."

Along these lines Brody developed four null hypotheses as follows:

1. There is no difference between children who have experienced parental divorce and those in intact families, as shown by the Hansburg S.A.T. (ten patterns and total) scores. There would also be no difference on Child's Behavior Rating Scale (CBT) (five subscales and total) scores.
2. Children of divorce are not more knowledgeable about divorce than children in intact families, as shown by pretest scores.
3. The term "custody" is not better understood by children of divorce than by children in intact homes, as shown by a particular item on the pretest.
4. The divorce education program had no effect on the children's knowledge of divorce, as shown by a comparison of pretest and posttest results.

Only the first null hypothesis will be considered in this presentation since it is more germane to the theme of this book.

Brody arranged for the participation of 141 third-grade children from four Catholic elementary schools in the Phoenix area. She states that she focused on children of this age (7, 8, and 9) because of the lack of research concerning the effects of divorce on these children. The participating schools were selected by the Superintendent of Catholic Schools in the Phoenix Diocese, who used socioeconomic factors as the basis for her choices. One school, located in an upper-socioeconomic-status (SES) area, had two third-grade classes, both of which took part. The three other cooperating schools were in lower-SES areas. Each of these schools had one third-grade class. The two third-grade classes in the upper-SES school and the three third-grade classes from the lower-SES schools constituted the sample. The three classes in the lower-SES schools were randomly assigned to the experimental or control group, as were the two classes in the upper-SES school. The children were simply told that the researcher was studying third graders' opinions and needed their help. Eight out of the original sample of children had to be omitted because they were unable to complete valid tests, either because of unwillingness to cooperate, a lack of sufficient English-language skills, or school absence.

Scores on the S.A.T. and the CBT were gathered for 133 children. Finally, thirteen more children were eliminated because of a number of irregularities in the testing procedures. Table 5.1 provides a picture of the children taking part in the study.

Unfortunately, because of the considerable dependency on the validity of the teachers' judgment with regard to the marital status of the children's families, Brody was forced to evaluate her data with some trepidation. She stated: "Parts of this study are focused on School #2 because the participating teacher there was confident of her knowledge of her students' family situations." As will be seen later, School #2 became an important indicator for Brody with regard to the significance of differences between the children of divorce and those from intact families. Since she was concerned with the educational aspects of a divorce program, Brody introduced pre- and posttests with regard to the children's knowledge of divorce and developed a divorce education program subsequently which was the subject of the posttest later. Thus, this experiment was intermingled with her other experiment with regard to her first hypothesis. What is interesting is the procedure that Brody adopted for the administration of the S.A.T., which was given before any of the other tests. Her description of this procedure is provided below in its entirety.

This researcher tape-recorded the seventeen statements following each picture, enabling the child to hear the statements while he or she was reading

Table 5.1

A NUMERICAL DESCRIPTION OF CHILDREN IN THE STUDY

Subjects	Experimental	Control	
Male	29	26	
Female	24	41	
Lower-SES	21	30	
Upper-SES	32	37	
Total	53	67	120

them silently. The tapes were made in order to lessen the effects of the child's reading ability on the test results. Each child was told to select as many of the seventeen statements as he or she believed represented how the child in the picture felt. The child indicated his or her choice of a statement as soon as it was heard by saying "yes, that one" or the number of the statement. When all seventeen statements had been read, the child was asked if he or she had anything to add about how the child in the picture felt. The child's responses were recorded on a recording chart.

Before giving this test to the children in the sample, this researcher practiced its administration with two other third grade classes. At that time it was learned that some children needed help in understanding the vocabulary of the test. The tape recorder was stopped in order to explain those words that needed explanation. Two words "institution" and "suicide" were routinely defined for all the children. Others needed help with such words as "permanently," "transferred," and "coffin."

Testing took place in a variety of settings including a storeroom, assembly hall, lunch room, and an outside corridor. All these areas were unused (by the school) while testing was taking place, which provided a quiet testing setting with a minimum of distractions. Each child was with this researcher for approximately a half hour. No direct questioning of the child about his or her parents' marital situation was allowed, but some freely gave this information without being asked. Two of the children were absent too often to be tested and six of them were unable to be tested either because of an inadequate knowledge of English or because of a refusal to cooperate.

Following this administration of the S.A.T., the CBT was completed by the teacher for each child.

The scores on the SAT and the CBT were compared for those children whose parents were divorced and who lived with the mother as one group and those whose parents were married and living together with the children. Children who were omitted from the study included those who had suffered the death of one parent, or whose mothers were never married, or whose parents were just separated without being divorced, or who lived with the father or who did not live with their natural parents.

The teachers were aware of present family situations of their students, but were not certain that they knew what took place years before, such as a divorce and remarriage which could make the child appear to be in an intact family. The teacher in School #2 was more confident than the other teachers, that she had correctly identified all children of parental divorce in her class because of her work with her students' families. Because of this . . . a more thorough individual analysis of the test protocols for the children of divorce in School #2 was also done to see if any systematic patterns emerged.

Brody presented the following analysis of the scores on the S.A.T.

The S.A.T. scores were analyzed in three ways . . . the mean scores of the children of divorce were compared with the mean scores of children of intact families for children in all participating classes. Second, the mean scores of children of divorce were compared with the mean scores of children from intact families for just those children in the third grade from School #2. Third, individual evaluations of S.A.T. protocols for children in School #2 and identified as being children of divorce, were examined.

The analysis of variance appears in Table 5.2

This analysis of variance showed no statistical differences between children of divorce and children of intact families on the S.A.T. scores. Nevertheless, an examination of the scores for the girls as a group, regardless of home situation, scored below the adequate range on hostility, while the male children of divorce scored lower than the adequate range on reality avoidance.

The female children of divorce scored much higher in concentration impairment and sublimation percentage than ordinarily

Table 5.2

ANALYSIS OF VARIANCE RESULTS FOR S.A.T. RESPONSES

AND HOME SITUATIONS OF ALL SUBJECTS

	Type IV SS	F Value	PR > F
S.A.T. Total	23.5	.02	.88
Attachment	.00	.45	.50
Individuation	.01	.47	.49
Hostility	.00	.44	.51
Painful Tension	.00	.04	.84
Reality Avoidance	.00	.14	.71
Concentration Impairment and Sublimation	.01	1.84	.18
Self-Love Loss	.00	.46	.50
Identity Stress	.00	.50	.48
Attachment-Individuation Balance	.00	.00	.96
Mild-Strong Difference	.00	.45	.50

Note: df = 1.

should have been expected. Brody interpreted this as signifying feelings of ineffectuality, and she suggested that the female children of divorce were weakened in their feelings of effectiveness by the absence of the father. On the other hand, it appeared that male children of divorce were far below the norm in the attachment-individuation balance. She did not comment on this but indicated the necessity to explore this further for any significance.

An analysis of variance for School #2 resulted in one significant difference between children of divorce and children from intact families (see Table 5.3). The individuation score was high for children of divorce as a group, and even higher for male children of divorce. She suggested that these boys were moving toward an excessive self-sufficiency. The individuation percentage score when correlated with the children's home situation yielded an F value of 6.04 and a P value of .03.

An evaluation of the individual protocols of the ten children iden-

Table 5.3

ANALYSIS OF VARIANCE RESULTS FOR S.A.T. RESPONSES

AND HOME SITUATIONS OF CHILDREN IN SCHOOL #2

	Type IV SS	F Value	PR > F
S.A.T. Total	1504.30	.99	.37
Attachment	.00	.44	.52
Individuation	.06	6.04	.03
Hostility	.01	.66	.43
Painful Tension	.01	1.26	.28
Reality Avoidance	.00	.12	.73
Concentration Impairment and Sublimation	.01	1.18	.29
Self-Love Loss	.01	.96	.34
Identity Stress	.00	1.11	.31
Attachment-Individuation Balance	.11	1.00	.33
Mild-Strong Difference	.00	.01	.91

Note: df = 1.

tified as children of divorce in School #2 was made. Denial was evident in seven of the ten protocols, either in the form of a constricted protocol, affect blunting, or high reality avoidance scores. She interpreted this finding as representing the possibility of "some kind of emotional disorder." (It is likely that this patterning fits more closely the concepts of excessive self-sufficiency and/or detachment.)

There was evidence that the male children of divorce at this age level were repressing hostility since their scores were lower than the norms. Brody quoted *Adolescent Separation Anxiety*, Vol. II:

It is to be expected that degrees of resentment and anger will normally be aroused, as such normal hostilities should be expected in the test patterning and, when absent or low, should be considered with suspicion as evidence of attempts to repress normal resentments. (pp. 26–27)

I quote from Brody:

Male children of divorce from all the schools and also from School #2 had low reality avoidance scores. Hansburg (1976) explains such low scores saying "In a sense, a low level of separation denial could be called a denial of denial. This individual is saying, 'since I do not have any need to be concerned with separation problems, I have no need to deny them' " (p. 30). In addition, Hansburg says, "If such a low level of separation denial is accompanied by a high degree of individuation responses which are far above the attachment level, one would have to suspect that the individual must constantly deny that he is needful" (p. 30). The male children of divorce in School #2 fit this pattern . . . denial is one of the stages Hozman and Froiland (1977) say that children go through on the way to reaching acceptance of their parents' divorce.

When the scores of concentration impairment and sublimation are much higher than self-love loss, a feeling of being ineffective and lacking in self-confidence is suggested. Hansburg (1976) says this may be an "overdependence on a supportive figure whose absence reduces the feeling of effectiveness" (p. 36). This pattern is evident in female children of divorce in School #2. This is in keeping with Erikson (1950), who says that school age children are in the Industry vs. Inferiority stage of development and that without a stable family life, the crisis of this stage will not be resolved. Without successfully resolving this crisis, the child may develop feelings of inferiority and inadequacy.

The one statistically significant difference found between children of divorce and children of intact families in School #2 was the individuation score. This score was high for the children of divorce, and even higher for the male children of divorce. This could be an example of Despert's (1953) belief that children with divorced or divorcing parents often have a strong outward show of independence which is really just a compensation for a greater need to be dependent.

That one particular pattern of responding to the S.A.T. by all children of divorce did not emerge goes along with Anthony (1974), Kapit (1972), Kelly and Wallerstein (1977) and Mahler and Rabinovitch (1956), who said that there are many possible reactions to parental divorce, but these children are susceptible to psychological problems. Although there was not one specific response pattern, the individual protocols evaluated do indicate that these children do have problems pertaining to their separation experiences. This is not to say that all their problems have their origins in their parents' divorce, but it does mean that this age child does need help in dealing with divorce and should not be left out of the research into the effects of divorce on children.

Parenthetically, it should be noted that the CBT checklist completed by the classroom teachers did not show any significant differences between the children of divorce and those from intact families. Thus, this latter scale did not indicate any differences of a meaningful nature in behavior in children of divorce.

I have one comment with regard to the selection of the child population. It is well known that the Catholic Church does not sanction divorce, but despite this, four Catholic schools participated in the study and did institute a divorce education program, which, according to pre- and posttests devised by Brody, indicated considerable positive results for the children of all families. Even third graders whose parents were divorced were shown to have improved in their understanding of divorce. Brody strongly recommended that divorce education programs be instituted in elementary schools.

REFERENCES

Anthony, E. J. "Children At Risk From Divorce: A Review," in E. J. Anthony and C. Koupernik (eds.), *The Child in His Family: Children at Psychiatric Risk*, Vol. III. New York: John Wiley and Sons, 1974.

Bane, M. J. "Marital Disruption and the Lives of Children." *Journal of Social Issues*, 1976, 32, 103–117.

Black, K. "What about the Child from a One Parent Home?" *Teacher*, January 1979, 24–28.

Bowlby, J. *Attachment and Loss*, Vol. II: *Separation: Anxiety and Anger*. New York: Basic Books, 1973.

Boyer, S. "Tips for Working with Single Parents." *Instructor*, September 1979, p. 79.

Brody, N. P. *An Investigation of the Effects of Parental Divorce on Third Graders, etc.* Unpublished doctoral dissertation, Loyola University, Chicago, 1981.

Despert, J. L. *Children of Divorce.* Garden City, N.Y.: Doubleday, 1953.

Fisher, E. "A Guide to Divorce Counseling." *The Family Coordinator,* 1973, 22, 53–63.

Erikson, E. *Childhood and Society.* New York: W. W. Norton, 1950.

Freud, S. "Inhibition, Symptoms and Anxiety," in *The Complete Psychological Works of Sigmund Freud,* Vol. XX. London: Hogarth Press, 1926. (English translation, 1959.)

Froiland, D., and Hozman, T. Counseling for Constructive Divorce. *Personnel and Guidance Journal,* May 1977, 55, 525–529.

Gardner, R. A. *Psychotherapy with Children of Divorce.* New York: J. Aronson, 1976.

Gettleman, S., and Markowitz, J. *The Courage to Divorce.* New York: Simon and Schuster, 1974.

Glueck, E., and Glueck, S. *Unraveling Juvenile Delinquency.* Cambridge, Mass.: Harvard University Press, 1950.

Hammond, J. "A Comparison of Elementary Children from Divorced and Intact Families," *Phi Delta Kappan,* November 1979, 61(3), 219.

Hansburg, H. G. *Adolescent Separation Anxiety,* Vol. I: *A Method for the Study of Adolescent Problems.* Springfield, Ill.: C. C. Thomas, 1972. Reprinted, Melbourne, Fla.: R. E. Krieger, 1980.

Hansburg, H. G. *Adolescent Separation Anxiety,* Vol. II: *Separation Disorders.* Melbourne, Fla.: R. E. Krieger, 1980.

Kalter, N. "Children of Divorce in an Outpatient Population." *American Journal of Orthopsychiatry,* January 1977, 47, 40–41.

Kapit, H. E. "Help for Children of Separation and Divorce," in I. E. Stuart and L. E. Abt. (eds.), *Children of Separation and Divorce.* New York: Grossman Publishers, 1972.

Kelly, J., and Wallerstein, J. "Brief Intervention with Children in Divorcing Families." *American Journal of Orthopsychiatry,* January 1977, 47, 23–39.

Krantzler, M. *Creative Divorce.* New York: M. Evans, 1974.

Landis, J. T. "The Trauma of Children When Parents Divorce." *Marriage and Family Living,* 1960, 22, 7–13.

Magrab, P. "For the Sake of the Children: A Review of the Psychological Effects of Divorce." *Journal of Divorce,* Spring 1978, 1, 233–245.

Mahler, M. S., and Rabinovitch, R. "The Effects of Marital Conflict on Child Development," in V. W. Eisenstein (ed.), *Neurotic Interaction in Marriage*. New York: Basic Books, 1956.

McDermott, J. F. "Divorce and Its Psychiatric Sequelae in Children." *Archives of General Psychiatry*, November 1970, *23*, 421–428.

Morrison, J. R. "Parental Divorce as a Factor in Childhood Psychiatric Illness." *Comprehensive Psychiatry*, 1974, *15*, 95–102.

Nye, I. F. "Child Adjustment in Broken and in Unhappy Unbroken Homes." *Marriage and Family Living*, 1957, *19*, 356–361.

Parks, A. "Children and Youth of Divorce in Parents without Partners, Inc." *Journal of Clinical Psychology*, Summer 1977, 44–47.

Ricci, I. "Divorce, Remarriage and the Schools." *Phi Delta Kappan*, March 1979, *60*(7), 509–511.

Rohrlich, J., Ranier, R., Berg-Cross, L., and Berg-Cross, G. "The Effects of Divorce: A Research Review with a Developmental Perspective." *Journal of Clinical Child Psychology*, Summer 1977, 15–20.

Rubin, L., and Price, J. H. "Divorce and Its Effects on Children." *The Journal of School Health*, December 1979, 552–556.

Wilkinson, G., and Bleck, R. "The Children's Divorce Groups." *Elementary School Guidance and Counseling*, February 1977, *11*, 204–213.

6

Burger's Application of Attachment Theory to Separated and Divorced Males

Further research on divorce was reported by Dr. Donald G. Burger of San Diego, California, entitled "Bowlby's Theory of Separation as It Applies to Separated and Divorced Males." This doctoral study was completed at the San Diego branch of the California School of Professional Psychology in 1981. The study was concerned with the effects of divorce on ninety young adult males divided into three groups of thirty each, one divorced for zero to two months, a second divorced for two to twelve months, and a third for twelve to twenty-four months. Using a revision of the S.A.T. picturing young adult males rather than children in separating situations, and replicating the response patterns of the original (Hansburg, 1972), Dr. Burger made comparisons of the results of the test for the three groups, thus studying the effects of the passage of time on the reactions to the divorce.

In this research study the S.A.T. was adapted to young adult males who had been divorced and were not remarried. The pictures of the original Hansburg test were redrawn with the central figure as a young adult male, and adjustments were made to the phrases so that they would be more applicable to this group. Although this resulted in a new test, the similarity was so considerable as to suggest that normative data could readily be developed along similar lines. (The newly created instrument may be found in Chapter 23.)

Burger was concerned with the reactions of his subjects to various stages subsequent to the separation or divorce. For this reason he obtained three groups of young male adults who had been separated from zero to two months, from two to twelve months, and from twelve months to two years. Using Bowlby's concept of three stages of reaction—protest, despair, and detachment (which Bowlby developed for infants and young children)—Burger assumed that each group of young adult males for the three divorced periods corresponded to Bowlby's concepts, with some overlap between the groups.

Burger selected the S.A.T. because he believed that certain significant differences in this test would appear at different stages of the divorce process. He addressed himself to the question of what happens to the intensity of the attachment that a man has developed for his wife subsequent to a divorce. If Bowlby's theory is correct, he reasoned, there should follow a strong emotional protest against the break, followed subsequently by a despairing feeling that the attachment cannot be recouped, and then finally by a detachment from the wife and a redirection of this attachment elsewhere. He hypothesized that the degree of attachment need would be greatest in the despair phase, less in the protest phase, and least in the detachment phase. Accordingly, he expected to see the attachment percentage on the S.A.T. fall, rise, and then fall again.

Burger further hypothesized that separation hostility would be most severe in the protest phase, less so in the despair phase, and least in the detachment phase. This concept was based on the notion that affective reactions, especially resentment and anger, would be quite prevalent in the initial stages of the divorce, whether induced by the previous marital struggles or the frustration of inconveniences thrust upon the male as a result of the separation. It was theorized that, as time progressed, a new adjustment would take place and that by the end of the second year (as indicated by previous researches), the hostile reactions would have subsided to a normal level.

Burger also assumed that defensive denial of the separation would be greatest in the protest phase but gradually decrease through the following stages of despair and detachment. The theoretical assumption was that the early shock wave of the separation and divorce would be more difficult to accept than in the later phases of the separation. Thus, the necessity for defensive denial would have receded considerably after two years from the time of the initial divorce.

For obvious reasons it was theorized that the stress of the separation, as measured by the fear-anxiety-pain syndrome on the

S.A.T., would be greatest in the despair phase (assuming hostility would be greatest in the initial protest phase), less in the protest phase, and still less in the detachment phase. It was assumed that as time proceeded, the major stress reaction would be reduced and other patterns would become more dominant.

Burger then hypothesized that the identity stress response would be greatest in the despair phase, assuming that the shock to the sense of self would be greatest later rather than earlier. During the protest phase he did not expect the sense of identity to be so affected and that the least effect would appear in the third or detachment period.

Following the course of this thinking, he assumed that self-love loss would not be as intense in the first few months but, like identity stress, would be most intense during the later months (two to twelve) and would then wear off during the period of detachment (twelve to twenty-four months). Thus, he assumed that depressive reactions on the S.A.T. would correspond to Bowlby's concept of despair. (Burger did not take into account the relationship between the self-esteem-preoccupation percentage score and the self-love loss level, which is more likely to indicate a depressive syndrome.)

Referring to the individuation index, Burger considered the likelihood that the progression of the effect on this pattern would be a gradual decrease in the first phase (protest), a continued decrease in the second phase (despair), and a recovery in the third phase (detachment). He reasoned that in the early stages of the divorce, the man would be more vulnerable to a loss of personal resourcefulness and would reach the depths of this somewhere between two and twelve months and then in the second year would make a recovery.

Finally, he hypothesized that the pattern of self-esteem preoccupation would show its greatest frequency in the period between two and twelve months and would be less affected initially. He presumed that the least would occur in the third or detachment phase. (Burger made no use of other factors in the test, including total number of responses, responses to mild pictures, responses to strong pictures, absurd responses, differences between mild and strong picture responses, responses to mental set questions, etc. He also did not use the clinical evaluations available in *Adolescent Separation Anxiety*, Vol. II. To this degree the full richness of the method was not utilized in preference for the statistical analysis of the eight patterns.)

Burger obtained his subjects, ninety in number, from white, middle-class males who lived in San Diego County in California. They were all participants in support groups for the separated and divorced in local Protestant churches. The men fit the criteria for participation in this study—they had all been married at least two years and were physically separated from their spouses. Some subjects were merely separated, and others were already divorced. None of the subjects who had children had been given custody of them.

The men were divided into three groups: one group of thirty had been separated from their wives up to two months, another group of thirty separated from two to twelve months, and a third group of thirty separated for one to two years. The author states, "The time period was based on the research done by Adam and Adam (1979), Fisher (1974), personal consultation with Hansburg (1980), Hetherington, et al (1976), Krantzer (1974), Thweatt (1980) and Wallerstein and Kelly (1980)." The following demographic information about the subjects is summarized in Table 6.1. (In his dissertation Burger does not comment on the demographic data, although there are some differences among the groups which could create problems for the interpretation of the results. For example, in group 1, only 17% of the men initiated the separation, while in groups 2 and 3, 40% were the initiators. Further, 87% of group 2 had children, while 70% and 73%, respectively, had children in groups 1 and 3. Apparently, Burger did not consider these differences to be meaningful.)

Burger describes the creation of his revision of the S.A.T. for use with divorced males. The twelve new pictures, with a description of each and its method of development, appear in Section Four of this book. It is suggested that the reader refer to this material in that section.

Table 6.1

DEMOGRAPHIC INFORMATION ON ALL SUBJECTS

Group	Age		Years of Marriage		Percent of Men with Children	Separation Initiated by		
30 in Each	Mean	Range	Mean	Range	Percentage	Self	Spouse	Mutual
0–2 mos.	35.6	25–46	12.3	3–25	70%	17%	43%	40%
2–12 mos.	38.9	26–49	12.1	2–28	87%	40%	43%	17%
12–24 mos.	38.7	28–49	13.2	3–26	73%	40%	47%	13%

The statistical evaluation of the data on the three groups of divorced males was accomplished by a one-way analysis of covariance of the adjusted group means, and individual two-tail t tests were used to determine the individual mean differences. The level of significance was established at .01.

Each of the eight hypotheses was tested by using a one-way analysis of covariance for the three adjusted group means while controlling for age, length of marriage, number of children and who initiated the separation. Individual two-tail t tests were used to determine the individual mean differences. Since multiple tests were performed on the same sample, there is an increased likelihood of making a Type I error. In an attempt to control for this, the level of significance was established at .01.

Every subject responded to all twelve pictures on the Separation Anxiety Test. The mean number of responses for group 1 (0–2 mos. separated) was 46.7 with a range of 23–82; the mean number of responses for group 2 (2–12 mos.) was 47.4 with a range of 27–84; and the mean number of responses for group 3 (12–24 mos.) was 47.1 with a range of 24–81. An F test for equality of variance was computed for the three groups and was found not to be significant, which indicates that the data met the assumptions on which the analysis of covariance was performed.

Table 6.2 provides a summary of Burger's data on his revision of the S.A.T. for eight patterns of that test and for each of the three groups.

An analysis of the above data suggested that none of the hypotheses previously noted were found to be correct in terms of significance at the .01 level. Nevertheless, many of them were found to be in the correct direction. For example, attachment need showed a definite rise during the interim period of two to twelve months, which has been referred to as despair, and a drop back to a lower level in the third phase, referred to as detachment. Hostility appeared to be strongest in the first phase and was lower in the second and third phases. The pain of separation appeared much stronger in the second phase and dropped considerably in the second year of the divorce. Thus, the fear-anxiety-pain syndrome seemed to be strongest during the middle period and apparently subsided in the second year. What is very striking in these data is the very large increase in the individuation level in the third or detachment period. While this was predicted, the extent of this increase was surprisingly strong.

Thus, we see two important trends in the data. The first trend in-

dicates that the period from two to twelve months has a stronger degree
of attachment need, separation pain, identity stress, and self-love loss.
These are all characteristics of a depressive syndrome and suggest that
the characterization of this period as one of despair has some validity.
The second and even more significant factor lies in the twelve- to twen-
ty-four-month period, in which there was the very extensive increase in
the individuation level and a considerable drop in self-love loss, self-
esteem preoccupation, and separation pain. This adaptation and adjustment to the separation is very suggestive and gives further credence
to Bowlby's concept of detachment. (The original report of this study
contains a number of graphs and tables which provide covariance [AN-
COVA] data and an analysis of trends. They have not been reproduced
here for reasons of space.)

Burger provided the following composite view with regard to the
meaning of his findings; I quote it verbatim:

Another way of looking at the results of this study is an examination of the eight
psychological patterns or systems in combination with each other as seen in
each phase. The eight patterns represent emotions, cognition and defenses
which combine to form a distinctive pattern in each phase. Although these may
not represent a strict linear progression from phase to phase, these are the
trends that generally would be expected.

Table 6.2
ADJUSTED GROUP MEAN NUMBER OF RESPONSES FOR EACH PERIOD
SUBSEQUENT TO SEPARATION ON EIGHT PATTERNS OF THE S.A.T.

S.A.T. Pattern	Group 1 (0–2 mos.)	Group 2 (2–12 mos.)	Group 3 (12–24 mos.)
Separation Denial	6.4	6.1	6.2
Attachment Need	9.7	11.4	9.2
Separation Hostility	7.6	5.8	6.0
Separation Pain	5.4	8.6	3.4
Identity Stress	3.7	4.6	2.3
Self-Love Loss	4.1	5.2	3.5
Individuation	10.9	9.0	18.0
Self-Esteem Preoccupation	.24	1.0	-2.7

The man in the protest phase reacts to his recent separation with anger and hostility. Even though he feels pain, it is overshadowed by his anger at being alone. He is aware of his need to be with his wife and cannot quite believe that his marriage is over. In the absence of his major relationship, he is aware of his feeling of not being loved and at the same time begins to question if he is lovable. He experiences difficulties in concentration as he begins to mull over these questions about himself and his place in the world. His problems with concentration may affect his job performance, which in turn affects his feelings of competence. Alternating with these negative feelings, there may also be a sense of self-reliance and a new-found feeling of freedom.

The move into the despair phase is marked by a large drop in anger as it was experienced in the protest phase. In its place is anger that is directed inward. The pain of separation reaches its most intense level as the man experiences severe doubts about his lovability, his competence in relationships, and even his competence in areas unrelated to the separation. His need of others becomes much more intense as his feelings of self-reliance decrease. The overriding characteristic of this phase is an overall feeling of despair and doubt.

A major characteristic of the detachment phase (the second year) is a significant increase in feelings of self-reliance and a generally improved sense of well-being. As he feels much greater confidence in himself, the energy that was previously spent in self-examination is now available for work and other activities. He rarely feels the self-blame and despair he experienced in the despair phase (2–12 months) and again is more able to direct his anger outward. His need for others is less than in the despair phase and his ability to rely on his own resources increases.

It is obvious that these generalizations cannot all be attributed to a single individual; they represent a composite of a person who actually does not exist. Burger was making a point about general trends which has some validity from his data but is not clinically applicable to any single person. Burger went on to discuss the limitations of his study and some of the practical implications which follow.

A limitation in the generalizability of this study is related to sampling procedures. All of the subjects were white, middle-class males in southern California. Although there is no research that would suggest that the process would be different for men from other socioeconomic classes and other races, generalizations of these results should be limited to men similar to those used in this study.

Another important characteristic of the subjects is that all had been married only once. Again, there is no evidence to indicate that a different process would take place in a second or third separation and divorce, but the possibility cannot be ruled out. The sampling procedure used in this study should also be considered. . . . The subjects were those who volunteered to participate. It is not known how they might differ from men who were aware of the study and chose not to participate.

This sample came from groups for the separated and divorced that were sponsored by religious denominations. It has been found that persons reporting moderate to high religious involvement and activity show worse adjustment to separation and divorce than those low on religious involvement (Chiriboga et al., 1979; Peterson, 1978; Raschke, 1974; White, 1979). Thus, the results of this study may reflect more severe reactions than might be found in a non-religious sample. It should also be considered, however, that there was no measurement of religious involvement and activity among the subjects . . . and so it cannot be assumed that their religious involvement extends beyond participation in these groups.

. . . [T]hat these men participated in groups to help them deal with separation and divorce must be taken into account. There are several kinds of speculations that could be made about the difference between these men and men who do not seek group support, but it is impossible to know what the differences are and how they might affect these results.

An uncontrolled variable in this study was the presence or absence of new attachment figures. There is ambiguity as to the role new attachment figures may play in the process of adjustment to separation and divorce (Ainsworth, 1978; Bowlby, 1969; Cohen, 1974; Gewirtz, 1972; Lamb, 1974; Weiss, 1973, 1976). This author [Burger] decided not to deal with this variable because of problems in determining the intensity and meaning of new relationships.

Two methodological factors that may have affected the results of this study are the cross-sectional design and the absence of a control group for comparison. Implicit in the cross-sectional design was the assumption that each group of subjects had gone or would go through each of the three phases of separation. Because of the two year time-line, it was impractical to measure the three phases longitudinally. Because of the use of the cross-sectional design, this study did not provide variables that could be associated with failure to go through the three phases or with the length of time an individual might take to go through the three phases. Because a control group was not used for comparison, it was not known whether these responses are unique to the separation experience.

Finally, questions arise with regard to the Separation Anxiety Test. Projective techniques are clearly found wanting when evaluated by test standards. They usually lack standardization of administration and scoring procedures; there is a lack of adequate norms, reliability and validity (Anastasi, 1976). The Separation Anxiety Test could be called a "quasi-test" (Anastasi, 1976, p. 586) in that, although it is a projective instrument, efforts have been made to utilize test standards (Hansburg, 1972). Standardization of administration and scoring procedures are available. Normative data have been calculated on children, adolescents and adults with attempts to determine reliability and validity.

Certain practical implications arise from the results of this study and suggest that separated and divorced men can be expected to experience changes in several areas of emotional functioning as they work towards resolution of the separation experience. In addition, the results suggest that the effects on the man's functioning may be more far-reaching than may have been previously thought. Common sense would lead one to believe that during separation the man would experience doubts and concerns about establishing a new place for himself socially and about the possibility of being in love again. It is somewhat surprising, however, that these doubts may generalize to other areas of his life unrelated to the separation.

What is most interesting about Burger's data is the increase in attachment need in the first year of the divorce and its decrease in the second year, while the exact opposite appears in the second year in the area of individuation. The latter shows a mild drop in the first year and a soaring increase in the second year. This seesawing of the attachment-individuation balance from the first to the second year of the divorce indicates the most likely effect of divorce on the typical male undergoing this experience. This reaction was also accompanied by the rise and then considerable fall in the separation pain index.

Such findings are of great importance to the (psycho)therapist who works with separated and divorced men. The (psycho)therapist's awareness of what emotional issues are affected by separation, the intensity of the feelings, and the anticipated progression towards resolution will help to determine appropriate interventions. This may be particularly important since there is evidence that separated and divorced men, when compared to widowers, are less articulate about their feelings and seem not to know how they ought to feel (George & Wilding, 1972).

As with other phase theories there is the danger of expecting a strict linear progression through the phases. Those making interventions must allow for individual reactions and movement back and forth between phases. Lastly, the support for Bowlby's theory provided by this research may give direction for future research. This modification of Hansburg's Separation Anxiety Test could prove useful in other research about adult separation.

REFERENCES

Adam, J. H., and Adam, N. W. *Divorce: How and When to Let Go.* Englewood Cliffs, N.J.: Prentice Hall, 1979.

Ainsworth, M. D. *Patterns of Attachment: A Psychological Study of the Strange Situation.* Hillsdale, N.J.: Lawrence Erlbaum Associates, 1978.

Anastasi, A. *Psychological Testing.* New York: Macmillan Publishing Co., 1976.

Bloom, B. L., and White, S. W. "Factors Related to the Adjustment of Divorcing Men." *Family Relations*, in press.

Bowlby, J. *Attachment and Loss*, Vol. I: *Attachment*. New York: Basic Books, 1969.

Bowlby, J. *Attachment and Loss*, Vol. II: *Separation*. New York: Basic Books, 1973.

Bowlby, J. *Attachment and Loss*, Vol. III: *Loss*. New York: Basic Books, 1980.

Burger, D. G. *Bowlby's Theory of Separation As It Applies to Separated and Divorced Males*. Unpublished doctoral dissertation, California School of Professional Psychology, San Diego, 1981.

Chiriboga, D. A., and Cutler, L. "Stress Responses among Divorcing Men and Women." *Journal of Divorce*, 1978, *1*(2), 95–106.

Cohen, L. J. "The Operational Definition of Human Attachment." *Psychological Bulletin*, 1974, *81*, 207–217.

Fisher, E. O. *Divorce: The New Freedom, a Guide to Divorcing and Divorce Counseling*. New York: Harper and Row, 1974.

George, V., and Wilding, P. *Motherless Families*. Boston: Routledge and Kegan Paul, 1972.

Gewirtz, J. L. *Attachment and Dependency*. Washington, D.C.: V. H. Winston & Sons, 1972.

Hansburg, H. G. *Adolescent Separation Anxiety*, Vol. I: *A Method for the Study of Adolescent Separation Problems*. Springfield, Ill.: C. C. Thomas, 1972. Reprinted, Melbourne, Fla.: R. E. Krieger, 1980.

Hansburg, H. G. *Adolescent Separation Anxiety*, Vol. II: *Separation Disorders*. Melbourne, Fla.: R. E. Krieger, 1980.

Hansburg, H. G. Personal communication, May 1980.

Hetherington, E. M., Cox, M., and Cox, R. "Divorced Fathers." *The Family Coordinator*, 1976, *25*, 417–428.

Krantzler, M. *Creative Divorce: A New Opportunity for Personal Growth*. New York: M. Evans & Co., 1974.

Parkes, C. M. *Bereavement: Studies of Grief in Adult Life*. New York: International Universities Press, 1972.

Peterson, L. C. "Guilt, Attribution of Responsibility, and Resolution of the Divorce Crisis (doctoral dissertation, University of Massachusetts, 1978)." *Dissertation Abstracts*, 1978, *39*, 1703B.

Raschke, H. J. "Social and Psychological Factors in Voluntary, Post-Marital Dissolution Adjustment (doctoral dissertation, University of Minnesota, 1974)." *Dissertation Abstracts*, 1974, *35*, 5549A.

Thweatt, R. W. "Divorce: Crisis Intervention Guided by Attachment
    Theory." *American Journal of Psychotherapy*, 1980, 34(2), 240–245.
Wallerstein, J. S., and Kelly, J. B. *Surviving the Breakup: How Children and
    Parents Cope with Divorce*. New York: Basic Books, 1980.
Weiss, R. S. *Loneliness: The Experience of Emotional and Social Isolation*.
    Cambridge, Mass.: MIT Press, 1973.
Weiss, R. S. *Marital Separation*. New York: Basic Books, 1975.
Weiss, R. S. "The Emotional Impact of Marital Separation." *Journal of Social
    Issues*, 1976, 32(1), 135–145.

FURTHER STUDIES OF
MOTHERS AND CHILDREN

7

Varela's Study of Separation Anxiety in Mothers and Hospitalized Young Children

The following three studies of mothers and children are varied in a number of ways. In one, the mothers and young children were both studied; in another, the mothers were the subject of study; and in a third, the children alone were studied.

The first study, presented here, is by Dr. Lynn Millikin Varela, entitled "The Relationship between the Hospitalized Child's Separation Anxiety and Maternal Separation Anxiety." It was completed in 1982 at the California School of Professional Psychology in Los Angeles. The mothers and young children were both examined but with similar instruments which were differentiated for age. The study demonstrates the possibility of relating reactions to separation in a parent and child simultaneously.

This study was conducted at the Los Angeles branch of the California School of Professional Psychology and was completed in 1982. What was most interesting was Varela's attempt to study the relationship between the separation anxiety of the young child (aged 4–7) and maternal reactions to separation. Varela used a series of tests and interviews for both child and mother, but for the purposes of this summary we shall be concerned largely with two tests—the Hansburg (1972) S.A.T. (adult administration), given to the mothers, and the Klagsbrun-Bowlby (1976) revision of the Hansburg test for young children, entitled "A Clinical Test for Young Children," which Varela revised further for her use in this study.

In general, Varela (p. 8) was concerned with the frequency with which

. . . hospitalized children are removed from their parents during particularly stressful periods. Children continue to experience examinations and painful medical procedures without the support of their parents. Furthermore, pediatric surgical patients experience sudden separation from their parents when they are taken to surgery. Subsequently, they experience the waiting period outside the operating room immediately prior to surgery, the induction of anesthesia and the awakening period in the recovery room without the comfort of their parents' presence.

Varela pointed out that despite newer practices by many hospitals consisting of unrestricted visiting hours, rooming-in for parents and reduction in the length of hospital stays,

. . . the serious problem of parent-child separation within the hospital is far from resolved. . . . It has been suggested in the literature (Fagin, 1964; Mason, 1978; and Oremland and Oremland, 1973) that the sudden separation from parents at this time is exceptionally difficult for children because it is in conjunction with surgery, a severe stress.

It is the period of the child's separation from the mother at the time the child is taken to surgery and subsequently reunited with the mother that Varela was interested in exploring in this study. This was in contrast to the many other studies which were concerned with the child's in-hospital separation either at some time during the hospitalization or during the posthospitalization.

Varela defined separation according to Bowlby's and Ainsworth's usage of the term. Quoting Bowlby (1973, p. 405), she stated:

Anxiety (separation) is "how we feel when our attachment behavior is activated and we are seeking an attachment figure but without success." Also, Bowlby stated that anxiety is "how we feel when for any reason we are uncertain whether an attachment figure(s) will be available should we want one." The first denotation reflects the way in which the term separation anxiety is used in the present study.

Varela combined two aspects of anxiety: one deals with the child's apprehension of the danger which the oncoming surgery represents, and the other deals with the separation from the mother under these circumstances. It is the confluence of these two experiences which is the separation anxiety that Varela deals with in this study.

Varela also pointed to Stayton, Ainsworth and Main (1973), in which the term separation anxiety is used the way Varela herself uses it. The two characteristics of protest and apprehension are presented: one is the child's protest at leave-taking from the mother, and the other is the apprehension with regard to the potential inaccessibility of the mother. Varela emphasizes the arousal of attachment need and the protest at not obtaining proximity to the attachment figure. Perhaps it can be best stated as follows: (a) potential surgery is a signal of danger ahead, (b) anxiety is aroused and protection from the attachment figure is sought, and (c) the child is unable to achieve proximity to the attachment figure. Separation anxiety is then intensified. (I suggest that a period of subsequent anxious attachment might then be expected.)

Varela provided an intensive and extensive review of the literature dealing with the effects of hospitalization experiences on young children, such as studies by Fagin (1964), Brain and Maclay (1968), and Branstetter (1969). Varela was especially impressed by Branstetter's contribution, in which it was shown that the use of substitute or surrogate mother care was highly salutary and prevented disturbances in the child subsequent to hospitalization. She also noted that rooming-in arrangements for the real mother in Fagin's study were highly effective in preventing problems. Brain and Maclay arrived at a similar conclusion. Varela stated that previous studies of this problem did not deal sufficiently with the separation from the mother but rather with the fear of surgery and the strange environment.

While Varela developed nine hypotheses for her complete study, only five will be discussed here because they deal with the two tests of separation anxiety—the Hansburg S.A.T. and the Varela version of the Klagsbrun-Bowlby test. Varela hypothesized that there would be positive relationships between the following sets of variables:

1. Varela's Interview with Mother Scale and the child's separation anxiety as measured by Varela's version of the Klagsbrun-Bowlby Scale.
2. Varela's Interview with Mother Scale and the mother's level of separation anxiety as measured by the Hansburg S.A.T.

3. The child's level of separation anxiety as measured by
   Varela's version of the Klagsbrun-Bowlby Scale and
   the mother's level of separation anxiety as measured by
   the Hansburg S.A.T.

4. The child's level of separation anxiety as measured by
   Varela's version of the Klagsbrun-Bowlby Scale and
   the number of affectional bond disruptions in the
   child's attachment history as measured by certain
   items included in a Parent's Attachment History
   Questionnaire.

5. The child's level of separation anxiety as measured by
   Varela's version of the Klagsbrun-Bowlby Scale and
   the number of affectional bond disruptions in the
   mother's attachment history as measured by such
   items in the Parent's Attachment History Questionnaire.

Varela's population sample consisted of thirty children aged 4 through 7. Tables 7.1 and 7.2 are provided so that background data on the child and the mother may be seen in an overall picture.

As may be seen from Table 7.1, the children averaged 5½ years in age, two thirds were males, two thirds were white, more than two thirds were preschool or kindergarten, almost all had never been in psychotherapy or counseling, half had had a previous hospitalization averaging a stay of about 2½ days, most had had hospital preparation from parents and many had had further preparation from physicians and/or hospital staff members, and 80% of them were operated on in private hospitals. From Table 7.2 it may be noted that the mothers ranged in age from 22 to 38, with an average age of close to 31, a background of education averaging first year of college, more than half married and living with their husbands, with incomes ranging from $5,300 to $60,000 a year, with an average of $25,603, half of whom were working outside the home, nearly half of whom had been in psychotherapy, who reported a very high degree of closeness with their children, and half of whom stayed overnight in the hospital with their children during the operation. We can see from these tables that the children and their mothers have some degree of homogeneity, but con- siderable variations exist in some areas. For the children the variations appear mainly in the areas of previous hospitalization and preparation for the hospitalization period under study. For the

Table 7.1

DEMOGRAPHIC DATA ON CHILDREN

Characteristic	Data
Age	
Range	4-2 to 7-7
Average	5-6
Sex	
Male	21
Female	9
Race or Nationality	
Caucasian	22
Hispanic	7
Black	1
Schooling	
Pre-School or Kg.	23
1st or 2nd grade	7
Therapy or Counseling	
Yes	2
No	28
Previous Hospitalization	
Yes	15
Average length of stay	2.4 days
No	15
Present Hosp. Preparation	
Mother and/or father	9
Mother and/or father and physician and/or nurse	13
Mother and/or father and hosp. staff member	5
Physician and/or hosp. staff member only	3
Type of Hospital	
Private	24
Public Teach. Hosp.	6

mothers the variations exist in many areas such as education, marital status, employment, psychotherapy, and, what may be crucial, the overnight stay with the child in the hospital. What effect these variables might have had on the study is problematic.

Varela describes in considerable detail the procedures that were followed in the administration of the various tests, but these are not discussed here. However, I provide a detailed quote of the research design and statistical analysis used by Varela so that those students and

Table 7.2

DEMOGRAPHIC DATA ON MOTHERS

Characteristic	Data
Age	
Range	22–38
Average	30.71
Education	
Range	8th grade to 5 yrs. post-grad.
Average	13.5
Marital Status	
Married	17
Separated	4
Divorced	7
Single (never married)	2
Children	2 or more
Income	
Range	5,300 to 60,000
Average	25,603
Working Status	
Outside home	15
Homemakers	10
Assorted housework	5
Psychotherapy	
None	17
Yes	13
Degree of closeness to child (1–100)	
Average	93.2
Maximum rating (100)	18 mothers
Overnight stay in hosp.	
Stayed	13
Did not stay	8
Hosp. didn't allow stay	7
Missing data	2

psychologists who wish to utilize this material in their own studies can obtain a definitive picture.

This study utilized a single group design and the group was composed of mother-child dyads. Since no experimental manipulation occurred, all collected data were descriptive and correlational. After the completion of data collection, the data were coded for computer analysis. In all cases where feasible, data were coded on a linear scale to permit correlational analysis. Data analyses were performed through the utilization of the Statistical Package for the Social Sciences (SPSS) (Nie, Hull, Jenkins, Steinbrenner, and Bent, 1975).

Frequency distributions were obtained for all variables. The characteristics of the mother-child pairs as well as the variables relevant to the hypothesis testing are based on these frequency distributions. Measures of central tendency (mean, median and mode) and variability (range and standard deviation) were utilized to describe the data obtained.

In addition, simple correlational analysis was utilized. This approach enabled the measurement of the strength and direction of the relation between two variables. Pearson product-moment correlation coefficients were calculated for all of the variables of interest in the . . . study. The correlation coefficients provided initial clues regarding the nature of the relationship between variables.

The major statistic utilized in the testing of the hypotheses was multiple regression and correlation. This statistic enabled an examination of the unique contributions of a number of mother and child independent variables as they related to the two dependent variables of interest, the hospitalized child's response to separation from mother and the child's level of separation anxiety. (p. 146)

Varela developed a statistical score which she referred to as the "Separation Test Index Score." This score proved to be a highly effective method for the study of the relationship between the mother's separation difficulties and the corresponding level of the child's separation stress. I quote:

. . . the subsequent results in regard to the testing of Hypothesis 3 point to the Separation Test Index Score as being the most effective measure of the relationship between the child's and the mother's levels of separation anxiety. . . . The biggest difference between the Separation Test Index Score and both the Attachment Detachment Score and the Attachment Individuation Balance Score is that the Separation Test Index Score comprises a larger number of components than the other two scores. In contrast to the other scores, it reflects different facets of response to separation. The Separation Test Index Score is the sum of the following indices: (1) Attachment-Self Reliance Balance, (2) Hostility-Attachment Ratio, (3) Hostility-Anxiety Ratio, (4) Anxiety Ratio, (5) Avoidant Responses and (6) Responses showing Loss of Self-Esteem [on the S.A.T. Varela uses Self-Love Loss here].

Actually, Varela used three scores for the measurement of the child's level of separation anxiety which were all based on the child's responses to Varela's revision of the Klagsbrun-Bowlby Scale (1976), entitled "A Clinical Test for Young Children." These scores were as follows:

1. The first score was the Attachment-Detachment Score, which was calculated by adding the attachment per-

centage and the painful tension (fear-anxiety, pain system) percentage and then subtracting from this the sum of the individuation (self-reliant) percentage and the hostility percentage.

2. The second score was the child's Attachment-Individuation Balance Score, which represented a comparison between the child's attachment and individuation responses on the mild pictures. This method of scoring was based on the Klagsbrun and Bowlby method for the calculation of Index I. As more individuation responses than attachment responses are expected on the separation situations which are mild and frequent in childhood experience, one positive point was given for each individuation response and one negative point was given for each attachment response obtained on the mild pictures. The child's Attachment-Individuation Balance Score represents the sum of the negative and positive points obtained.

3. The third score was the Separation Test Index Score, which has already been described above. The six indices of this score were obtained on the Varela Scale while the similar six indices for the mother were obtained from the Hansburg Separation Anxiety Test.

Thus, there were three types of scores for both mother and child which could be compared to each other.

The mother's report of the child's level of anxiety as the mother noted it on the child's behavior scale was correlated with each of the three scores on the Klagsbrun-Bowlby Scale and similar correlations with the child's Separation Difficulty Score, which was also part of the interview with the mother. Only 25 parent-child dyads were available for these calculations. While Varela provided twelve massive tables of correlations, both simple and multiple, with their t scores and significance levels, we shall provide here only those relevant to the five hypotheses referred to previously because they relate to the two scales of separation anxiety used in the study. Table 7.3 provides those data referrable to the Attachment-Detachment Scores.

Table 7.4 provides similar data for the mother.

Table 7.5 provides data relative to the Attachment-Individuation Balance Score Method.

Table 7.6 presents the data on the mother's Attachment-Individuation Balance Scores and the correlations with significant factors.

Actually, the data demonstrated that neither Hypothesis 1 nor Hypothesis 2 was confirmed because the child's reactions to the separation as reported by the mother did not accord with either the child's separation anxiety level as found on the Varela version of the Klagsbrun-Bowlby Scale or the mother's level of separation anxiety as

Table 7.3

ATTACHMENT-DETACHMENT SCORES CORRELATIONS WITH
OTHER SIGNIFICANT FACTORS
(The Child Only)

Predictor Variable	Simple r	Multiple R	R^2	R^2 Change	t	p
Child's Separation Behavior Score	.05	.37	.134	.008	-.45	.66
Child's Separation Difficulty Score	.09	.36	.131	.004	-.32	.75
Mother's Attachment-Detachment Score	.36	.36	.127	.127	1.87	.08

Table 7.4

ATTACHMENT-DETACHMENT SCORES CORRELATIONS WITH
OTHER SIGNIFICANT FACTORS
(The Mother Only)

Predictor Variable	Simple r	Multiple R	R^2	R^2 Change	t	p
Child's Separation Behavior Score	.30	.31	.097	.095	1.52	.14
Child's Separation Difficulty Score	.36	.36	.129	.121	1.75	.09
Child's Attachment-Detachment Score	(see Table 7.1)					

found on the Hansburg Scale. The reasons appeared to lie in the subjective nature of the mother's reporting of the child's anxiety, which has been known to often conflict with what the child really feels. It was only when the S.A.T. indices for both mother and child were correlated that the real relationships between the mother's and the child's level of separation anxiety were revealed. I quote Varela (p. 231) relative to her discussion of Tables 7.7 and 7.8.

Table 7.5

ATTACHMENT-INDIVIDUATION BALANCE SCORES CORRELATIONS
WITH OTHER SIGNIFICANT FACTORS
(The Child Only)

Predictor Variable	Simple r	Multiple R	R^2	R^2 Change	t	p
Child's Separation Behavior Score	-.12	.11	.012	.012	-.52	.61
Child's Separation Difficulty Score	-.16	.16	.026	.026	-.78	.44
Mother's Attachment Indiv. Bal.	(see Table 7.6)					

Table 7.6

ATTACHMENT-INDIVIDUATION BALANCE SCORES CORRELATIONS
WITH OTHER SIGNIFICANT FACTORS
(The Mother Only)

Predictor Variable	Simple r	Multiple R	R^2	R^2 Change	t	p
Child's Separation Behavior Score	-.19	.24	.056	.045	-1.02	.32
Child's Separation Difficulty Score	-.10	.21	.042	.016	-.61	.55
Child's Attachment-Individu. Balance Score	-.19	.19	.037	.037	-.96	.35

It is indeed interesting that the maternal separation anxiety score that accounted for the largest proportion of the variance of the child's separation anxiety (i.e., the Separation Test Index Score) is based on the largest number of components. Furthermore, the scores which explained smaller proportions of the variance of the child's separation anxiety score are based on correspondingly fewer components. Based on the results of the testing of Hypothesis three, it appears that a score which measures a diverse number of facets relating to response to separation may be the most effective measure of tapping the relationship between child and maternal separation anxiety. It may be that the larger number of diverse components included in the Separation Test Index Score enables measurement of facets of response to separation that are excluded—or reduced in importance—in the Attachment-Detachment Score and Attachment Individuation Balance Score. The utilization of the Separation Test Index Score as a measure of child and maternal level of separation anxiety is but an exploratory first step. Future studies would do well to further explore its potential. Clearly, the finding that the Mother's Separation Test Index Score accounts for almost 22% of the child's level of separation anxiety gives rise to hopes that this first step will spark further research regarding the precise nature of the relationship between child and maternal separation anxiety and its antecedents within the context of family life.

By way of editorial comment, it should be pointed out that in connection with Hypothesis 2, the mother's Attachment-Detachment Score did indeed reflect some definitive influence on the child's Separation Difficulty Score. The Separation Difficulty Score was obtained on the mother's interview scale, in which she reported her sub-

Table 7.7

SEPARATION TEST INDEX SCORES CORRELATIONS
WITH OTHER SIGNIFICANT FACTORS
(The Child Only)

Predictor Variable	Simple r	Multiple R	R^2	R^2 Change	t	p
Child's Separation Behavior Score	.12	.12	.014	.014	.57	.57
Child's Separation Difficulty Score	.30	.30	.088	.088	1.49	.15
Mother's Separation Test Index Score	.47	.47	.219	.219	2.59	.02[a]

[a]Significance level = $p < .05$.

jective reactions to the child's difficulty in separating from her. For this
reason it would be premature to discard this method of calculating the
child's separation anxiety level as a useful tool since it has proved useful
in other studies (see Chapters 4 and 19).

Nevertheless, we see in the one result in connection with
Hypothesis 3 an important contribution to the study of measurement of
both maternal and child separation anxiety. One aspect of this result is
the development of the S.A.T. Index for both mother and child. The
second aspect is the definitive relationship obtained when the same
method is applied to both mother and child, even though the instruments used are not strictly comparable. Many of the concepts of the
instruments are the same in the sense that the pictures represent
separation experiences and there is provision for similar types of
responses. Varela provided similar interpretive structures for using the
responses which made it possible to do the comparative studies.

In the study of the relationship between these two tests and the experiences of past disruptions of attachment for both mother and child
as mentioned in Hypotheses 4 and 5, Varela made certain correlations
between the three scores for separation anxiety and the two scores for
attachment disruptions in the child's history and the mother's history.
These data are provided in Tables 7.9 to 7.11.

None of the above data show any relationship between the three
measures of separation anxiety and the measures of child and mother's

Table 7.8

SEPARATION TEST INDEX SCORES CORRELATIONS
WITH OTHER SIGNIFICANT FACTORS
(The Mother Only)

Predictor Variable	Simple r	Multiple R	R^2	R^2 Change	t	p
Child's Separation Behavior Score	.28	.28	.080	.066	1.26	.22
Child's Separation Difficulty Score	.27	.33	.110	.022	.74	.47
Child's Separation Test Index Score	(see Table 7.7)					

disruptions in their attachment life obtained from their histories. This left Hypotheses 4 and 5 previously referred to as unsupported by the data. However, Varela reported some simple correlations which shed further light on the hospitalized child's anxiety which should be considered.

She stated:

The findings indicated a significant positive relationship ($r = .52$, $p = .003$) between the number of the hospitalized child's anxiety related behaviors observed by the mother (recorded in the mother's interview, i.e., Separation Behavior Score) at the time of separation and the mother's score on the attachment response pattern as measured by Hansburg's (1972) Separation Anxiety Test. The positive simple correlation indicates mothers with higher attachment percentages describe their children as showing significantly more anxiety related behaviors at the time of pre-surgery separation from the mother. Similarly, findings indicated a significant positive relationship between mother's rating of her child's separation difficulty (recorded in the mother's interview, i.e. Separation Difficulty Score) and mother's score on the attachment response pattern derived from the Separation Anxiety Test ($r = .58$, $p < .001$). The correlation indicates that mothers with higher attachment percentages report more separation difficulty in their children when the children have to leave the mothers to go for surgery.

The results lend support to the possibility that the mother with a heightened attachment need has a greater responsiveness to her child's needs and concern about what happens to him/her, and, therefore, is more likely to respond to his/her fears and uncertainties than the mother with a lower attachment percentage. Consequently, she would be more likely to be highly sensitive to the child's response to separation. If this is the case, the significant positive relationship may represent the degree to which the mother's sensitivity to her child's behaviors and feelings enables her to note the smallest signs of distress expressed by her child.

Table 7.9

THE CHILD'S ATTACHMENT-INDIVIDUATION BALANCE SCORES
CORRELATED WITH ATTACHMENT DISRUPTIONS IN THE
CHILD'S AND MOTHER'S HISTORY

Predictor	Simple r	Multiple R	R^2	R^2 Change	t	p
Child's Attachment Disruptions	-.12	.21	.046	.007	-.40	.69
Mother's Attachment Disruptions	.04	.22	.050	.005	.32	.76

The hospitalized child's response to separation appeared not to be linked to the child's attachment need. In this study, the child's attachment percentage, derived from responses on the revised (Varela's) Klagsbrun-Bowlby (1976) scale, is not significantly related to the Separation Behavior Score ($r = -.06$, $p = .39$). Similarly, the child's attachment percentage is not related to the Separation Difficulty Score ($r = -.12$, $p = .28$). Furthermore, the child's attachment percentage is not related to the mother's attachment percentage ($r = -.14$, $p = .24$).

In summary, the findings suggest that the mother's report of her child's response to pre-surgery separation is significantly linked to her attachment need, but there is no evidence that the child's separation response, as reported by the mother, is related to the child's attachment need. It is possible [that] the significant positive correlation reflects the mother's heightened sensitivity and responsiveness to her child's response to separation. (pp. 261–263)

There is evidence in this study that the child is considerably influenced by the level of the maternal separation stress reactions as demonstrated by the correlations between the Separation Test Indices from the child's test and the mother's test. Further, there is evidence that the mother's attachment needs influence her reporting of the child's separation behaviors and difficulties. Why the child's observed behaviors and difficulties did not relate to the child's responses to Varela's revision of Klagsbrun-Bowlby's Separation Test is more likely explainable by the mother's subjective reporting. It was unfortunate that Varela's efforts to tape the hospital scenes between the mother and child prior to the surgery proved to be prematurely abortive. It might have proved useful to have had a more objective measure of the child's behavioral and separation difficulties before surgery by having a research experimenter make the observations in the manner that was done by Ainsworth, Main and their associates as reported in their work

Table 7.10

THE CHILD'S ATTACHMENT-DETACHMENT SCORES CORRELATED WITH
ATTACHMENT DISRUPTIONS IN THE CHILD'S AND MOTHER"S HISTORY

Predictor	Simple r	Multiple R	R^2	R^2 Change	t	p
Child's Attachment Disruptions	-.18	.36	.131	.000	-.13	.90
Mother's Attachment Disruptions	-.11	.36	.131	.000	-.02	.98

Table 7.11

THE CHILD'S SEPARATION TEST INDEX SCORES CORRELATED WITH
ATTACHMENT DISRUPTIONS IN THE CHILD'S AND MOTHER'S HISTORY

Predictor	Simple r	Multiple R	R^2	R^2 Change	t	p
Child's Attachment Disruptions	-.03	.49	.244	.010	.54	.59
Mother's Attachment Disruptions	-.01	.50	.246	.002	.21	.84

(*Patterns of Attachment*, 1979). The fact that Klagsbrun found a good correlation between the teacher's ratings of the child's adjustment and the child's reactions to the Klagsbrun-Bowlby Scale for Young Children certainly suggests that a more objective observation of child behavior than the mother's reports is likely to show more positive correlations with the child's responses to the test. Nevertheless, it is my impression that this study provides us with significant evidence that a child's reactions to separation bear considerable relationship to the mother's reactions. Another important contribution is the development of the Separation Test Index, which may become a highly useful method in future research.

REFERENCES

Black, H. M. *Trait Anxiety and Separation Distress: An Analysis of Two Measures in Parents and Their Adolescent Children.* Unpublished doctoral dissertation, California School of Professional Psychology, Los Angeles, 1981.

Bowlby, J. *Attachment and Loss*, Vol. II: *Separation: Anxiety and Anger.* New York: Basic Books, 1973.

Bowlby, J. "Attachment Theory, Separation Anxiety and Mourning," in S. Arieti (ed.), *American Handbook of Psychiatry* (2nd ed.), Vol. VI. New York: Basic Books, 1975.

Bowlby, J., Robertson, J., and Rosenbluth, D. "A Two-Year-Old Goes to the Hospital." *The Psychoanalytic Study of the Child*, 1952, 82–94.

Brain, D. J., and Maclay, I. "Controlled Study of Mothers and Children in Hospital." *British Medical Journal*, 1968, *1*, 278–280.

Branstetter, E. "The Young Child's Response to Hospitalization: Separation Anxiety or Lack of Mothering Care?" *American Journal of Public Health*, 1969, *59*, 92–97.

Cohen, L. J. "The Operational Definition of Human Attachment." *Psychological Bulletin*, 1974, *81*, 206–217.

DeLozier, P. P. *"An Application of Attachment Theory to the Study of Child Abuse."* Unpublished doctoral dissertation, California School of Professional Psychology, Los Angeles, 1979.

Hansburg, H. G. *Adolescent Separation Anxiety*, Vol. I: *A Method for the Study of Adolescent Separation Problems.* Springfield, Ill.: C. C. Thomas, 1972. Reprinted, Melbourne, Fla.: R. E. Krieger, 1980.

Hansburg, H. G. *Adolescent Separation Anxiety*, Vol. II: *Separation Disorders.* Melbourne, Fla.: R. E. Krieger, 1980.

Heinecke, C., and Westheimer, I. *Brief Separations.* New York: International Universities Press, 1965.

Klagsbrun, M., and Bowlby, J. "Responses to Separation From Parents: A Clinical Test for Young Children." *The British Journal of Projective Psychology and Personality Study*, 1976, *21*, 7–27.

Mason, E. A. "Hospital and Family Cooperating to Reduce Psychological Trauma." *Community Mental Health Journal*, 1978, *14*, 153–159.

Miller, J. *The Effects of Separation on Latency Age Children as a Consequence of Separation/Divorce.* Unpublished doctoral dissertation, California School of Professional Psychology, Los Angeles, 1980.

Nie, N., Holl, C., Jenkins, J., Steinbrenner, K., and Bent, D. *SPSS Statistical Package for the Social Sciences.* New York: McGraw-Hill, 1975.

Oremland, E. K., and Oremland, J. D. (eds.). *The Effects of Hospitalization on Children.* Springfield, Ill.: Charles C. Thomas, 1973.

Parness, E. "Effects of Experiences with Loss and Death among Pre-school Children." *Children Today*, 1975, *4*, 2–7.

Stayton, D. J., Ainsworth, M. D., and Main, M. G. "Development of Separation Behavior in the First Year of Life: Protest, Following and Greeting." *Developmental Psychology*, 1973, 9, 213–225.

Varela, L. M. *The Relationship between the Hospitalized Child's Separation Anxiety and Maternal Separation Anxiety.* Unpublished doctoral dissertation, California School of Professional Psychology, Los Angeles, 1982.

Wallace, A. *An Application of Attachment Theory to the Study of a Population of Divorced People.* Unpublished doctoral dissertation, California School of Professional Psychology, Los Angeles, 1977.

8

Kelly's Study of Attachment Reactions in Mothers of Hyperactive Boys

A second study with regard to children dealt with the mothers of boys who had been diagnosed as hyperactive. The study was done by Dr. Anne-Marie Ciminel Kelly. Entitled "The Relationship of Maternal Attachment Factors to the Hyperactive Behavior Disorder in a Sub-Group of Hyperactive Boys," it was completed at the California School of Professional Psychology in 1981. This study is interesting because it studied the mothers of children considered to have a handicap.

This study was undertaken to determine whether a significant number of mothers of children diagnosed as hyperactive demonstrated more degrees of dysfunctional attachment than that found among mothers whose children are considered to be relatively well adjusted. Kelly was interested in two sub-groups of hyperactive children, one of which she described as aggressive hyperactive. In a very extensive review of the literature (pp. 26–89) she found that this group of hyperactive youngsters had been described as displaying deficits in control and judgment, excessive demands for attention, temper outbursts and decreased self-esteem in addition to over-activity and inappropriate response to social stimuli. She inferred that "these behaviors bear a startling resemblance to the 'anxiously attached' behaviors as outlined by Hansburg (1972, 1979 and in a seminar Oct. 20–21, 1979)." Kelly described hyperactivity as a primary phenomenon and the aggressive factor as secondary, implying that the latter occurred largely as a result

95

of exposure to noxious influences in the family while the former was an innate phenomenon either genetic or acquired in gestation.

The general hypothesis of the study that followed from this reasoning was that mothers of the aggressive, hyperactive youngsters would show more dysfunctional attachment patterns than either the mothers of only primarily hyperactive children or the mothers of relatively intact children. Further, that mothers of primarily hyperactive (non-aggressive) children would show more dysfunctional attachment patterns than the mothers of the intact group. She presumed that these differences would be demonstrated on the Separation Anxiety Test.

Seven more hypotheses related to differences Kelly assumed would be shown on a test called Parent Report (Dibble and Cohen, 1974) and on the Wallace Attachment History Questionnaire. The Conners Teacher Rating Questionnaire was used to determine the group of hyperactive children to which each case would be assigned.

Kelly obtained the cooperation of 63 mothers of elementary school boys whose ages ranged from 6.0 to 11.5 years. All mothers in the sample were biological mothers and all families were relatively intact with father or father substitutes either present in the home or having regular and continued contact with the boys. In an effort to control for the confounding effects of other disorders, all boys with diagnosed neurological or sensory deficits were excluded from the study. Likewise all boys with a history suggestive of major psychological impairment, such as autism or childhood thought disorders, were excluded. All boys were required to have demonstrated at least average intellectual ability on psychometric evaluation or teacher evaluation of academic achievement. Additionally, because psychotropic medications, including CNS stimulants, affect classroom behavior, only boys who were observed while medication-free for at least a period of seven to ten days prior to the teacher's rating were included in the present study.

Forty-one mothers were identified as mothers of hyperactive children, based on previous physician, clinic or school evaluation of their boys. This designation was confirmed through Kelly's use of the Conner's Teacher Rating Questionnaire (1969). All boys identified as hyperactive met or exceeded the cut-off score of 15 on the 10 CTRS items discriminative for hyperactivity (Sprague, 1977). Of the 41 mothers comprising the hyperactive group, 16 were designated as mothers of primary (exclusive) hyperactive children and 25 were designated as mothers of secondary (aggressive/hyperactive) hyperactive children. This distinction was based on independent scale screening scores using the CTRS as established by Loney and Milich (1980).

The remaining twenty-two mothers were identified as mothers of a non-hyperactive comparison group. For the children of these mothers, an absence of previous history of hyperactive behavior and a score of less than 15 on the CTRS were essential criteria for inclusion in this group. The total population was obtained from various sources in the Los Angeles area including schools, pediatricians, clinics, etc., and often newspaper advertising was necessary. The sixty-three subjects were selected from eighty-three respondents. A very careful work-up of demographic data along socioeconomic, education, age of parents and youngsters, ethnic background, marital status, and occupational levels was developed by Kelly. There were no significant differences in any of these areas.

One factor about this selection stands out. The differential diagnosis afforded by medical personnel is often inaccurate and inferential. There is still no solid way in which hyperactivity can be diagnosed as either genetically organic or familial experienced through tension and anxiety. Hyperactivity, even when justifiably defined by medical and teacher personnel, has many subtle implications not adequately understood. For this reason it would be difficult to be certain of the differences and contamination could easily result. Further, it is probable that many of Kelly's subjects are victims of both areas of origination.

The procedure for examining the mothers is described as follows by Kelly:

All mothers whose children met the requirements for inclusion in the study were contacted by telephone to schedule an appointment with a trained research assistant who administered the instruments to them. Research assistants remained "blind" to the child's group designation until the completion of the study. In all cases appointments for the interview were conducted in the homes of the subjects at a mutually agreeable time during which mothers were relatively free of other demands. The interviews lasted approximately one and a half hours. At the time of the scheduled interview, after a brief period of introduction and encouragement of rapport, subjects were presented with the instruments in the following invariant order. First, the Attachment History Questionnaire, including demographic data, followed by the Parent Report and finally, the Hansburg Separation Anxiety Test were presented for mother's completion. This fixed order of presentation was based on the results of two previous studies using alternative forms of the Attachment History Questionnaire and the S.A.T. (DeLozier, 1979, and Mitchell, 1980). These studies indicated that the S.A.T., when administered first, tended to influence responses to the Attachment History Questionnaire and increase test anxiety due to its projective qualities. Thus, to minimize anxiety and provide a balance of potentially emotionally arousing tasks with more objective tasks, the instruments were presented in the order described above. After all three instruments were administered, mothers were given the opportunity to ask questions related to both the study and to any concerns which may have arisen as a result of the tests at the completion of the interview. (pp. 107–108)

Statistical analyses of the data were often accomplished by nonparametric methods. Kelly used the Krushal-Wallis statistical technique where the data were not at an interval or ratio level and three grouped rank comparisons were made. In the use of two group comparisons with non-interval level data, the Mann-Whitney U Test, a variant of chi-square analysis, was used. One-way analyses of variance were used to determine possible differences among the three groups on selected variables. In addition, in order to compare all possible group means, Scheffe tests were performed for all analyses of variance, which demonstrated differences among the groups at the .05 level and below.

One hypothesis—that mothers demonstrating severe dysfunctional attachment (on the Hansburg S.A.T.) would report parenting styles (on the Parent Report of Dibble and Cohen) more significantly dysfunctional—was tested with a t test statistic since only two groups were compared (mild and severe anxious attachment groups) on parenting style, an interval scale variable.

There were no significant differences among the three groups of mothers in terms of dysfunctional attachment scores. Then a post-hoc analysis was performed to ascertain whether the combined experimental group of mothers of hyperactive children achieved significantly different scores in dysfunctional attachment than the comparison group of mothers of the nonhyperactive group. The Mann-Whitney U statistical test was used to assess possible differences between these two groups but no significant results were obtained. It should be noted that Kelly used only three items of the anxious attachment scale on the S.A.T. to measure the presence or absence of anxious attachment (p. 118). Actually, DeLozier used five or more, as did Mitchell in their studies. Then a second post-hoc analysis was performed, examining all six factors comprising anxious attachment on the S.A.T. (It would have been interesting to see whether the number of both anxious attachment cases on all six factors and the number of detachment cases added together as a pathological number would have shown differences between the groups.)

Kelly did find a significant difference on one of the patterns of the six alluded to above, that is, the defensive system. Table 8.1 presents this finding. It is shown that mothers of the aggressive hyperactive children reported a higher incidence of defensive system responses than did mothers of the nonaggressive comparison group.

When a two-group analysis of defensive system responses was performed using the Mann-Whitney U statistical test, the difference between the combined groups of mothers of hyperactive children and mothers of the nonhyperactive comparison group was also significant at the $p = .01$ level. Further inspection of the data revealed that the mothers of the hyperactive children responded to the S.A.T. with greater defensive system responses than did mothers of the nonhyperactive comparison group (see Table 8.2).

No other factors of anxious attachment or detachment from the S.A.T. were found to significantly discriminate between any of the three groups of mothers. (An interesting result was obtained on the Parent's Report on which the mothers of hyperactive children portrayed themselves as implementing less desirable child-rearing prac-

Table 8.1

KRUSHAL-WALLIS ANALYSIS SUMMARY FOR COMPARISON OF THREE GROUPS ON S.A.T. FACTOR DEFENSIVE SYSTEM RESPONSES $>$ 13%

Group Mothers of	N	Mean Rank[a]	Corrected y^2	p
1. Nonhyperactive	22	38.81		
2. Aggressive hyperactive	25	27.34		
3. Exclusive hyperactive	16	30.10		
			6.63	.036[b]

[a]Rank numbers corrected for ties.

[b]$p < .05$.

tices even though they reported being aware of more acceptable parenting styles.) However, separation frequency reported on the S.A.T. and discrepant with occurrence of separations on the Attachment History Questionnaire proved to be of significance. Table 8.3 presents the findings of discrepant versus nondiscrepant reports for the three groups of mothers.

It appears that the mothers of aggressive hyperactive children show very high levels of discrepancy between reports of separation frequency on the S.A.T. and the Attachment History Questionnaire. This accords with their defensive reactions in the dysfunctional attachment area on the S.A.T. In Kelly's discussion of the S.A.T. results, she makes the following statements and comments, which I quote verbatim:

On the post hoc analysis, the S.A.T. (Hansburg 1972) identified significant differences only in the defensive responses between mothers of combined hyperactive and aggressive hyperactive children and mothers of non-hyperactive children. Mothers of the identified hyperactive groups responded to the projective stimuli of the S.A.T. with a higher frequency of defensive responses than did mothers of the comparison group.

An additional post hoc analysis compared mothers' discrepant reports of the same separation experiences reported on the S.A.T. and the Attachment History Questionnaire. A statistically significant difference among the groups on discrepant reports (χ^2 = 8.58, df = 2, p = .025) was found. Visual inspection of the chi-square table (see Table 8.3) showed that mothers of aggressive hyperactive children reported greater discrepancies regarding separation experiences than did mothers in the comparison group. When an additional chi-square analysis of the discrepancy data was performed, com-

Table 8.2

FREQUENCY DISTRIBUTION FOR THE PRESENCE OF S.A.T. DEFENSIVE
SYSTEM RESPONSE FACTOR DETECTED IN SAMPLES OF MOTHERS

Group Mothers of	Absolute Frequency		Relative Frequency (%)		Cumulative Frequency (%)	
	Yes	No	Yes	No	Yes	No
1. Nonhyperactive	6	16	27.3	72.7	27.3	100
2. Aggressive hyperactive	16	9	64.0	36.0	64.0	100
3. Exclusive hyperactive	9	7	56.3	48.7	56.3	100
Total	31	32	49.2	50.8		

paring mothers of the combined hyperactive group with mothers of the non-hyperactive group of children, this same difference was obtained ($\chi^2 = 6.53$, $df = 1$, $p < .025$) in the same direction. A most interesting finding was that mothers of aggressive hyperactive children tended to report specific incidents of separation experiences when faced with the projective instrument (S.A.T.), which were denied or omitted on the Attachment History Questionnaire. Their responses to these separations on the S.A.T., however, reflected an aroused defensiveness. It may be speculated that a function of this observed defensiveness may have been to ward off the emotional impact of the separation stimuli.

Elevated defensiveness in the attachment responses of the mothers of more behaviorally disturbed children are entirely consistent with an attachment theory perspective. Bowlby (1973) points out that defensive processes aimed against recognition or disclosure of disturbing family relations occurs most frequently in those who have experienced such disruptions. He suggests (1980) that the operation of blame and guilt inducing behaviors observed in parents of these children accounts for the development of "defensive exclusion" of past separation experiences and often prevents realistic clinical or research appraisal of the strong emotional components (anxiety, fear) associated with these disruptions.

The finding of defensiveness among these two groups of mothers of hyperactive children raises a number of possible explanations for the null results found (with the remainder of the S.A.T. factors). First, mothers of these hyperactive children may have dysfunctional patterns of attachment that the S.A.T. failed to reveal, due to extreme defensiveness. . . . Or, alternatively, these mothers are defensive for reasons that cannot be explained by the present study *and* they are *not* experiencing dysfunctional patterns of attachment. In this case, since there were no differences reported among groups on the variable of dysfunctional attachment, it might be assumed that the S.A.T. is

Table 8.3

CHI-SQUARE ANALYSIS OF OCCURRENCE OF DISCREPANT REPORTS OF
SEPARATION ON THE HANSBURG S.A.T. AND ATTACHMENT HISTORY
QUESTIONNAIRE BY THREE GROUPS OF MOTHERS

Group Mothers of		Discrepant Reports		Nondiscrepant Reports		df	χ^2
	N	*N*	%	*N*	%		
1. Non-hyperactive	22	4	18.2	18	81.8		
2. Aggressive hyperactive	25	15	60.0	10	40.0		
3. Exclusive hyperactive	16	6	37.5	10	62.5		
						2	8.58

Note: $p = < .05$.

validly measuring what it purports to measure. If this is so, then the hypotheses which associate maternal attachment factors with aggressive hyperactivity in children are not correct.

However, it must be asked why these mothers of hyperactive children were defensive on inquiries into their child-rearing behaviors. These same groups reported poorer parenting practices despite an expressed understanding of more desirable caretaking behaviors. Bowlby's (1980) interpretation of the development of defensive exclusion suggests one explanation for the specificity of defensive responses with respect to separation stimuli. The present findings suggest that these mothers are more defensive with regard to separation experiences in their own childhoods than regarding their child rearing practices, thus providing evidence for the specificity of defensive responses with respect to separation experiences.

There were other interesting findings in this study, especially on the Parent Report Test. The mothers of aggressive hyperactive children as well as the undifferentiated hyperactive group reported significantly poorer parenting styles than the comparison group, although expected differences between the two major subgroup mothers were not forthcoming. Kelly discusses at length the effect that hyperactivity in the child may have on the parenting behavior of the mother. In this connection she refers often to the studies of Thomas, Chess and Birch (1968) and Bell (1968) that

. . . child variables significantly influence the quality of mother-child interaction, as well as the converse. Mothers of exclusive hyperactive children were not significantly different from the mothers of aggressive hyperactive children in respect to parenting style. This finding is consistent with Thomas, Chess and Birch's formulation, since exclusive hyperactive children would also be expected to be somewhat more difficult to manage than the non-hyperactive children.

She refers to Wender (1971), who suggests that

. . . some severely disturbed hyperactive children may be extremely difficult to handle, elicit poor parenting, and at the same time may be living in families where the predisposing parental pathology, as noted by Cantwell (1972), reinforces the child's disturbed behaviors, causing a vicious cycle. (p. 172)

Kelly concludes her discussion with the following:

Both animal (Harlow and Harlow, 1970) and human studies (Bowlby, 1969; Frommer and O'Shea, 1973) amply demonstrate that the repertoire of parenting behaviors is greatly influenced by the quality of care parents received as children. The use of control through guilt and anxiety by mothers of aggressive hyperactive children might be, in part, a reflection of the kind of care they received as children. The demonstrated defensiveness that these mothers show in relationship to attachment factors may be, in fact, a defensiveness against blame and guilt associated with possible previous pathogenic family relationships. However, since there are no substantive data in the present study to implicate dysfunctional attachment factors as influencing parental style, further research is needed to understand more fully the implications of specific child rearing factors in families of hyperactive children. It seems reasonable to conclude that the weight of the data supports the proposition that the child's behavioral characteristics may significantly shape the quality of parental caregiving behaviors.

REFERENCES

Bell, R. Q. "A Reinterpretation of the Direction of Effects in Studies of Socialization." *Psychological Review*, 1968, 75, 81–95.

Bowlby, J. *Attachment and Loss*, Vol. II: *Separation*. New York: Basic Books, 1973.

Bowlby, J. *Attachment and Loss*, Vol. III: *Loss*. New York: Basic Books, 1980.

Cantwell, D. P. "Psychiatric Illness in the Families of Hyperactive Children." *Archives of General Psychiatry*, 1972, 27, 414–417.

Conners, C. K. "A Teacher's Rating Scale for Use in Drug Studies with Children." *American Journal of Psychiatry*, 1969, *126*, 884–888.

DeLozier, P. P. An Application of Attachment Theory to the Study of Child Abuse. Unpublished doctoral dissertation, California School of Professional Psychology, Los Angeles, 1979.

Dibble, E., and Cohen, D. "Companion Instruments for Measuring Children's Competence and Parental Style." *Archives of General Psychiatry*, 1974, *30*, 805–815.

Frommer, E., and O'Shea, G. "The Importance of Childhood Experience in Relation to Problems of Marriage and Family Building." *British Journal of Psychiatry*, 1973, *123*, 157–160.

Hansburg, H. G. *Adolescent Separation Anxiety*, Vol. I: *A Method for the Study of Adolescent Separation Problems*. Springfield, Ill.: C. C. Thomas, 1972. Reprinted, Melbourne, Fla.: R. E. Krieger, 1980.

Hansburg, H. G. Seminar at California School of Professional Psychology, Los Angeles, October 1979.

Hansburg, H. G. "Psychological Systems and Separation Disorders," paper presented at the American Psychological Association Convention, New York, 1979.

Harlow, H., and Harlow, M. "Developmental Aspects of Emotional Behavior," in P. Black (ed.), *Physiological Correlates of Emotion.* New York: Academic Press, 1970.

Kelly, A. M. C. *The Relationship of Maternal Attachment Factors to the Hyperactive Behavior Disorder in a Sub-group of Hyperactive Boys.* Unpublished doctoral dissertation, California School of Professional Psychology, Los Angeles, 1981.

Loney, J., and Milich, R. "Hyperactivity, Inattention and Aggression in Clinical Practice," paper presented at the Meeting of the American Psychological Association, Montreal, 1980.

Mitchell, M. *An Application of Attachment Theory to a Socio-Cultural Perspective of Physical Child Abuse in the Mexican-American Community.* Unpublished doctoral dissertation, California School of Professional Psychology, Los Angeles, 1980.

Sprague, R. L. "Psychopharmaco Therapy in Children," in M. F. McMillan and S. Henae (eds.), *Child Psychiatry: Treatment and Research.* New York: Brunner/Mazel, 1977.

Thomas, A., Chess, S., and Birch, H. *Temperament and Behavior Disorders in Children.* New York: University Press, 1968.

Wallace, A. S. *An Application of Attachment Theory to the Study of A Population of Court-Referred Divorced People.* Unpublished doctoral dissertation, California School of Professional Psychology, Los Angeles, 1977.

Wender, P. *Minimal Brain Dysfunction in Children.* New York: Wiley-Interscience, 1971.

9

Duplak's Study of Attachment/Separation Reactions of Learning Disabled Boys

A third study of latency-age children dealt with those who were largely suffering from reading disability and who therefore could not handle the reading requirement of the test. This study, entitled "Attachment Patterns and Arousal of Separation Reactions in Learning Disabled Boys," was completed by Dr. Christine Duplak for the Graduate School of School Psychology at New York University in 1982. It demonstrated another method for recording and studying the reactions to the S.A.T. pictures.

This study arose out of Dr. Duplak's contact with the original research with the Separation Anxiety Test and her cooperation in developing it as a clinical instrument. (See acknowledgments in *Adolescent Separation Anxiety*, Vols. I and II.) In her later years of work at the Jewish Child Care Association she took charge of the program for learning disabled youngsters and became involved with many of their problems of living and adjustment. The contiguity of these two separate experiences in the Mental Hygiene Clinic of that agency contributed to her interest in doing a doctoral dissertation on the attachment-separation problems of these children. However, Duplak did not use the children at the agency because they were placed youngsters and therefore derived her population of learning disabled children from two public junior high schools in New York City.

Duplak did not use the S.A.T. in the usual way in her research, although she had originally planned to do so. The Education Department at her university wanted her to utilize a technique which would

provide a less complicated method of administration, recording and
scoring and also wanted proof that the S.A.T. actually produced
separation anxiety reactions in children. To this end a compromise was
reached and the S.A.T. pictures were used simply to stimulate reactions in the subjects of her study as well as a demonstration project or
pilot study. It is this compromise study which is reported here. The
resultant over-simplification of the problems of attachment and
separation will be apprehended later when we discuss the results of the
study.

Duplak's examination of the literature provided ample evidence
that children with learning disabilities are often characterized by ego
deficits, maturational delays associated with neurological immaturities
and consequent difficulties in social relationships (Bryan, 1974, 1976,
1978; Connolly, 1971). Consensus among various researchers included
the following observations. These youngsters are more egocentric and
less competent in perceiving the affective states of others; they tend to
have particular difficulties with organized patterning of perceptual experiences which influence their social judgment (DeHirsch, 1975,
Buchholz, 1978). Emery (1975) refers to a "social learning disability"
in these children. They are reported to be vulnerable to typical
developmental stresses (Buchholz, 1977). Bachara (1977) noted that
children 10 to 12 years old with learning disabilities display more concomitant emotional problems than their peers. Wender (1971) found
that these youngsters have weaker ties to their parents and have
ongoing frustrations in the social-academic sphere. (Also see Hansburg,
1956, on emotional problems of the reading-disabled.) Although not
discussed by Duplak, the emotional and social problems of children
with reading disability began to be noted in the literature at the turn of
the century and were later considered of significance by many of the
famous students in the field, such as Blanchard (1946), Fernald (1943),
Gates (1947), Monroe (1932), and Liss (1949).

Leaning heavily on the work of Hansburg (1972) and Bowlby
(1977), Duplak discusses the effect of attachment and separation experiences on the personality development of children and adolescents.
She suggests that the usual problems centering on the development of
close relationships with others may become accentuated in the learning
disabled youngster. She assumes, hypothetically, that the solution to
separation experiences in the learning disabled would be to turn away
from the usual attachment seeking behavior and adopt avoidant reac-

tions. Therefore, she hypothecated that the learning disabled would show detached patterns of interaction and, when exposed to separation stimuli, would become even more detached.

In her selection of subjects Duplak defined learning disabled children as meeting three criteria: (a) academic achievement two years below mental age expectations with certain learning deficits associated with subtle neurological dysfunction, (b) I.Q. between 85 and 119, and (c) not having serious emotional disturbance, primary behavior disturbance, gross cerebral damage, marked sensory handicaps or extreme cultural deprivation. She defined separation stimuli as follows:

Separation anxiety or stress will be defined in accordance with Hansburg's (1972) work in which he conceptualizes it as that anxiety related to separation from a significant attachment figure. Hansburg's work includes a series of twelve pictures depicting children in various separation situations. These pictures have been found to arouse reactions to separation, namely separation anxiety in children.

She based her concept of attachment pattern on attachment styles described by Horney (1945). While there were three such styles, Duplak included only two in her study, namely moving toward others and moving away from others. This was defined operationally by a series of cartoons which depicted either one of these two styles. From these she was able to refer to either attachment or detachment. Despite this acceptance of Horney's descriptive attachment styles, Duplak gives a great deal of attention to attachment theory (Bowlby's formulation, 1969). She applies this theory to learning disabled children, postulating that "if for both internal (ego deficits of child) and external reasons (mother unpredictable) the attachment figure is not seen as available or accessible, anxiety can intensify in an attempt to restore closeness." Of course, Bowlby's theory stresses the mother's level of accessibility rather than the child's deficits. Duplak, however suggests that the child's deficits may frustrate the mother and "she may then tend to turn off or pull away in frustration and ignorance."

Duplak concludes her discussion of attachment and separation in the following way:

Attachment and separation are universal themes in each child's emotional life as he/she grows and develops. What each individual brings to these experiences genetically, neurologically, emotionally and historically modifies the quality of the attachments formed and the ease with which separation experiences are handled. It is more of a struggle for some than for others. This study attempted to highlight these issues in showing that not only do more vulnerable children form different kinds of attachments but that they are also more vulnerable to the developmental stresses of life, including the stress of separation. This investigation explored whether learning-disabled and non-learning-disabled children generally moved "toward" or "away" from others and if this kind of attaching or non-attaching behavior increases when the stress of separation is involved.

Using the criteria referred to above, Duplak selected a total of 64 children who were learning disabled and 64 children of comparable age who were not so disabled from the 7th and 8th grades of two public junior high schools. Table 9.1 provides the demographic data limited to I.Q. and age. According to Duplak the differences noted between the means were not significant. The experimental groups were exposed to the separation stimuli (the twelve pictures of the S.A.T.) two weeks after the teachers had completed a rating scale and the children had been prepared for the experiment by parental consent.

At the time the study was begun all of the children had been requested to sort a deck of 30 attachment pattern cartoons (see Section Four, Chapter 22) consisting of stick figures in various attitude positions. Each child was given two envelopes, one of which was marked "like me" and the other one, "not like me." They were asked to place those cartoons which they believed were "like me" in one envelope and those which they believed to be "not like me" in the other envelope. In this manner they were characterizing their responses as going toward the other person or going away from the other person, i.e., attachment or detachment.

Table 9.1

DEMOGRAPHIC CHARACTERISTICS OF THE CHILDREN

	Learning-Disabled		Non-Learning-Disabled	
	Experimental	Control	Experimental	Control
Mean I.Q.	90.2	92.3	106.5	102.4
Standard Deviation I.Q.	2.1	1.9	2.0	1.5
Mean Age	11.4	11.9	11.2	11.8
Standard Deviation Age	1.4	1.6	1.1	.9

Two weeks after this sorting took place, the investigators returned and administered the separation arousal condition only to the experimental groups. The controls were sent elsewhere. (The manner of giving the Hansburg S.A.T. pictures is described in Section Four.) After viewing these slides, the children of the experimental groups were joined by the control children and all were again requested to sort the 30 cartoons into the "like me" and "not like me" envelopes. At this second request for sorting of the cartoons, the children were given the explanation that by sorting the cards again, more information about how children learn would be obtained. Ostensibly, this procedure was devised to determine the effect of producing attachment or detachment reactions in the experimental groups after having been subjected to vicarious separation experiences through the medium of the S.A.T. pictures. The cartoons were the method of measuring attachment and detachment reactions before and after the stimulus of separation.

While the teacher rating scale used in this study is less pertinent to the purposes of this volume, it should be pointed out that Duplak's avowed intention was to determine the degree of agreement between the child's perception of his attachment style and the teacher's perception of this style. Material on this is included in the original study with statistics, but this material will not be provided here. Suffice it to say Duplak found considerable agreement in this area.

The pre-experimental cartoon testing provided some interesting statistics on the comparative attachment and detachment scores of the learning disabled and non-learning disabled youngsters. These are presented in Table 9.2. Note that Duplak uses t value scores.

Table 9.2

ATTACHMENT AND DETACHMENT PRETEST MEANS, STANDARD DEVIATIONS AND t VALUES FOR LEARNING-DISABLED AND NON-LEARNING-DISABLED

Attachment Pattern	Group	(N = 128) M	S.D.	t
Attachment	Learning-Disabled	2.14	1.34	18.88[a]
	Non-Learning Disabled	6.92	1.50	18.88[a]
Detachment	Learning-Disabled	5.92	1.52	20.36[a]
	Non-Learning-Disabled	1.38	1.38	20.36[a]

[a] $p < .05$.

The data present striking evidence of the greater trend to detachment among the learning disabled youngsters and a greater tendency to attachment among the non-learning-disabled boys. All the differences were significant at the .05 level. The greater detachment behavior of the learning disabled had already been shown on the teacher rating scale.

The subsequent data dealing with the influence of the Separation Anxiety Test pictures on both the learning disabled and non-learning-disabled groups is depicted in Table 9.3 and further in Table 9.4.

The attachment reactions of the learning disabled group moved further in the direction of detachment while the reactions of the non-learning-disabled group moved toward attachment. The data were significant at the .01 level. Differences between experimentals and controls were also significant at the same level. These calculations demonstrate that the learning disabled group were influenced by the separation pictures toward greater detachment while the non-learning-disabled group moved in the direction of attachment. The general direction of movement under stress appears to be related to an already acquired tendency.

An analysis of variance of the mean change scores on attachment for both groups under experimental and control conditions demonstrated that the two independent variables (learning disabled and non-learning-disabled under control and experimental conditions) were found to be significant at the .01 level. Similar analyses were made for the detachment means. In the table for the means on pre- and posttest scores for detachment it was obvious that the learning disabled group showed more detachment on the second testing than on the first which was significant at the .01 level while the non-learning-disabled group showed no change. The table for the mean change scores on detachment indicated a significant change in the direction of detachment for

Table 9.3

ATTACHMENT MEANS ON PRE- AND POSTTEST SCORES

(N = 128)		Control	Experimental
Learning-Disabled	Pretest	2.56	1.70
	Posttest	2.59	1.29
Non-Learning-Disabled	Pretest	7.90	6.93
	Posttest	7.78	8.25

Table 9.4

MEAN CHANGE SCORES ON ATTACHMENT FOR BOTH GROUPS
IN CONTROL AND EXPERIMENTAL CONDITIONS

(N = 128)	Control	Experimental
Learning-Disabled	+.03	-.41
Non-Learning-Disabled	-.125	+1.31

the learning disabled group while the mean change in detachment for the non-learning-disabled showed a significant movement in the minus direction for detachment. Analyses of the variance were all significant at the .01 level. Actually, all of the data were corroborative of the hypothesis that separations experienced vicariously through pictures would induce decreasing attachment and increasing detachment in the learning disabled group while producing increasing attachment and decreasing detachment for the non-learning-disabled group (tables from the study are not repeated here).

In her discussion of this experiment Duplak notes that the data support the contention of Buchholz (1978) that the ego deficits which accompany learning disabilities affect the learning disabled child's object relations and the development of attachment as well.

The learning disabled child's reaction to the attachment instrument of this current study, consisting of cartoons of stick figures, reflected his fearfulness and sense of vulnerability. A typical learning disabled child's statement included concern over "being hit" or "pushed away" when the hands of a stick figure were outstretched. On the other hand, the typical non-learning-disabled child's comment consisted of "reaching out" or being "included," i.e., "they're asking him to play."

Duplak continues an extensive discussion on attachment in learning disabled children and its relationship to social and emotional maturity.

With regard to her second hypothesis relative to the effect of separation stimuli, Duplak has the following to say:

. . . attachment patterns (of the learning disabled) are intensified under exposure to separation stimuli. . . . Learning-disabled boys become even more detached in their interpersonal style. Non-learning-disabled boys become even more attached under the stress conditions. This is consistent with Schachter's

(1959) results. He studied affiliation in the adult population reporting that when an adult is subjected to stress, affiliation behavior intensifies. Hansburg (1972) also discusses the increased need for contact with others in relation to induced separation stress. He suggests that, in the normal course of development it is the intensity of the separation that is related to the intensity of the need for contact.

Youngsters with learning disability have developed an attitude that other people are not reliable. This factor relates to their difficulty with object constancy and prevents them from turning to others for support in stressful situations. They have apparently developed a defensive pattern of withdrawal, and this increases in intensity under stressful conditions. "Moving away from others" is a way of avoiding the anxiety of being rejected by others. Ultimately, these children, in attempting to avoid anxiety, pay the cost of losing the support and attention of others had they been able to recruit it as non-learning-disabled children do.

In line with my statement at the beginning of this chapter that the use of the measurement method of the stick figures on the separation reactions of the learning disabled boys would lead to oversimplification of the attachment-detachment concept, Duplak states (p. 52) that one of the limitations of the study was

. . . the narrowness of the instrument measuring attachment patterns. While the pilot study was extremely helpful in refining the instrument so that it was relevant and of interest to learning-disabled children, an aggressive mode of relating is also pertinent to this population and should be examined.

Actually, there is far more involved in the attachment phenomenon than even this concept, although Duplak recognized from her experience with the S.A.T. that attachment and separation were highly complicated phenomena. There are attachments which are highly loaded with fear, pain and anxiety and there are attachments strongly loaded with hostility. Additionally, strong defensiveness may characterize some attachments and not others. Individuation factors, identity, self-love loss and preoccupation with self-esteem are of significance. The attempt to simplify the concept of attachment or detachment may lead to some conclusions which may misrepresent the kind of detachment manifested by learning disabled boys.

Further, the factors studied in the S.A.T. also include the significant aspect of depression. Would the avoidant learning disabled have demonstrated a stronger depressive syndrome than their non-learning-disabled peers, that is, associated with their detachment?

How would the learning disabled have handled the differences in attachment on mild and strong stimuli? How might they have handled the feeling of rejection response included in the S.A.T.? These and other questions linger on in considering this study, and it is my impression that we might have obtained some better answers if Dr. Duplak had been able to carry out her original intention.

REFERENCES

Bachara, G. H. "Empathy in Learning Disabled Children." *Journal of Learning Disabilities*, 1977, *10*(8), 42–43.

Blanchard, P. "Psychoanalytic Contributions to the Problem of Reading Disabilities," in *Psychoanalytic Study of the Child*, Vol. II. New York: International Universities Press, 1946.

Bowlby, J. *Attachment and Loss*, Vol. I: *Attachment*. New York: Basic Books, 1969.

Bowlby, J. "The Making and Breaking of Affectional Bonds." *British Journal of Psychiatry*, 1977, *130*, 1–28.

Bryan, T., Wheeler, R., Felcan, J., and Henek, T. " 'Come on Dummy': An Observational Study of Children's Communications." *Journal of Learning Disabilities*, 1974, 7(5), 26–43.

Bryan, T. H. "Learning Disability—A New Stereotype." *Journal of Learning Disabilities*, 1974, 7(5), 46–51.

Bryan, T. H. "Peer Popularity of Learning Disabled Children: A Replication." *Journal of Learning Disabilities*, 1976, 9(5), 621–625.

Bryan, T. H. "Social Relationships and Verbal Interactions of Learning Disabled Children." *Journal of Learning Disabilities*, 1978, *11*(2), 58–66.

Buchholz, E. "Emotional Development and Controls of Learning Disabled," paper presented at the Meeting of the Orton Society, New York, Spring 1977. (Manuscript available from Professor Buchholz, New York University, Department of Educational Psychology.)

Buchholz, E. "Emotional Development in Learning Disabled Children," paper presented at the fall meeting of the CEC/ADAR, November 1978.

Connolly, C. "Social and Emotional Factors in Learning Disabilities," in *Progress in Learning Disabilities*, Vol. II. New York: Grune and Stratton, 1971.

DeHirsch, K. "Language Deficits in Children with Developmental Lags." *Psychoanalytic Study of the Child*, 1975, *30*, 95–126.

Duplak, C. *Attachment Patterns and Arousal of Separation Reactions in Learning Disabled and Non-Learning Disabled Boys.* Unpublished doctoral dissertation, New York University, 1982.

Emery, E. J. *Social Perception Processes in Normal and Learning Disabled Children.* Unpublished doctoral dissertation, New York University, Department of School Psychology, 1975.

Fernald, G. *Remedial Techniques in Basic School Subjects.* New York: McGraw-Hill, 1943.

Gates, A. I. *The Improvement of Reading.* New York: Macmillan, 1947.

Hansburg, H. G. "A Reformulation of the Problem of Reading Disability." *American Journal of Child Psychiatry*, 1956, 3(2), August 1956.

Hansburg, H. G. *Adolescent Separation Anxiety*, Vol. I. *A Method for the Study of Adolescent Separation Problems.* Springfield, Ill.: C. C. Thomas, 1972. Reprinted, Melbourne, Fla.: R. E. Krieger, 1980.

Hansburg, H. G. *Adolescent Separation Anxiety*, Vol. II: *Separation Disorders: A Manual for the Interpretation of the Separation Anxiety Test.* Melbourne, Fla.: R. E. Krieger, 1980.

Horney, K. *Our Inner Conflicts: A Constructive Theory of Neurosis.* New York: W. W. Norton & Co., 1945.

Liss, E. "Psychiatric Implications of the Failing Student." *American Journal of Orthopsychiatry*, 1949, *19*, 501–505.

Monroe, M. *Children Who Cannot Read.* Chicago: University of Chicago Press, 1932.

Schachter, S. *The Psychology of Affiliation.* Stanford, Cal.: Stanford University Press, 1959.

Wender, P. *Minimal Brain Dysfunction in Children.* New York: John Wiley and Sons, 1971.

STUDIES OF COLLEGE STUDENTS

10

Sherry's Study of Separation Reactions
in College Freshmen

College students are frequently the subjects of various kinds of psychological studies and experiments. This is often the case because they are students at universities where teachers and professors in the fields of psychology and allied fields are interested in studying their emotional, mental, and social reactions to all kinds of situations and problems. Thus, a very large number of dissertations are concerned with this age group. Among these studies are such problems as intimate relations, drug use, religious activities, separation from parents, and school achievement.

In a few of these studies the S.A.T. has been used to understand some of the complex problems which are involved in the college students' inner lives. Dr. Michael Sherry, working out of Michigan State University as a counselor to students, completed a study in 1980, entitled "Father Absence and Separation Anxiety Reactions in College Freshmen." In one group the loss of the father by death or divorce was a focus of the inquiry. Dr. Sherry compared students from this background with those from intact families.

This study was undertaken at Michigan State University by Dr. Sherry when he was a consultant at the counseling center of that college. While working with entering students at the center, he noticed that a number of students having difficulties in adjusting to college life had experienced serious separations earlier in their lives, including loss of parents by death or divorce. He hypothesized that prior problem separations that engendered feelings that cannot be mastered would

115

predispose a person to react with undue stress to current separations. He then investigated a larger group of students than was available to him in the clinic and confined his study to those freshmen whose homes were at least 60 miles away and who, therefore, found it necessary to take up residence at the school.

From this population he chose to confine his study to those who had lost a father through death and/or divorce earlier in their lives. Sherry did not explain why he selected father absence rather than maternal absence but it nevertheless was a welcome diversion from the usual concern with the child's relationship with the mother. Thus he used three groups of students: (a) father absent because of death, (b) father absent because of divorce, and (c) father not absent.

Sherry further hypothesized that (a) college freshmen who left home to attend college would be more anxious than those from intact families, (b) father-absent freshmen would seek attachments more often and would be less self-sufficient than intact-family freshmen, (c) father-absent freshmen would respond with more hostility following separations than those from intact families, and (d) father-absent freshmen would attempt more strongly to avoid the reality of a separation than those from intact families.

Sherry was able to obtain 90 students—80 from Michigan and 10 from out of state. All had begun college in September of 1979 and were tested in January of their freshman year after they had been at the University for five to six months. The subjects consisted of 45 males and 45 females (although in his report Sherry does not present separate data on sex differences). The subjects ranged in age from 18 to 19, with an average age of 18.6 years, and males and females were equally distributed among the three groups of students.

In order to evaluate current levels of general anxiety as well as the trait designating vulnerability to anxiety, the author selected the Spielberger State Anxiety Inventory. For the remainder of his study he concentrated on the data derived from the Hansburg Separation Anxiety Test. The State Trait Anxiety inventories (Spielberger, Gorsuch, and Lushene, 1972) are two self-reporting measures of trait and state anxiety. The Trait Scale is a highly reliable and valid measure of relatively stable individual proneness to anxiety. The State Scale measures validly and reliably transient feelings of tension, nervousness, worry and apprehension. When completing the State Scale, subjects were asked to imagine how they felt on their first day alone at

Michigan State University. (The data on the Spielberger Tests are not included in this summary, although Sherry concluded that the absence of the father from the home did not predispose freshmen students to anxiety in general. Some interpretations of the STAI data are, however, discussed here.)

Sherry explains that giving his tests after the freshmen students had had an opportunity to adjust for the period of approximately five to six months may have lost the advantage of detecting the immediate effects of separation if the students had been tested in September of that year. In spite of this handicap Sherry felt that at least vulnerability to disturbance might be still manifested in the father-absent students.

Sherry confined his study to only certain aspects of the results on the Hansburg S.A.T. The first of his presentations referred to individuation and attachment percentage results. Table 10.1 presents his findings in this area.

A two-by-two analysis of variance for the individuation measure produced an F of 4.82, significant at a .03 level. The same statistical measure of attachment produced an F of 3.58, significant at a .06 level. These results suggested that father-absent subjects differed significantly from intact family subjects, indicating that they were definitely less self-sufficient and not as tolerant of separation. Further, the results demonstrated that the father-absent freshmen were more needful in the attachment area than those from intact families. This trend appeared to support the hypothesis relating to these factors and that father-absent college freshmen tend to be more anxiously attached and less self-sufficient.

Another aspect of the S.A.T. studied by Sherry referred to the

Table 10.1

MEANS, F RATIOS AND SIGNIFICANCE LEVELS FOR PERCENTAGE
OF INDIVIDUATION AND ATTACHMENT RESPONSES FOR
FATHER-ABSENT (FA) AND INTACT-FAMILY (IF) SUBJECTS

	FA (N = 60) Mean % Score	IF (N = 30) Mean % Score	F	Significance
Individuation Percentage	18.3	22.9	4.82	.03
Attachment Percentage	24.1	21.9	3.58	.06

defensive patterning, or what was earlier referred to as avoiding the reality of a separation, termed separation denial (see *Adolescent Separation Anxiety*, Vol. I, Chap. 7; Vol. II, pp. 8–9, 52–54). Sherry provides Table 10.2, indicating the results obtained in a comparative study of two groups on the responses of withdrawal, evasion and fantasy.

The mean scores refer to the mean percentage of reality-avoidant responses selected on the S.A.T. For father-absent subjects 15.8% of their S.A.T. responses were reality-avoidant responses, while 12.4% of the S.A.T. responses for intact family subjects were reality-avoidant. An analysis of variance for the reality-avoidant measure produced an *F* of 6.32, significant at the .01 level. Defensive denial of separation patterning seemed to be more often characteristic of the students from father-absent families than the students from intact families.

Sherry decided to study a symbiotic index in the test by selecting all those students from both groups who scored above 25% on the attachment pattern and below 16% on the individuation pattern. After selecting these students, he performed a two-by-two chi-square comparing father-absent and intact-family subjects for the symbiotic measure. This produced a value of 1.86, significant at the .17 level. Table 10.3 presents these results.

The results do not show significance although they are in the expected direction. (Sherry might have found a better measure of the symbiotic phenomenon by using the factors of severe anxious attachment as described elsewhere.)

Analyzing his results further, he made a study of those who chose more than 15% responses to the reality avoidant pattern. He made a two-by-two chi-square comparing father-absent and intact-family subjects for the reality-avoidant measure, producing a value of 7.4 significant at less than a .01 level. Table 10.4 presents these results.

Table 10.2

MEANS, *F* RATIOS AND SIGNIFICANT LEVELS FOR PERCENTAGES
OF REALITY AVOIDANT RESPONSES FOR FATHER-ABSENT (FA)
AND INTACT-FAMILY (IF) SUBJECTS

	FA (*N* = 60)	IF (*N* = 30)	*F*	Significance
Reality-Avoidant Percentage	15.8	12.4	6.32	.01

Table 10.3

CHI-SQUARE FOR NUMBER OF FATHER-ABSENT (FA) AND INTACT-FAMILY (IF)
SUBJECTS RESPONDING SYMBIOTICALLY

	FA	IF	χ^2	Significance
Symbiotic	18	5		
			1.86	.17
Nonsymbiotic	42	25		

Table 10.4

CHI-SQUARE FOR NUMBER OF FATHER-ABSENT (FA) AND INTACT-FAMILY (IF)
SUBJECTS SHOWING REALITY AVOIDANT SEPARATON RESPONSES (RAVO)

	FA	IF	
RAVO	30	6	
			$\chi^2 = 7.4$, significant at .01 level
Non-RAVO	30	24	

These data seemed to support the hypothesis that father-absent subjects attempted to avoid the reality of the test depicted separations more than intact-family subjects. In an attempt to link symbiotic factors with reality-avoidant factors, Sherry tried to determine whether symbiotic father-absent subjects avoid the reality of a new separation more than symbiotic intact-family subjects. He performed a two-by-two chi-square comparing such subjects for the reality-avoidant measure. Table 10.5 presents the findings.

The above evidence strongly confirmed the thesis that symbiotic father-absent subjects are more avoidant of the reality of separation than symbiotic intact-family subjects. (The same problem applies to these data as was mentioned previously. It should also be noted that a high reality-avoidance level is one of the six factors of the S.A.T. anxious attachment category and therefore does correlate with the symbiotic index used by Sherry.)

In a study of the hostility pattern, Sherry did not find any significant differences between father-absent subjects and intact-family subjects. The mean percentage of hostile responses for the former was 13.8 (range of 11 to 16), while intact family subjects showed a mean percentage of 13.2 (range of 9 to 16).

Sherry further reported that data for college freshmen were con-

Table 10.5

CHI-SQUARE FOR NUMBER OF SYMBIOTIC FATHER-ABSENT (SFA)
AND SYMBIOTIC INTACT-FAMILY (SIF) SUBJECTS AVOIDING
THE REALITY OF A SEPARATION (RAVO)

	SFA	SIF	
RAVO	12	0	$\chi^2 = 6.97$
Non-RAVO	6	5	significant at $< .01$ level

sistent with the norms for the test as published in Volume II of *Adolescent Separation Anxiety*.

The following discussion of his findings on the Spielberger tests is of interest:

The data (from these tests) did not support the hypothesis that College freshmen from father absent families who have left home (for school) are more anxious than those from intact families. . . . This finding is consistent with results in other studies that college students who have lost a parent by death are no more anxious than non-bereaved college students.

The absence of elevated anxiety scores, in particular, the State Anxiety scores, for father absent subjects may be because of two methodological considerations related to the date of testing. Freshmen were tested in January after they had had four months to adjust to the separation. As a result the intensity of the separation was probably diminishing. Consequently, their reactions to the separation were probably lessening, manifested by the absence of elevated State Anxiety scores for the father absent group. Secondly, freshmen with the most aggravated separation reactions may have already dropped out of college. Thus, the extremes of the sample may have been lost by the relatively late date of the testing.

As was predicted by Sherry's hypothesis, father absence was found to be related to lessened individuation following a separation. The data strongly indicated that father-absent subjects were less inclined to use separations as springboards for independent, exploratory, self-developing activities than freshmen from intact families. Furthermore, a trend was present in which father absence was related to increased attachment-seeking.

These results suggested that college freshmen who have experienced father absence are, in Bowlby's (1973) terms, "anxiously attached." Anxious attachment occurs when an individual who has experienced traumatic separations in the past fears the repetition of a separation from a new attachment figure. The interpersonal strategy of father-absent subjects is to find new attachment figures upon whom they can become extremely dependent. This strategy appears to be at the expense of self-developing activities.

The data did not support the hypothesis that father absent subjects are more hostile following separations than those from intact families. Three possible explanations are offered for the lack of support for this hypothesis. First, hostility as a response to separation may have been exaggerated by Bowlby (1973) and Hansburg (1972). Prior loss may not predispose an individual to react angrily to a new separation; in fact, a depressive reaction rather than an angry one may be anticipated. However, dismissing the importance of hostility as a key response, when its presence has been thoroughly documented (Bowlby 1973, Hansburg, 1972, and Wolfenstein, 1969) would be premature.

A second possible explanation of a methodological nature suggests that the hostility measure of the S.A.T. appears to lack discriminating power. A look at the S.A.T. shows that some of the situations depicted [the judge is placing the child in an institution] are of such an infuriating nature that most, if not all, subjects would respond hostilely; other situations are so benign [the mother has just put the child to bed] that an angry response is most unlikely. Hansburg developed this measure by differentiating between adolescents from intact families and those who were institutionalized [children disturbed and unhappy and not necessarily delinquent and also in foster homes and group residences] for delinquency. One would surmise that those [thus] institutionalized were extremely angry and therefore, often responded with hostility on the test. Within a functioning college population, such hostility, for the most part is either channeled or absent. Hence, the S.A.T. may adequately measure hostility differences only when comparing excessively angry and normally functioning individuals.

A third possible explanation allows for the importance of hostility as a response to separation when the separation is of a particular kind. When separation is forced upon a person, he will probably react angrily (Bowlby 1973); the S.A.T. depicts forced, involuntary separations [not all the pictures]. However, the subjects in the present study probably chose to separate at this time in their lives. Consequently, their separation was of a voluntary nature. As a result they may not have responded angrily to the test stimuli because the separation pictures differed significantly from their experiences. [This explanation is not tenable because the subjects reported "yes" to many of the pictures when they were asked if the depicted situations had ever happened to them.] More importantly, the subjects may not have been angry at their new separation because they initiated it.

Sherry seemed concerned that the father-absent subjects did not show more separation hostility than the intact-family subjects. Actually separation hostility may not be a characteristic of college freshmen who come from broken homes, and there may be more likelihood that intrapunitiveness and feelings of rejection (depressive syndrome) would be present as Sherry stated earlier. This would suggest that feelings of hostility were turned inward against the self.

Sherry continued:

The results of this study confirmed the hypothesis that father-absent subjects tend to a significant degree to select avoidant and defensive responses on the S.A.T. more than intact-family subjects. There were more withdrawal, fantasy and evasive responses in the records of the former than the latter. These findings were consistent with Rochlin's (1965) and Hansburg's (1972, 1980) suggestion that the reality of a new separation may be avoided more often by those who have experienced traumatic past separations. It would appear that the father-absent subjects reacted more readily with avoidant defenses and that minor separations are frequently reacted to as though they were major ones.

Defensive reactions of this sort have been found to be stimulated much more readily in persons who are anxiously attached. This was shown by the interesting relationship that Sherry found between symbiotic reactions and reality-avoidant responses. "Symbiotic behavior" (Hansburg 1972) refers to the simultaneous presence of strong attachment and weak individuation tendencies. The data showed that symbiotic father-absent subjects avoided the reality of separations more than symbiotic family-intact subjects. Father absence for a symbiotic subject appears to encourage a predisposition to deny the reality of a new separation. This finding is understandable when we consider the child's vulnerability to loss. Wolfenstein (1966), Cantalupo (1978) and Furman (1974) suggested that bereaved children established the denial of a loss as a major way of coping with the trauma. Wolfenstein viewed children as incapable of accepting the reality of a loss; along with Furman and Cantalupo, she believed that bereaved children are "arrested" in their development at the stage in which they were at the time of their parent's death. . . . In an effort to deny the reality of the loss, the child attempts to keep the parents alive by continuing to be the child associated with the alive parent. Thus, although father absence does not predispose more individuals to be symbiotic, it clearly encourages those who are symbiotic to be reality avoidant. A good example of this is Case #3, *Adolescent Separation Anxiety*, Vol. I, pp. 117–120.

The hypotheses concerned exclusively with reactions to separation as measured by the S.A.T. tended to be confirmed in this study. The hypotheses concerned with general anxiety as measured by the STAI were not supported. We may hypothesize that Spielberg's STAI and Hansburg's S.A.T. are tapping two different types of anxiety. [See Black, 1981.] The STAI measures general anxiety both transitory and stable but, nevertheless not specific to any particular anxiety-provoking situation. On the other hand, the S.A.T. measures reactions to anxiety exclusively related to separation experiences. The absence of a general anxiety and the presence of a more particular separation anxiety in father-absent subjects suggest that 1) prior father absence does not influence the susceptibility to general anxiety in these subjects, but 2) it does predispose them to react anxiously to possible separation experiences.

Numerous studies have not found a clear relationship between parental absence and subsequent personality difficulties. Some studies reported a positive relationship between these two variables; other studies were more equivocal. A factor in the contradictory findings may be related to how the psychopathology tapped the particular vulnerability to separations of the parentally absent subjects. The results of this study suggest that father-absent children will be no more anxious than those from intact families, but they will be more anxious [or more disturbed or avoidant] when experiencing a separation. Therefore, the degree of separation implied in an event may determine whether those exposed to prior loss react anxiously [with disorder].

There is another possible explanation that may account for the support of hypotheses tested with the S.A.T. and the lack of support for hypotheses tested with the STAI. The STAI is a self-report measure in which subjects can easily defend against their feelings; they may attempt to present themselves in a socially more favorable, less anxious light. The S.A.T. however, is projective in nature. Like most projective tests, the S.A.T. offers less opportunity to defend consciously against the expression of deeper anxieties. For the subjects there are no right or wrong answers on the S.A.T. Thus, the hypotheses with regard to the latter test were generally supported because the test elicits a less defended picture of the subject's internal reaction patterns to separation.

In general, then this study has suggested that individuals who had experienced prior life losses (in particular the absence of the father) may be predisposed to react with the various forms of separation distress to new separations. This seems to be most characteristic for those with father absence between the ages of 4 and 14. These individuals demonstrated more attachment seeking, less individuation and more reality avoidance upon going away to college than subjects from intact families.

REFERENCES

Bowlby, J. "The Adolf Meyer Lecture: Childhood Mourning and its Implications for Psychiatry." *American Psychiatry*, 1961, *118*, 481–498.

Bowlby, J. *Separation: Anxiety and Anger*. New York: Basic Books, 1973.

Cantalupo, P. "Psychological Problems and Parental Loss," *Science News*, January 14, 1978, *113*(2), 21.

Furman, E. *A Child's Parent Dies: Studies in Childhood Bereavement*. New Haven: Yale University Press, 1974.

Hansburg, H. G. *Adolescent Separation Anxiety*, Vol. I: *A Method for the Study of Adolescent Separation Problems*. Springfield, Ill.: Charles C. Thomas, 1972.

Hansburg, H. G. "Adolescent Separation Hostility: A Prelude to Violence," *Abstract Guide to XXth International Congress of Psychology*, Tokyo, 1972, p. 599.

Hansburg, H. G. "The Use of the Separation Anxiety Test in the Detection of Self-Destructive Tendencies in Early Adolescence," in D. V. Sankar (ed.), *Mental Health in Children*, Vol. III. New York: P. J. D. Publications, 1976.

Rochlin, G. "The Dread of Abandonment—A Contribution to the Etiology of the Loss Complex and to Depression," *Psychoanalytic Study of the Child*, 1961, *16*, 451–470.

Sherry, M. *Father Absence and Separation Anxiety Reactions in College Freshmen*. Doctoral dissertation, Michigan State University, 1980.

Spielberger, C. D., Gorsuch, R. L., and Lushene, R. E. *Manual for the State-Trait Anxiety Inventory*. Palo Alto, Cal.: Consulting Psychologist Press, 1970.

Wolfenstein, M. "Loss, Rage and Repetition." *Psychoanalytic Study of the Child*, 1969, *24*, 432–460.

11

Levitz's Study of Separation-Individuation and Intimacy in College Women

Working out of the University of Missouri, Dr. Ellen M. Levitz used the S.A.T. in a study in 1982, entitled "Separation-Individuation Resolution and Intimacy Capacity in College Women." The groups totaled eighty-nine college women within the age range of 18–25, most of whom were in their freshman year and aged 18 or 19. They were studied for attachment or detachment disorders in relation to their degree of intimacy as measured by the Orlofsky Intimacy Status Interview.

In this study Dr. Levitz was interested in determining the relationship between the capacity for intimacy in college women and the development and experience of separation-individuation—a term coined by Margaret Mahler in her work on early childhood development. Levitz states (p. 1): "Separation and intimacy are two ostensibly antithetical concepts. While the former considers the individual and his growth as an essentially singular, unique entity in the world, the latter concerns his need to establish emotional connections or bonds with other individuals. A number of theorists on love and intimacy, however, have emphasized the paradox that the capacity for mature love and intimacy in adulthood becomes possible only after an acceptance and coming to terms with one's separateness has been achieved (Bak, 1973; Bergmann, 1971; Boesky, 1980; Fromm, 1956; Kernberg, 1974). Particular emphasis has been placed on the separation involved in growing away from a state of symbiosis or oneness with the mothering figure and on the separation involved in growing up and relinquishing childhood attachments and dependencies."

With this in mind, Levitz decided to assess levels of intimacy of a group of 89 college women, the majority of whom were freshmen at the University of Missouri, and completed her study for her doctorate in 1982. She used the Intimacy Status Interview developed by Orlofsky et al. in 1973. Three major intimacy statuses were defined: (a) high intimacy characterized by open communication, mutuality, affection, caring and respect; (b) merger status indicated by high involvement to the point of enmeshment, dependency and possessiveness; and (c) low intimacy suggested by superficial relationships and a lack of openness or deep emotional involvement. To determine the characteristic Separation-Individuation patterns, Levitz used the S.A.T. Lastly, she administered the adapted, revised version of the Wallace Attachment History Questionnaire developed by DeLozier (1978) with some changes of her own.

Levitz was strongly influenced by Mahler's conceptual framework with regard to the development of the separation-individuation process. She described in considerable detail for eleven pages this developmental process as seen by Mahler in early infancy and childhood and quoted extensively from her works. Utilizing this theory as a foundation stone, she proceeded to discuss those psychological theorists who followed this sequence into adolescence, including Blos (1967), whom she also quoted at length, and Wolfenstein (1969) as well as Masterson (1968). The essential aspects of this theory devolve around the growth from the autistic level, through the phases of separation-individuation and the achievement of object constancy. This object constancy is continuously challenged by childhood and later experiences, especially during adolescence, which Blos characterized as the second individuation process.

Levitz gives much attention to how the conceptual formulations of Erikson (1968), Blos (1967) and Jacobson (1964) apply to the problem of ego ideals, identity formation and individuation. Much emphasis is given to psychoanalytic explanations of these developmental problems and the reasons for growth failures. Levitz states:

In conclusion, psychoanalytic theorists perceive adolescent individuation as a complex, intrapsychic process, involving the capacity to gradually separate and mourn the loss of infantile attachments, wishes and supports and accompanied by a reorganization of the psychic structure based largely on new identifications with independent, responsible and sexually active adults. This process, however, may be prolonged, sidestepped or aborted in individuals lacking the ego strength to intrapsychically separate from infantile dependencies and securities. The final relinquishment of childhood attachments and the attainment of psychic independence have been emphasized as a prerequisite for the capacity to invest in new intimate relationships on an adult level.

Levitz then launches into a discussion of the separation process and its assessment, which she considers crucial to her study. She states:

By the time an individual reaches young adulthood, he has, in theory, achieved some degree of resolution of his own separateness and autonomy. Degree of separateness achieved, however, is a difficult concept to measure empirically, particularly beyond the earliest years of life. Such information is usually obtained from clinical impressions via interviews, projective techniques and course of psychotherapy or from observations of the mourning course undertaken by bereaved individuals.

Levitz presents an extensive description and analysis of the Separation Anxiety Test and some of the research that had been conducted with the instrument. The results of her examination of the data that were available to her brought her to the conclusion that the Separation Anxiety Test was a—

. . . sensitive and valid measure of an individual's reactions to separation experiences. In particular, it has been able to differentiate groups of individuals with pathology suggestive of unresolved attachment-separation issues from normal controls.

On the question of intimacy Levitz states:

The establishment of relatively enduring intimate relationships and commitment to a heterosexual love relationship is generally regarded as one of the major tasks of young adulthood. Erikson (1959, 1963), for example, stresses that the core psycho-social conflict which follows the adolescent crisis of identity vs. identity diffusion is that of intimacy vs. isolation. According to him, following the attainment of ego identity, the young adult seeks to fuse as well as counterpoint his identity with those of others (1968). . . . Erikson defines intimacy as "the capacity to commit (oneself) to concrete affiliations and partnerships and to develop the ethical strength to abide by such commitments even though they may call for significant sacrifices and compromises" (1963, p. 293). He further describes the intimate relationship as involving repeated openness, sharing, responsibility and a mutual trust. Erikson stresses that intimacy or "true engagement with others is the result and test of firm self-delineation" (1959, p. 124). True intimacy thus calls for a strong sense of self—capable of self-abandon and experiences approximating fusion without fear of boundary or ego loss. The individual lacking a firm sense of separateness or identity will find the fusion-like experiences of intimacy frightening rather than gratifying, since fusion and closeness become associated with the loss of identity (Erikson, 1959).

Levitz points out that other writers extended and further delineated Erikson's concepts and these may be classified as "adult, equal, mature or genital and those which may be classified as immature, narcissistic, symbiotic or pre-genital (Altmann, 1977, Fromm, 1956, Goldberg, 1972 and Sager, 1977)." Levitz indicates that:

. . . a salient theme running through the literature on love and intimacy is that to achieve mature intimacy, two individuals must have resolved their own separateness. Along with resolution of separateness comes an ability to perceive and accept the partner's real qualities and limitations (Modell, 1968). Correspondingly, there is less of a need to project qualities onto the partner which stem from unresolved developmental struggles with objects of the past. Closeness and commitment can be sought and enjoyed, since they pose no threat to autonomy. Likewise, mutual growth as separate individuals within and outside the partnership can be furthered, since such growth does not awaken overwhelming fears of loss and abandonment.

Turning to the assessment of intimacy, Levitz studied a variety of instruments (Yufit, 1956, Rubin, 1970 and Driscoll, et al., 1972) and finally settled on Orlofsky, et al. (1973). This classification system extended and elaborated upon Erikson's polar concepts of intimacy and isolation and included a broader range of intimacy resolutions. This semi-structured interview which was scored according to three major criteria, defined five intimacy statuses—intimate, preintimate, stereotyped, pseudointimate and isolate. Levitz provides a brief description of these statuses as follows:

The intimate individual forms deep relationships with male and female friends and is involved in an enduring, committed heterosexual relationship. The preintimate also forms deep and close relationships with friends; however, she is ambivalent about heterosexual commitment. The stereotyped individual typically maintains many relationships; however, they are superficial and lacking in closeness. The pseudointimate, like the stereotyped individual, forms relationships which lack depth; however, unlike the stereotype, the pseudointimate has entered into a heterosexual commitment. This relationship, too, is lacking in closeness or depth. The isolate is either completely or nearly completely withdrawn from social situations and relationships with peers (Orlofsky, et al., 1973.)

A long discussion of the various researches with the Orlofsky Intimacy Status Interview is followed by an attempt to define how women develop identity and intimacy capacity. She concluded that an investigation of women's reactions to separation and loss, an interpersonal issue, may be a more fruitful means of understanding their capacity for intimacy. She therefore hypothesized:

. . . that women in the lower intimacy statuses (isolate, pseudointimate and stereotype) and women in the enmeshed intimacy statuses (merger uncommitted and merger committed) would present significantly more patterns indicative of separation disorders than women in the higher intimacy statuses (intimate and preintimate). More specifically, women in the lower intimacy status groups were expected to produce S.A.T. profiles suggestive of excessive self-sufficiency or detachment (i.e., low attachment need and high individuation capacity on strong pictures as well as low emotional turmoil and high defensiveness).
Women in the enmeshed intimacy groups, on the other hand, were expected to produce S.A.T. profiles suggestive of symbiotic trends or excessively high anxious attachment (i.e., high attachment need and low individuation capacity on mild pictures as well as high emotional turmoil, defensiveness and self-love loss). Finally women in the higher intimacy status groups were expected to demonstrate healthy or intact profiles (i.e., low attachment need and high individuation capacity on mild pictures as well as the reverse pattern on strong pictures, moderate defensiveness and emotional turmoil and adequate self-love).

Not to neglect Bowlby's attachment theory (1969 and 1973), Levitz describes the formulations involved and indicates why she therefore utilized DeLozier's Attachment History Questionnaire (1978) in her study. The purpose of adding this instrument to her examining schedule was to "determine the presence or absence of actual disruptions of early attachment bonds as well as the nature of internalized representations of attachment figures." After describing the differences between Bowlby's theory and the usual psychoanalytic approach to the problems of attachment and separation, she discusses Bowlby's concept of anxious attachment and its converse, compulsive self-reliance and detachment. She emphasizes Bowlby's concept of exposure to pathogenic patterns of parenting which result in various forms of anxious attachment. The mother's lack of sensitivity produces in the child an uncertainty that an attachment figure will be accessible when needed. This may lead to a constant state of anxious attachment or to eventual detachment and pseudo-independence. Levitz refers to Bowlby's postulate that a strong etiological relationship exists between the child's attachment experiences with his parents and his later capacity for intimacy.

Utilizing the three instruments and the theoretical formulations noted above, Levitz developed two hypotheses and their corollaries for her study. The first hypothesis stated that women in the low intimacy status group (isolate, stereotype and pseudointimate groups combined) and women in the merger status groups (merger committed and merger uncommitted groups combined) would demonstrate more disorders of separation-individuation, as compared with women in the high intimacy status groups (intimate and preintimate groups combined), as measured by the individual subscales of the S.A.T. The second hypothesis stated that women in the low intimacy status group and women in the merger status group would report more indicators of early inadequate attachment, as measured by the attachment questionnaire, than women in the high intimacy group. Attention will be given largely to the data on the first hypothesis since that is most pertinent to the theme of this volume.

The 89 undergraduate college women of this study ranged in age from 18–25 with the majority being 18- and 19-year-olds in their freshman year. The majority (83%) were white and of parents who on the average had completed high school and some college. Nearly all of the women (94%) were planning some kind of career, and a large percentage (83%) intended to marry and work. According to several demographic tables in her study, Levitz did not find any significant differences between the intimacy groups as measured by the Orlofsky Interview with regard to background material. Of the 89 young women 17 were classified as high in intimacy status, 52 as of merger status and 20 in the low intimacy group. Levitz then arranged the scores on eight scales of the S.A.T. (mild attachment, strong attachment, mild individuation, strong individuation, painful tension, hostility, defensiveness and self-love loss) with their means for the three intimacy groups.

The relationship between intimacy status and reactions to separation and loss was then analyzed using multivariate analysis of variance (MANOVA). An alpha level of .10 was set as the level of significance in order to avoid overlooking any significant univariate effects. The MANOVA reached significance, F (16, 158) = 1.54, $p5.10$, by the Wilkes Criterion. The results of the univariate analyses of variance and mean comparisons utilizing Duncan's multiple range test for each dependent variable included in this MANOVA are summarized in Table 11.1.

The data in Table 11.1 demonstrated that the individuation mean score on the mild pictures was significantly greater for the high intimacy group than for either the merger or low intimacy groups. At the same time the merger and low intimacy groups showed a significantly higher level of separation defensiveness. While there is no significantly greater self-love loss in the merger and low intimacy groups, there is a definite trend in that direction.

Three post-hoc analyses were carried out with the S.A.T. on the

Table 11.1

ANALYSIS OF VARIANCE AND MEAN COMPARISONS[a] OF
SEPARATION ANXIETY TEST SUBSCALES FOR INTIMACY STATUS

| S.A.T. Subscales | Row | Intimacy Status | | | F (2, 86) |
		High (N = 17)	Merger (N = 52)	Low (N = 20)	
Attachment (Mild)	1	6.00	7.75	7.50	2.13
Attachment (Strong)	2	18.58	17.33	18.85	1.30
Individuation (Mild)	3	13.52	9.00	9.40	4.35[b]
Individuation (Strong)	4	4.58	3.62	4.35	.81
Painful Tension	5	23.12	21.67	21.95	.49
Hostility	6	14.41	16.04	13.90	1.41
Defensiveness	7	11.59	14.71	14.85	3.23[c]
Self-Love Loss	8	8.82	11.00	11.00	1.82

[a]Means in rows 1, 2, 4, 5, 6 and 8 do not differ significantly from one another at the .05 level of confidence by Duncan's multiple range test.

[b]$p < .02$.

[c]$p < .05$.

basis of the results described above. The first of these analyses tested for interstatus differences on attachment need and individuation capacity for mild pictures. Any deviations from the expected pattern of high individuation capacity and low attachment need on mild pictures is suggestive of a symbiotic separation disorder (Hansburg, 1976). A 3 × 2 repeated measures analysis of variance with one between subjects factor (intimacy status) and one with subjects factor (attachment need and individuation capacity for mild pictures) revealed a significant interaction effect, F (1, 86) = 4.71, $p < .02$ (see Table 11.2). Mean comparisons utilizing Scheffe's post-hoc analysis of cell means revealed that only the high intimacy group demonstrated a significantly greater individuation capacity than attachment need on mild pictures, F (1, 86) = 24.14, $p < .01$. No significant differences between these patterns were found for the merger, F (1, 86) = .67, $p > .05$, or low intimacy group, F (1, 86) = 1.54, $p > .05$.

A repeated measures design was also utilized to test for group differences on self-love loss and self-esteem preoccupation. Additional information concerning self-regard may be obtained when the self-love loss pattern is examined in relation to the self-esteem pattern (Hansburg 1976). When self-love loss exceeds self-esteem preoccupation, a depressive trend in the personality may be indicated. A 3 × 2 repeated measures analysis of variance with one between subjects factor (intimacy status) and one within subjects factor (self-love loss and self-esteem preoccupation) revealed a significant interaction effect, F (1, 86) = 3.28, $p < .05$ (see Table 11.3). A Scheffe test applied to the group means indicated that whereas the merger group, F (1, 86) = 14.3, $p < .01$, demonstrated significantly greater levels of self-love loss than self-esteem preoccupation, no significant differences were found for the high intimacy group, F (1, 86) = .26, $p > .05$.

Table 11.2

MEAN ATTACHMENT AND INDIVIDUATION SCORES
FOR MILD PICTURES BY INTIMACY STATUS

	Intimacy Status		
	High (N = 17)	Merger (N = 52)	Low (N = 20)
Attachment (Mild)	6.00 (3.76)	7.75 (3.00)	7.50 (2.48)
Individuation (Mild)	13.53 (5.26)	9.00 (4.94)	9.40 (7.23)

Note: Numbers in parentheses indicate standard deviations.

In the final post-hoc analysis, individual protocols were scored for the presence of patterns indicating anxious attachment. Five S.A.T. patterns can be delineated which are indicative of anxious attachment in adults (Hansburg 1976). When all five patterns are present, severe anxious attachment may be posited. The presence of three to four patterns is indicative of strong anxious attachment, and the presence of one to two patterns signifies mild anxious attachment. The five anxious attachment patterns are as follows:

1. high attachment need (greater than 25%) accompanied by low individuation capacity (less than 16%),
2. attachment need on mild pictures greater than or equal to individuation capacity on mild pictures,
3. high hostility and/or painful tension percentages (greater than 30%),
4. strong reality avoidance or defensiveness (greater than 13%),
5. stronger levels of self-love loss (greater than 8%) and greater than self-esteem preoccupation.

Using chi-square (see Table 11.4), group differences for the presence of the various types of anxious attachment were tested for.

The significant chi-square indicated that whereas the high intimacy group was most accurately categorized as exhibiting mild anxious attachment (only two subjects indicated no anxious attachment), women in the merger and low intimacy groups were most likely to exhibit strong or severe anxious attachment. Whereas less than

Table 11.3

MEAN SELF-LOVE LOSS AND SELF-ESTEEM PREOCCUPATION
SCORES BY INTIMACY STATUS

	Intimacy Status		
	High (N = 17)	Merger (N = 52)	Low (N = 20)
Self-Love Loss	8.82 (4.30)	11.00 (4.27)	11.00 (4.04)
Self-Esteem Preoccupation	8.18 (4.25)	6.23 (3.25)	5.95 (3.49)

Note: Numbers in parentheses indicate standard deviations.

30% of the women in the high intimacy group demonstrated 3 or more anxious attachment patterns, 60% of the women in the low intimacy group and 69% of the women in the merger group did.

In her discussion of this data, Levitz pointed out that the women in the high intimacy group were definitively differentiated from the women in both merger and low intimacy groups on a number of facets of the S.A.T. She stated that there were more disorders of the separation-individuation process among the low intimacy and merger groups of women. The results suggested that the latter groups of women exhibited a lower capacity for self-reliance, a greater need to defend against the impact of separation and a greater trend toward (separation) depression than the women classified in the high intimacy group.

Inspection of individual S.A.T. protocols for the presence of patterns reflecting anxious attachment revealed that the majority of women in the merger and low intimacy groups demonstrated strong or severe anxious attachment. Referring to my study (1976), she indicated that although mild anxious attachment was included in separation disorders, she understood that this "disorder" was not a negative condition but rather a normative and adaptive reaction in threatened separations or loss. However, both strong and severe anxious attachment are pathological conditions.

According to Hansburg (1976) strong to severe anxious attachment is indicative of increasing degrees of a symbiotic separation disorder and reflect the individual's uncertainty that an attachment figure can be relied upon to be available when needed. Hansburg (1976) further maintains that the presence

Table 11.4

NUMBER OF SUBJECTS IN EACH INTIMACY STATUS GROUP DEMONSTRATING NO
OR MILD AND STRONG OR SEVERE ANXIOUS ATTACHMENT[a]

Anxious Attachment	Intimacy Status		
	High ($N = 17$)	Merger ($N = 52$)	Low ($N = 20$)
None or Mild	12	16	8
Strong or Severe	5	36	12

[a] χ^2 (2) = 8.4, $p < .02$.

of severe anxious attachment is indicative of a strong unconscious wish to feel completely merged with an attachment figure.

The data from the current study therefore, suggest that women in the merger and low intimacy groups are struggling to a greater extent with unresolved attachment or symbiotic needs. . . .

The high intimacy group showed three significant differentiating factors from the other groups: (a) stronger individuation reactions, (b) lower separation defensiveness, and (c) a lower level of the depressive syndrome. These three are discussed at length by Levitz, who stated as follows:

It thus appears that while all groups experience a similar degree of longing for contact and closeness with an attachment figure, only for high intimacy women is this need balanced by a strong drive toward autonomy and pleasure in independent functioning . . . women in the merger and low intimacy groups may be suffering from deficits in ego functioning and thus have a greater need to rely on the presence of a primary attachment figure to maintain feelings of well-being . . . adolescent individuation may be less successful for these groups. The disengagement from parental involvement and dependency may expose considerable ego impoverishment and feelings of emptiness and loss.

With regard to the results on defensiveness Levitz suggests that:

. . . separation and loss are highly threatening to the egos of women in the merger and low intimacy groups and they have a greater need to avoid facing separation experiences . . . (and) reflects some difficulty (in) accepting the reality that objects are separate and can be lost (Modell, 1968). Acceptance of this reality is an important outcome of the adolescent individuation process and a fundamental component of a true sense of autonomy.

With reference to the depressive trend which appeared so much stronger in the merger and low intimacy groups, Levitz has this to say:

According to Hansburg (1972, 1976), a higher level of self-love loss than self-esteem preoccupation on the S.A.T. . . . points to a depressive trend in the personality. In comparison studies between healthy and disturbed adolescents, Hansburg (1972, 1976) found healthier youngsters to have greater concerns with self-esteem than disturbed youngsters, who had higher levels of self-love loss than healthier youngsters. Whereas the self-love loss pattern reflects concerns with feeling rejected, uncared about and unwanted . . . the self-esteem pattern reflects concern over . . . feelings of competence in what one does. Hansburg (1976) maintains that feeling unwanted and unloved in a separation experience reflects an earlier and more profound disturbance of the personality than concern over loss of competency and effectiveness.

Levitz is of the opinion that greater capacity for intimacy is related to a stronger internal object constancy, a notion which she derives from Mahler's theory of separation-individuation. The fact that those with lower intimacy ratings show stronger tendencies to feel unwanted and uncared for than those with higher intimacy ratings reflects a greater need for the external object. While Levitz does not refer to Piaget's concept of object permanence, this theory may well have relevance. Further, it accords with Bowlby's theory of the firm feeling of the accessibility and/or availability of the object (usually maternal) even when not in sight. Thus, the achievement of a higher level of intimacy becomes to some degree dependent on this inner feeling of security derived from having experienced a fairly constant available and accessible object (usually maternal).

Levitz was concerned that she was unable to find differences on the S.A.T. between the merger and the low intimacy groups; she states:

This finding, although contrary to prediction, is not entirely surprising. Although the two groups demonstrated contrasting relationship styles, these styles may actually reflect "two sides of the same coin" or two different solutions to a similar dynamic problem . . . [however] further research is needed to determine why [these different styles do not react differently to projective studies of separation].

In a final comment, Levitz notes the following: " . . . the current study does point to the usefulness of the Separation Anxiety Test as a research instrument for non-clinical populations."

REFERENCES

Altmann, L. "Some Vicissitudes of Love." *Journal of the American Psychoanalytic Association*, 1977, 25, 25–52.

Bak, R. C. "Being in Love and Object Loss." *International Journal of Psychoanalysis*, 1973, 54(1), 1–8.

Bergmann, M. S. "Psychoanalytic Observations on the Capacity to Love," in J. B. McDevitt and C. F. Settlage (eds.), *Separation-Individuation: Essays in Honor of Margaret S. Mahler*. New York: International Universities Press, 1971.

Blos, P. "The Second Individuation Process of Adolescence." *Psychoanalytic Study of the Child*, 1967, 22, 162–186.

Boesky, D. "Introduction of Symposium on Object Relations Theory and Love." *Psychoanalytic Quarterly*, 1980, *49*, 48–55.

Bowlby, J. *Attachment and Loss*, Vol. I: *Attachment*. New York: Basic Books, 1969.

Bowlby, J. *Attachment and Loss*, Vol. II: *Separation: Anxiety and Anger*. New York: Basic Books, 1973.

Bowlby, J. "Attachment Theory, Separation Anxiety, and Mourning," in *American Handbook of Psychiatry* (2nd ed.), Vol. VI. New York: Basic Books, 1975.

DeLozier, P. P. *An Application of Attachment Theory to the Study of Child Abuse*. Unpublished doctoral dissertation, California School of Professional Psychology, Los Angeles, 1979.

Driscoll, R., Davis, K. B., and Lipetz, M. E. "Parental Interference and Romantic Love: The Romeo and Juliet Effect." *Journal of Personality and Social Psychology*, 1972, *24*, 1–10.

Erikson, E. "Identity and the Life Cycle." *Psychological Issues*, 1959, *1*, 1–171.

Erikson, E. *Childhood and Society* (2nd ed.). New York: Norton, 1963.

Erikson, E. *Identity: Youth and Crisis*. New York: Norton, 1968.

Fromm, E. *The Art of Loving*. New York: Harper and Row, 1956.

Goldberg, A. "On the Incapacity to Love." *AMA Archives of General Psychiatry*, 1972, *26*(1), 3–7.

Hansburg, H. G. *Adolescent Separation Anxiety*, Vol. I: *A Method for the Study of Adolescent Separation Problems*. Springfield, Ill.: Charles C. Thomas, 1972. Reprinted, Melbourne, Fla.: R. E. Krieger, 1980.

Hansburg, H. G. *Adolescent Separation Anxiety*, Vol. II: *Separation Disorders: A Manual for the Interpretation of Emotional Disorders Manifested by the Separation Anxiety Test*. Melbourne, Fla.: R. E. Krieger, 1980.

Hansburg, H. G. "The Use of the Separation Anxiety Test in the Detection of Self-Destructive Tendencies in Early Adolescence," in D.V. Siva Sankar (ed.), *Mental Health in Children*, Vol. III. New York: P. J. D. Publications, 1976.

Hansburg, H. G. *"Separation Disorders of the Elderly,"* unpublished study, 1978 (Now published in this book).

Jacobson, E. *The Self and the Object World*. New York: International Universities Press, 1964.

Kernberg, O. "Mature Love: Prerequisites and Characteristics." *Journal of the American Psychoanalytic Association*, 1974, *22*, 743–768.

Levitz, E. M. *Separation-Individuation Resolution and Intimacy Capacity in College Women.* Unpublished doctoral dissertation, University of Missouri, 1982.

Levitz-Jones, E. M., and Orlofsky, J. L. "Separation-Individuation and Intimacy Capacity in College Women," *Journal of Personality and Social Psychology*, 1985, 49, 156–169.

Mahler, M. S. "On Child Psychosis and Schizophrenia: Autistic and Symbiotic Infantile Psychosis." *Psychoanalytic Study of the Child*, 1952, 7, 286–305.

Mahler, M. S. "Thoughts about Development and Individuation." *Psychoanalytic Study of the Child*, 1963, *18*, 307–324.

Mahler, M. S., Pine, F., and Bergman, A. "The Mother's Reaction to Her Toddler's Drive toward Individuation," in E. J. Anthony and T. Benedek (eds.), *Parenthood: Its Psychology and Psychopathology.* Boston: Little, Brown, 1970.

Mahler, M. S., Pine, F., and Bergman, A. *The Psychological Birth of the Human Infant: Symbiosis and Individuation.* New York: Basic Books, 1975.

Masterson, J. "The Psychiatric Significance of Adolescent Turmoil." *American Journal of Psychiatry*, 1968, *124*(11), 107–112.

Modell, A. H. *Object Love and Reality.* New York: International Universities Press, 1968.

Orlofsky, J. L., Marcia, J. E., and Lesser, I. "Ego Identity Status and the Intimacy vs. Isolation Crisis of Young Adulthood." *Journal of Personality and Social Psychology*, 1973, 27(2), 211–219.

Rubin, Z. "Measurement of Romantic Love." *Journal of Personality and Social Psychology*, 1970, *16*, 265–273.

Sager, C. J. "A Typology of Intimate Relationships." *Journal of Sex and Marital Therapy*, 1977, *3*(2), 83–112.

Wallace, A. *An Application of Attachment Theory to the Study of Divorced People.* Unpublished doctoral dissertation, Los Angeles, California School of Professional Psychology, 1977.

Wolfenstein, M. "Loss, Rage and Repetition." *Psychoanalytic Study of the Child*, 1969, *24*, 432–460.

Yufit, R. *Intimacy and Isolation: Some Behavioral and Psychodynamic Correlates.* Unpublished doctoral dissertation, University of Chicago, 1956.

12

Schwartz's Study of Attachment/Separation and the Fear of Death

Dr. Pauline K. Schwartz obtained the cooperation of seventy-two students at a California university to study the fear of death. Her study, entitled "Attachment-Separation and the Fear of Death," was completed at the California School of Professional Psychology in 1980. She compared students' reactions on the S.A.T., the Attachment History Questionnaire (CSPP-LA), the Death Anxiety Scale, and a Word Association Test.

The fear of death is a phenomenon present in persons of all ages, persuasions, cultural levels and national groups. It is so pervasive that criminals use it to deprive others of their rights, material goods and dignity. The threat of death moves people to abandon their homes or their country. It shocks men and women into seeking medical aid, to search for dietary and physical care and to protect their young. It moves people into religious cults, to pray for salvation and to search for some final philosophical solution. The debacles and catastrophes of natural events including earthquakes, hurricanes, tidal waves and lightning storms cause people to seek shelter from the potential death that could readily engulf them. Our sciences are devoted to the pursuit of methods to extend life and to avoid death. Our concern with death is of such magnitude that in recent years psychologists have been giving considerable attention to the psychological problems surrounding it. The study presented here is another in the long series of examinations of the problem with special reference to the use of the Separation Anxiety Test.

Schwartz undertook this study to investigate the extent to which early attachment bonds and separation experiences contribute to the development of the fear of death. She conceived that factors, such as the loss of a caretaker due to illness in early attachment formation, separation between parents, divorce, death, parental inaccessibility and threats of abandonment, would be of significance in creating fears of death. The study was not intended as a treatise on death but rather as an extension of attachment theory (Bowlby, 1969).

To study this question Schwartz decided to examine a sizable group of adults in terms of their early attachment history, their current death anxiety, their patterns of reaction to separation experiences and their word associations. Toward this end she selected four psychological instruments: (a) the CSPP-LA Attachment-Separation History Questionnaire, (b) The S.A.T., (c) The Death Anxiety Scale, and (d) a Word Association Test.

A word of explanation should be given with regard to the selection of the two tests, the Death Anxiety Scale and the Word Association Test. Schwartz was concerned about the self-report on a conscious level of the DAS. Individuals are often moved to be defensive and to put their best foot forward. Thus, deeper reactions are often covered in such a way as to be incompletely revealing. It was Schwartz's reasoning that a test which would reach unconscious processes would reveal feelings which were not available on the DAS. For this purpose a word association test was chosen. As will be noted in the results, this reasoning proved to be meaningful.

Along the lines of attachment theory she adopted the following hypotheses:

1. that there is a significant relationship between distressing childhood separation experiences and the fear of death,
2. that a similar relationship exists between the fear of death and the experience of inaccessibility of the major caretaker (in most cases the mother),
3. that repeated childhood abandonments and threats of such abandonment are correlated with the fear of death, and
4. that the intensity of the fear of death is related to dis-

ordered patterns of separation anxiety (anxious attachment or detachment).

The author obtained the cooperation of 72 college students from a
number of psychology classes at a university. With half of the group
consisting of females and half males, she found ages ranged from 18 to
33 and their educational levels from the first to the fourth year of undergraduate work. After satisfying herself that the demographic data
obtained from the students were within the range of typical men and
women born in the United States and eliminating those who were not
adequately representative, Schwartz administered all four instruments
in random order to eliminate the possible bias of order of test administration. (The difference in this reasoning from that of DeLozier
(1979), Kelly (1981) and Mitchell (1980) with regard to a fixed order of
administration is quite striking. Refer to Kelly's paper for a discussion.)

The following description of the statistical procedures is provided
by Schwartz:

A "Frequencies" Subroutine of the SPSS program was used to determine the
basic descriptive characteristic of each of the variables. Pearson product
moment correlation coefficients were derived using the "Pearson Corr"
subroutine of the SPSS program. These correlations were performed to ascertain the strength of the relationships between each predictor variable and the
scores for the fear of death as measured by the Death Anxiety Scale and the
Word Association Test. Correlation indices were used because they are more
suited to non-continuous data.

To further describe relationships among variables, chi-square analyses
were conducted using the "Cross tabs" subroutine of the SPSS program. An
analysis of variance was employed using the "ANOVA" subroutine of the SPSS
program to determine the relationships between the percentages of total
responses from the complete protocol of the Separation Anxiety Test, and the
scores from the fear of death as measured by the Death Anxiety Scale and the
Word Association Test.

(For those who are not familiar with the statistical procedures
mentioned herein, it would be well to consult a standard statistical
manual describing the methods or to examine the original manuscript
of the study.)

I omit the results and conclusions with regard to the Attachment
History Questionnaire and its relationship to the Death Anxiety Scale
and the Word Association Test and confine the discussion to the
relationship of the SAT results and the DAS and WAT; those who wish

to acquaint themselves with the entire study are referred to the original dissertation. What Schwartz noted first was the significant relationship between the degree of fear of death and the higher level of the individuation percentage. Table 12.1 presents these findings.

The pattern of individuation consists of three responses—adaptation, well-being and sublimation. To refer strongly to this pattern represents a form of self-sufficiency especially when the attachment pattern is low. To correlate highly with scores on death anxiety on a conscious level in young people of the age level selected by Schwartz, would suggest an excessively self-sufficient attitude toward the possibility of dying.

Schwartz stated the following in connection with this result:

The further an individual passes beyond childhood, continuing on a developmental path characterized by extreme self-sufficiency and detachment, the more likely he will be cut off from strong affective expression of joy, love, emotional security, anger, grief, sadness and fear because these emotions are aroused primarily through activation and active functioning of his attachment system. As such, he can displace defensively, excluded affects of fear and anxiety onto death, which our culture, folklore and conventional wisdom view as the absence of all human contact. Therefore, within this context, if death comes to be perceived by an individual as a total and ultimate separation from life, then a significant relationship between an excessive level of individuation and the fear of death would be expected.

The results suggested that higher levels of self-sufficiency in the face of separation are not correlated with a fuller acceptance of death, as one might derive from personal observations. This result does seem contrary to what we expect from self-sufficient persons in daily life.

When Schwartz studied the relationship between DAS scores and the attachment (loneliness, feeling of rejection and empathy—

Table 12.1

ANALYSIS OF VARIANCE FOR THE INDIVIDUATION
RESPONSE PATTERN AND THE DAS MEASURE

Source of Variation	Sum of Squares	D.F.	Mean Square	F	P Level
Main Effect					
DAS	1.417	2	0.709	2.912	.05
Error	16.548	68	0.243		

reactions to separation which indicate the intensity of attachment need) pattern, she did not find a significant correlation, but the results were in the predicted direction. No explanation is offered for this result, although later material suggests ambivalence as more importantly related.

On the other hand, Schwartz's data on the hostility (anger, projection and intrapunitiveness) pattern indicates a significant relationship with the fear of death on a conscious level. Table 12.2 presents the findings on this pattern as related to the DAS scale.

Hostility on the SAT is viewed as a response to deal with threat or fear of painful effects and in various forms will be expressed during and after separation experiences (Hansburg 1972). When the emotional conflict arises and intensified feelings of anxiety and anger increase without mitigation by responsiveness from an attachment figure, hostility overrides painful tension and eventually weakens the attachment bond. However, the anxiety and hostility do not dissipate. They continue to be active in the personality, often becoming repressed or displaced elsewhere. Hence, when these feelings are unable to be directly expressed, they begin to influence behavior in disturbing ways (Bowlby, 1973, 1975). Therefore, in light of these considerations, if the fear of death is perceived of as an outcome of separation experiences that involve threat or fear of pain, then the significant relationship between the heightened level of hostility and the DAS can be considered as a confirmation of these variables.

Along the lines of Schwartz's reasoning, the DAS did not correlate with the fear-anxiety-pain pattern on the S.A.T. As noted previously, Schwartz points out that the DAS is a measure of the conscious awareness of the fear of death. However, the fear-anxiety-pain system showed a definite relationship with the fear of death when it was

Table 12.2

ANALYSIS OF VARIANCE FOR THE HOSTILITY
RESPONSE PATTERN AND THE DAS MEASURE

Source of Variation	Sum of Squares	D.F.	Mean Square	F	P Level
Main Effect					
DAS	1.488	2	0.744	3.109	.05
Error	16.512	69	0.239		

correlated with the scores on the WAT which gave a measure of the unconscious fear of death. Table 12.3 presents these results.

It is apparent that while hostility was more consciously related to
death anxiety, the fear-anxiety-pain system (separation pain or painful
tension) was definitely related to death fears which are on a more unconscious level. How does Schwartz explain this? She states:

Separation from an attachment figure when the ego is not developed enough to
tolerate degrees of painful tension within limits, must eventually create pain
that can result in either bodily manifestations, intrapsychic conflict or both.
Although tolerance of a somewhat stronger painful tension level is considered
evidence of better health and adjustment, prolonged excessive painful tension
. . . can . . . be transferred into hostility (Hansburg, 1972).

These data strongly suggest that unconscious awareness of the fear of
death is more related to the fear-anxiety-pain system while on a conscious level it is more related to hostility.

Schwartz then raises the issue of the reality avoidance pattern or
what may be referred to as the defensive system—the system of
avoidance. Here the data which she presents suggest a relationship to
the unconscious reactions to death fear. The data follow in Table 12.4.

Schwartz's explanation for this result is as follows:

There are times when the ego is not sufficiently ready for the realities of
separation, hostility and painful tension. When pain is too overwhelming and
hostility unacceptable, the ego can avoid the impact of the reality of a
separation experience by using such maneuvers as withdrawal, evasion and
fantasy (denial). These three reactions are combined on the S.A.T. to form an
index for the avoidance of reality or defensive exclusion (Hansburg, 1972;
Bowlby, 1980). Until recently, death in America has been one of avoidance

Table 12.3

ANALYSIS OF VARIANCE FOR THE PAINFUL TENSION
RESPONSE PATTERN AND THE WAT MEASURE

Source of Variation	Sum of Squares	D.F.	Mean Square	F	P Level
Main Effect					
WAT Measure	2.910	2	1.455	3.229	.05
Error	31.090	69	0.451		

and denial. However, ultimately we all must face the reality that some day we will die (Feifel, 1959; Kubler-Ross, 1969). Therefore, in light of this evidence if death is commonly feared by those who respond to separation experiences by avoiding the reality of separations, then the significant relationship demonstrated between an elevated level (percentage) of reality avoidance and the WAT can be considered as a confirmation.

Schwartz thought that the unconscious fear of death demonstrated on the WAT should be more related to defensive reactions and, therefore, did not show on the DAS, which is more productive of conscious anxiety.

On the other hand, the identity stress percentage showed a significant and positive relationship to the self-reported and consciously felt anxiety of the DAS. Table 12.5 presents the data. That death anxiety on a conscious level should be related to identity stress seems logical if death itself represents the loss of identity. Those persons who have the greatest death anxiety would be much more likely to feel the threat of the loss of the identity of the self in many types of separation experiences. In these data we have a simple proof of this hypothesis. In passing, it is of interest that elderly persons who are close to death and confined to a hospital should show very high percentages of identity stress responses on the S.A.T., as was seen in my study of the elderly (see Chapter 18).

In studying the categories ranging from severe anxious attachment to detachment, Schwartz made some interesting observations about her data with regard to the DAS and WAT. After an analysis of the S.A.T. protocols, she found that those subjects who obtained high death anxiety scores showed classified patterns of hostile-anxious attachment while subjects with low death anxiety scores demonstrated a

Table 12.4

ANALYSIS OF VARIANCE FOR THE REALITY
AVOIDANCE PATTERN AND THE WAT MEASURE

Source of Variation	Sum of Squares	D.F.	Mean Square	F	P Level
Main Effect					
WAT Measure	3.987	2	1.993	3.207	.05
Error	42.888	69	.622		

patterned separation disorder of excessive self-sufficiency. Subjects whose DAS scores were within the normal range showed response patterns of mild anxious attachment.

Schwartz does not explain the latter results, but they are worth examining. Hostile-anxious attachment was defined (*Adolescent Separation Anxiety*, Vol. II, pp. 17–19) as a pattern in which hostility dominated the affect and in which there is strong attachment present. I quote: "(it) refers mostly to youngsters whose attachment to their parents is not only filled with uncertainty but is also permeated by intense mutually provoking interactions." Ainsworth (1982, p. 7), in discussing such a pattern in very early childhood, states, ". . . using the strange situation procedure, most infants can be classified as securely (Group B) or anxiously attached to their mothers, and that the anxiously attached infants can be further classified as avoidant (Group A) or ambivalent (Group C)." She referred here to those anxiously attached infants who also alternate with avoidant behavior. This is quoted from Ainsworth (1972, p. 119):

"They seek to gain and maintain contact and they also resist it. They seek to be picked up by the mother, but then hit, kick or push away from her; if put down, they tend to resist release and struggle to gain contact again."

It would appear from Schwartz's data that persons with strong ambivalent reactions to attachment figures may have greater conscious fear of death than persons who are more securely attached.

The real question at this point is twofold: (a) is this reaction in infancy eventually found in adults in the manner in which it appears on the Separation Anxiety Test or is it manifested differently in the personality, and (b) is this one of the more likely origins of death

Table 12.5

ANALYSIS OF VARIANCE FOR THE IDENTITY STRESS
RESPONSE PATTERN AND THE DAS MEASURE

Source of Variation	Sum of Squares	D.F.	Mean Square	F	P Level
DAS	1.343	2	0.672	2.782	.05
Error	16.657	69	0.241		

anxiety—that is, the uncertainty and ambivalence with regard to the earliest attachment figure? It would appear from Schwarz's study that some such characteristic dominates those who have the greatest death anxiety.

In the study of the categories, the second result referred to those with low levels of death anxiety who tended to show excessive self-sufficiency. One would assume that those individuals who show little death anxiety would demonstrate a capacity to use their resources with a minimum of anxiety in other areas. The result fits the lower death anxiety levels of men or women who enter occupations in which there is a constant threat of death, such as policemen, firemen, soldiers, deep-sea divers, parachutists and the like. A study of persons in these occupations with both the DAS and the SAT would be of interest in order to corroborate this theory.

It was also of interest that Schwartz found medium scores on the DAS to be associated with mild anxious attachment. This result seems to accord with my study of mothers of young children (see Chapter 19), in which mild anxious attachment was seen to be typical for a considerable percentage of the population. It is presumed that moderate levels of anxious attachment not only are common in the general population but are a likely natural base for many kinds of anxiety, especially separation anxiety. Perhaps that is why it is associated with moderate degrees of death anxiety.

From this study it would appear that patterns of separation reaction derived from the S.A.T. may be predictive of the level of death anxiety. Perhaps, to restate this in another way, high levels of death anxiety are most characteristic of persons who show serious ambivalence and insecurity in their attachment to close persons. It suggests, further, that when severe hostility and anxiety are involved in a close attachment, the acceptance of death becomes a much more difficult task than when hostility is less in evidence.

Schwartz considered many hypotheses in this study and derived considerable data from other tests and questionnaires but it was not intended to discuss these in this short report. The readers are referred to the original study (Schwartz, 1980) for a fuller discussion of all the issues which she researched.

REFERENCES

Ainsworth, M. D. S. "Attachment Dependency: A Comparison," in J. L. Gewirtz (ed.), *Attachment and Dependency*. Washington, D.C.: Winston and Sons, 1972.

Ainsworth, M. D. S. "Attachment: Retrospect and Prospect," in C. M. Parkes and J. Stevenson-Hinde (eds.), *The Place of Attachment in Human Behavior*. New York: Basic Books, 1982.

Anthony, S. *The Child's Discovery of Death*. New York: Harcourt, Brace & Co., 1940.

Becker, E. *The Denial of Death*. New York: Free Press, 1973.

Boulding, K. *The Image*. Ann Arbor: University of Michigan Press, 1956.

Bowlby, J. "The Nature of the Child's Tie to His Mother." *International Journal of Psychoanalysis*, 1958, *39*, 350–373.

Bowlby, J. "Separation Anxiety." *International Journal of Psychoanalysis*, 1960, *41*, 89–113.

Bowlby, J. "Grief and Mourning in Infancy and Early Childhood." *Psychoanalytic Study of the Child*, 1960, *15*, 9–52.

Bowlby, J. *Attachment and Loss*, Vol. I: *Attachment*. New York: Basic Books, 1969.

Bowlby, J. *Attachment and Loss*, Vol. II: *Separation: Anxiety and Anger*. New York: Basic Books, 1973.

Bowlby, J. *Attachment and Loss*, Vol. III: *Loss, Sadness and Depression*. New York: Basic Books, 1980.

Dumont, R., and Foss, D. *The American View of Death*. Cambridge, Mass.: Schenkman Publishing Company, 1972.

Feifel, H. *The Meaning of Death*. New York: McGraw-Hill, 1959.

Feifel, H. *New Meanings of Death*. New York: McGraw-Hill, 1977.

Feifel, H., and Branscomb, A. B. "Who's Afraid of Death?" *Journal of Abnormal Psychology*, 1973, *81*, 282–288.

Fulton, R. "The Sacred and the Secular: Attitudes of the American Public toward Death, Funerals and Funeral Directors," in R. Fulton (ed.), *Death and Identity*. New York: John Wiley and Sons, 1965.

Hansburg, H. *Adolescent Separation Anxiety*, Vol. I. Springfield, Ill.: Charles C. Thomas, 1972. Reprinted, Melbourne, Fla.: R. E. Krieger, 1980.

Hansburg, H. "Psychological Systems and Separation Disorders," a paper read at the meetings of the American Psychological Association, New York, 1979.

Kastenbaum, R., and Aisenberg, R. *The Psychology of Death*. New York: Springer, 1972.

Kubler-Ross, E. *On Death and Dying.* New York: Macmillan, 1969.

Lester, D. "Experimental and Correlational Studies of the Fear of Death." *Psychological Bulletin*, 1967, *67*, 27–36.

Lester, D. "Relation of Fear of Death in Subjects to Fear of Death in Their Parents." *Psychological Record*, 1970, *20*, 541–543.

Lifton, R. J. *The Life of the Self.* New York: Simon and Schuster, 1976.

Nagy, M. H. "The Child's Theories Concerning Death." *Journal of Genetic Psychology*, 1948, *73*, 3–27.

Parkes, C. M. *Bereavement: Studies of Grief in Adult Life.* New York: International Universities Press, 1972.

Pattison, E. M. *The Experience of Dying.* Englewood Cliffs, N.J.: Prentice-Hall, 1977.

Schwartz, P. K. *A Study of the Relationship between Attachment-Separation and the Fear of Death.* Unpublished doctoral dissertation, California School of Professional Psychology, Los Angeles, 1980.

Templer, D. I. "The Construction and Validation of a Death Anxiety Scale." *Journal of General Psychology*, 1970, *82*, 165–177.

Templer, D. I., Ruff, C. F., and Franks, C. M. "Death Anxiety: Age, Sex and Parental Resemblance in Diverse Populations." *Developmental Psychology*, 1971, *4*, 108.

Weiss, R. *Loneliness: The Experience of Emotional and Social Isolation.* Cambridge, Mass.: Massachusetts International Press, 1973.

13

Noble's Study of Separation Reactions in Marginal Religious Cult Participants

A study by Dr. Arlene Noble, entitled "Separation/Individuation Patterns and Participation in Marginal Religious Groups," was completed at the Professional School of Psychology in San Francisco in 1984. While the main groups were either cult joiners or visitors to cults, the comparison group consisted of twenty-five college students, all of whom were tested with the S.A.T., a personal data sheet, a Modified Children's Report of Parental Behavior, and the Assessment of Qualitative and Structural Dimensions of Object Representations. She made comparisons between the Moonies, the Krishnas, the visitors, and the college group on five S.A.T. patterns.

This study was conceived by Dr. Noble with the intention of furthering the understanding of the personalities of those young people who seek out cultist groups as a solution to their growth problems. It examines

. . . how adolescent separation/individuation from parents is related to joining a marginal religious group. Previous life separations and attachments, as well as current object relations, influence the degree of turmoil in adolescent experiences during the separation process (Blos, 1967; Bowlby, 1969; Hansburg, 1972). The research will examine how the interplay between the desire for further separation and autonomy and the pressure of strong attachment needs are related to joining a communal religious group.

Research on the psychological condition of those who join new religious groups reveals various findings. Some scholars have found abnormal personality traits such as excessive narcissism, borderline disorders and high

151

hostility among recruits (Olsson, 1980; Kriegman, 1980; E. Levine, 1980). However, the majority of researchers note that, although these groups do attract individuals who are experiencing "painful feelings" and depression prior to joining, they are not a clinically more disturbed group (Levine, 1979; Singer, 1979). According to most observers, these new religious groups promise a solution to the distress of the developmental crisis endemic to this life stage. They reach those who are between affiliations (Singer, 1979); older adolescents who have left the family unit through residential campus living or travel, and have not yet committed to beliefs and life philosophies of their own (Marciano, 1982).

Dr. Noble discusses some of the philosophical and social issues which have given birth to the nearly 5000 marginal religious groups in existence (Ahlstrom, 1972), each extremely varied in ideology, leadership, organization, size, doctrine, and ritual.

Marginal religious groups refer to contemporary movements which include sects which have emerged within established churches, non-church-related cults or quasi-religious communities (Lukas, 1982). The concept of cult has been increasingly used as an equivalent term. Nelson (1969) defined cults as religious movements which make a fundamental break with the religious tradition of the culture . . . they are composed of individuals who have had or seek mystical, psychic or ecstatic experiences and they purport to be concerned with the problems of individuals. For the purpose of this study, the focus will be further narrowed to groups that entail communal lifestyle, charismatic leadership, submission to authority and rigid ideology.

Noble further concerns herself with the second individuation process of adolescence and the later commitment stage. She describes the theories of Blos (1962), Erikson (1958), A. Freud (1958), et al., and leans heavily on Blos (1962, 1970):

When the adolescent's internalized representations of parents are relinquished and replaced by new external identificatory figures, . . . the parents are deidealized and seen in a more realistic fashion and self-esteem is consolidated with the formation of a reliable, stable, more realistic sense of self.

She continues with the notion that the full achievement of ego identity and individuation often becomes an issue even when the adolescent arrives in the early twenties or post-adolesence. From this material and from many of the studies of the marginal religious groups, especially Schwartz and Kaslow (1979) and Lukas (1982), it was found that

. . . the parents of marginal religious group joiners were perceived by their children as exhibiting a lack of control and expectations, which may indicate permissiveness, . . . the lack of parental structure and limits which may lead a person to seek structure through participation in these religious groups.

Noble describes a number of studies indicating predisposing factors in the adolescents who are moved to join these groups. Barker (1981), Judah (1978), and Galanter (1979), while focusing on the nature of group pressure, imply that those who join are more passively accepting of manipulation and make few judgments. Clark (1979) and Singer (1979) describe these young people as being "between affiliations, depressed and confused, with a sense that life is meaningless." Clark found 40% of a group studied had no long-standing emotional problems but had become situationally depressed and frightened on beginning the true separation from the family. The second group were more troubled and trying to find other avenues for personal affiliation, while a third group, small in number, were delinquent and sociopathic. Clark cited such factors as personal distress, a low tolerance for ambiguity, susceptibility to trance states, dependency and a tendency to conceptualize problems in religious terms.

Noble provides an intensive examination of the literature dealing with the sociological factors which relate to the cultist groups and their attraction to some late adolescents. This will not be discussed here except to point out that a group used in Noble's study were from the British Unification Church (Moonies) and she discusses Barker's (1981) extensive study of this church cult. She indicates that a large percentage of these come from comfortable middle-class homes where there has been considerable emphasis on religion as a cultural and psychological force. However, Barker had found that less than 10% had described their relationship with parents as "poor." Barker also noted that extremes of happiness and unhappiness had characterized the Moonie joiners. Barker's statistics pointed to stress before joining and a variation or possibly a slower rate of adolescent development.

Noble points out that the literature dealing with the mental health problems of cult joiners often emphasizes the healing characteristics of the cultist group. A study by Galanter and Buckley (1978)

. . . of 119 members of the Divine Light Mission . . . found a significant decline in the incidence of neurotic symptoms and of alcohol and drug use immediately after joining . . . Galanter attributed ritual meditation and group related activities and attitudes as significant in ameliorating symptoms.

Later, Galanter et al. (1979)

. . . administered a neurotic distress scale, a religiosity scale and a general wellbeing schedule to 237 members of the Unification Church and to a matched comparison group of 305 persons. They reported that for church affiliates, 39% had serious emotional problems prior to joining, 30% sought professional help and 6% were hospitalized for psychiatric disturbance; in addition 23% had serious drug problems in the past. The findings that 91% had a lower distress score right after conversion, and a much higher religiosity scale score, emphasized the considerable and sustained relief from neurotic distress that the group provided . . . (however) over time the joiners reported a decline in work satisfaction and religious commitment, and tended to return to previous levels of distress. Thus, the symptom improvement seems to be transitory and the seeming personality defects are not substantially altered.

Levine's studies (1976, 1979) concluded that cults do attract individuals who feel alienated, depressed and anxious prior to joining and some are clearly borderline in functioning (32 had a crisis before membership). Generally, Levine felt that the disturbances were situationally rather than clinically based. Noble reports that Levine believes that the cults fulfill the basic needs of believing and belonging "which leads to a rise of self-esteem for its members."

Simmonds's (1977) study of 96 members of a Jesus commune had found dependency to be a strong factor. The nature of the dependency was often switched from drugs to a rigid religious belief system, and he characterized the participants as "addictive personalities." Deutsch and Miller (1979) from an intensive study of an individual Moonie suggested that repressed dependency, hostility and sexual conflict played a role. " . . . the clinging to the old values and to the new authority suggests the inadequate accomplishment of the adolescent tasks of separation, individuation and super-ego reorganization." The search appeared to be for a new and higher authority, a good ideal father who can serve to reduce ambivalence. Ungelieder and Wellisch (1979) in a test study of 50 subjects found them to be using participation as an externalized superego substitute, especially in areas of hostility management, a problem which had existed before they joined the group. Gitelson and Reed (1981), using Erikson's formulation of identity, found a diffused and moratorium status of identity in the joiners and with protracted involvement, development of identity was arrested. In a comprehensive study Lukas (1982) corroborated this finding and added lower self-esteem and distorted self-appraisal, functioning in the preconventional and conventional stages of moral development, less responsible, less autonomous, more passive and permitting lower levels of intimacy. Lukas also found further evidence of parental permissiveness and less family structure. One further aspect of the latter study was the corroboration of Offer and Offer (1969, 1971, 1975) that there were significantly more deaths among parents than in comparison groups.

Kriegman (1980) in a test study found cult members to be more constricted and defensive, with more immature object relations and a greater narcissistic pathology of self-objects. No severe psychopathology was present. Using Kohut's (1966, 1971) concepts, Kriegman posits that a relatively healthy adult does not build his entire life around the idealized object. It is no longer age-appropriate to do so, and cult joiners tend to maintain primitive narcissistic ties to the idealized parental image. Numbers of studies focusing on family systems have found a lack of family direction and weak fathers. Of interest was Kaslow and Schwartz's findings that "those who resisted cult affiliation successfully, showed evidence of inner direction and a strong bond with their fathers. . . ."

Noble integrates her general interest in those adolescents who join cultist groups with theories and research studies of adolescent development with specific reference to concepts of separation/individuation. She has a long and intensive discussion (16 pages) of this issue in which she goes into details with special description of Mahler's (1975) theories as further developed by Blos (1967) and Bowlby (1969) in his attachment theory. Her evidence from the literature suggests that while adolescence is not necessarily filled with turmoil, there are crisis stages which need to be considered. It is during these crisis stages that adolescents and young adults are most prone to join these groups. She refers to the frequently accepted notion that adolescence produces a reworking of the infantile and early childhood problems and conflicts and the resultant movement toward "autonomous-relatedness," a term first coined by Bowlby and referred to by Murphy, Bilber, Coehlo, Hamburg and Greenberg (1963) in a study of this issue in 19 college-bound senior high school students. She quotes extensively from Mahler, Bowlby, Hansburg, Offer and Offer, and Stierlin (1974) to illustrate the developmental concepts that she presents. Noble documents her points with a host of studies on the separation/individuation process in late adolescence. The failures in either autonomy or relatedness or both, and the psychological factors responsible for these failures, become the focus of her discussion. The joining of the cultist group then represents one of the gambles or moves made to achieve the autonomy and shift relatedness to a new authority.

Noble sets up a series of five hypotheses with detailed corollaries for her study:

1. that there is a significant difference between the cultist and non-affiliated groups in separations and loss
2. that there is a significant difference between these two groups in their individuation and attachment system balance
3. that there will be a higher degree of self-love loss and depression as measured by the S.A.T. between the cultist and non-cultist groups
4. that there will be a significant difference in the perception of parents' variables of positive involvement, negative control, and lax discipline between the groups, and
5. that there will be a significant degree of grandiose idealizations of important people in the lives of the cultists as compared to the non-cultists.

Noble selected 50 young people who were affiliated with two marginal religious groups, 31 from the Unification Church (Moonies) and 19 from the International Society for Krishna Consciousness (ISKON or Hare Krishnas). I omit here the principles and behavioral tactics which characterize these groups, except to say that they both have communal lifestyle, charismatic leadership, submission to authority and rigid ideology, and both demand intense commitment to a systematic theology. The comparison group consisted of 18 individuals who visited a marginal religious group and chose not to join and 25 college students who were never members of any cult and never visited with one. The details of the extensive and intensive activities that went into obtaining the cooperation of these groups are omitted here for the sake of brevity, but all-out efforts were made to obtain an adequate and representative sample. The demographic data collected by Noble are presented in Table 13.1.

It can be seen that there were significant differences in age, the college group being younger and with more education. Noble describes these differences in detail and explains them. She presents further demographic tables on sex, race, family size, religious background, and type of community background raised, in which she found no meaningful differences. She also compared the Moonies and Krishnas with regard to the speed with which they were converted, and the data indicated a significant difference—the Moonies were converted in a much shorter time. The college group, which had never participated in any cult, cited having attended mainstream religious organizations significantly more often than the cult visitors, while numbers of the visitors had also visited or participated in other cult groups.

There were some revelations with regard to emotional disturbance. The Krishnas appeared to have had the largest number of all groups in previous treatment, although in this respect they were not that much different from the visitors. When the variable was treatment with prescribed medication, the Krishnas were significantly higher. Observational data confirmed that the Krishnas were, from the clinical point of view, a far more disturbed population—at least three members of that group were so emotionally upset that they could not complete the test battery. The Krishnas had shown a history of far more participation in communal living in other groups before joining ISKON, while this was far less true of the Moonies.

Table 13.1

MEANS, STANDARD DEVIATIONS, AND t-TEST
FOR AGE AND EDUCATION

Variable	Moonies ($N = 31$)		Krishnas ($N = 19$)		College ($N = 31$)		Visitors ($N = 18$)	
	M	S.D.	M	S.D.	M	S.D.	M	S.D.
Education	14.4	2.1	13.1	3.1	14.6	1.1	15.1	2.1
Age	26.5	4.3	27.58	5.04	23.5	4.27	25.5	6.5
Age Joined	22.5	3.0	23.1	6.3				

	Marginal Religious Group	Comparison Group	t
Education	13.96	14.82	-2.00[a]
Age	26.96	24.24	2.71[b]

[a] $p < .05.$

[b] $p < .005.$

In general, the Krishnas seemed on the whole to be significantly different in a number of respects with regard to their background than the other three groups.

Noble used the following instruments for her test battery which she describes in detail in her study: (a) a personal data sheet from which she derived the data referred to above, (b) the Hansburg S.A.T., (c) a Modified Children's Report of Parental Behavior Inventory (Raskin, Boothe, Reatig, Schulterbrant, and Odle, 1971), and (d) the Assessment of Qualitative and Structural Dimensions of Object Representations (Blatt, Chevron, Quinlan and Wein, 1981). Only the data on the S.A.T. will be referred to here, except where other data impinge on this test.

For the purposes of her study Noble divided the results on the Separation Anxiety Test into five groups: Minor Anxious Attachment, Major Anxious Attachment, Secure Attachment, Minor Detachment, and Major Detachment. Separation disorder percentages were arrived at by combining major attachment and detachment scores and then analyzing them with a chi-square for between-group differences. Since the two comparison groups scored much differently, the data were treated statistically with three separate cells: Cult, College sample and Visitors. Table 13.2 presents the percentages of the current attachment patterns as demonstrated by the Separation Anxiety Test for the four groups tested.

Both major attachment and major detachment disorders are much more prevalent to a significant degree among both the Moonies and the Krishnas than among the college or visitors groups. The difference between the college non-joiners and the other groups is statistically significant with the following data ($\chi^2 = 7.49$ (2), $p < .05$). When the three Visitors who were currently involved in cultlike groups were omitted, this population becomes more similar to the college sample. Comparison groups were then combined and contrasted to the marginal religious groups; the difference was statistically significant as follows: $\chi^2 = 5.976$, $p < .01$. In the case of the Moonie adherents, four of the ten individuals with major detachment disorders were categorized as Dependent detachment while there were none with this kind of disorder in the other groups, a significant difference. Major attachment disorders were found equally among the Krishnas, Moonies and Visitors, averaging 27.3%. Only 12% of the non-joiner college population was classified with this pattern. The college group also had the highest percentage of secure attachment patterns (20.8%), which contrasted with the Moonie followers (3%), with the Krishnas (13.3%) and with the Visitors (11%). Since three members of the Krishna group were unable to complete the test battery because of emotional upset, it is likely that the percentage of disorders in this group would have been higher.

Several other added factors in relation to Table 13.2 should be of note. Since the three Visitors who were members of other cults showed major separation disorders, the positive evidence of cult membership relationship to disturbed attachment patterns is manifested. Further, since the comparison groups were generally younger and better educated, a one-way analysis of variance for each of these demographic

Table 13.2

PERCENTAGES OF CURRENT ATTACHMENT PATTERNS

(Chi-Square on Differences between Cult
and Noncult Groups for Separation Disorders)

Current Attachment Patterns	Moonies (N = 29)	Krishnas (N = 15)	College (N = 24)	Visitors[a] (N = 15)
Major Attachment Disorder	27.5%	26.6%	12.5%	20%
Secure Attachment	3.4%	13.3%	20.8%	13.3%
Major Detachment	37.9%	33.3%	16.6%	26.6%
Dependent Detachment	13.8%	0	0	0
		$\chi^2 = 8.2$[b], $df = 3$		
Severe Detachment	24.1%			
Minor Attachment	13.8%	0	29.16	0
Minor Detachment	17.2%	26.6%	20.8%	40%
Total Major Separation Disorder	65.4%	60%	29.1%	46.7%
		$\chi^2 = 5.976$[b]		
Total Secure and Minor Disorders	33.8%	39.9%	71.3%	53.3%

[a]Three of the Visitors who were affiliated with other cultlike groups were omitted.

[b]$p < .01$.

variables was done. The results for this demonstrated no significant correlations with the combined major separation disorders. The f value for education was .47, $p = .4939$; and for age, $f = 1.23$, $p = .27$. We can be certain that the age and education differences were not related to the test results. Thus, the hypothesis listed as number 2 was confirmed.

The hypothesis listed under item 3 above related to self-love loss and depression. It was assumed that these problems would be more common to the cultist groups than to the non-joiners. Table 13.3 presents the results of the S.A.T. in the first of these areas. From the table it can be readily seen that there is a significant difference between the marginal religious group means of 9.08 and the nonjoiners, of 7.16 with the F (82) $= 4.08$, $p < .05$. In specific terms feelings of rejection and intrapunitiveness are significantly greater among the cult groups under separation stimulation.

Table 13.4 presents the results for the depressive syndrome which represents the relationship between the self-love loss percentage and the self-esteem preoccupation.

Table 13.4 gives a strong indication that depressive reactions were far more common in the cult groups than in the comparison population. The data show 51½% of the cult groups in the depressive syndrome category, while only 28½% of the nonaffiliated appear in that category. The difference was significant at the .03 level.

It was found that age and education were correlated with self-love loss and depression scores. Neither had an impact on self-love loss when

Table 13.3

MEANS, STANDARD DEVIATIONS, AND ANOVA-SELF-LOVE LOSS
MARGINAL RELIGIOUS GROUPS COMPARED TO NONAFFILIATED GROUPS

	Moonie		Krishna		College		Visitors		Marginal Groups[a]	Comparison Group
	M	S.D.	M	S.D.	M	S.D.	M	S.D.	M[a]	M
Self-Love Loss	9.2	5.2	8.9	3.6	7.0	3.9	7.4	4.34	9.0805[a]	7.16

	SS	df	MS	F
Source of Variance Between Group	78.65	1	78.65	4.08[a]

[a]$p < .05$.

analyzed with univariate analysis of variance (F value for age was .65 and p = .423, F = .42 for education and p = .5196.) The depression indicator yielded no significant difference on the age variable (f = .84, $p < .3614$), but demonstrated a distinct difference on the education variable. The lower the education level, the greater the possibility of depression in this population (f = 5.68, $p < .02$).

At this point I present Noble's discussion verbatim, since she provides a quite pertinent, extensive discussion of the two hypotheses on the results of the use of the S.A.T.

Hypothesis 2 affirmed that the members of marginal religious groups had more disturbance in their attachment system, either in the direction of detachment or anxious attachment, as measured by the Separation Anxiety Test (S.A.T.). The College group had, emotionally, the healthiest profiles, with over 70%, as compared to the cult groups' 37%. The cult group exhibited twice as many serious separation disorders.

The S.A.T. provided a wealth of information on psychological functioning and identified dysfunctional attachment systems for this study's population of cult members and non-joiners. The main focus for this research was on the current attachment patterns derived from the test.

Table 13.4

CHI-SQUARE ON DEPRESSION INDICATOR COMPARING
MARGINAL RELIGIOUS GROUPS TO NONAFFILIATED GROUPS

	Depression Indicator			
	No		Yes	
	#	%	#	%
Moonies (N = 30)	15	50	15	50
Krishnas (N = 15)	8	53	7	47
College (N = 25)	18	72	7	28
Visitors (N = 14)[a]	12	71	5	29
Marginal Groups (N = 45)[b]	22[b]	49	23[b]	$51\frac{1}{2}$
Comparison Group (N = 39)	27[b]	$71\frac{1}{2}$	12[b]	$28\frac{1}{2}$

$$\chi^2 = 4.79,[b] \quad df = 1$$

[a] Visitors = 14, omitting affiliates of cultlike groups;
when Visitors = 17, χ^2 = 3.77, $p < .052$.
[b] $p < .03$.

The separation pictures, both mild and severe, suggested possible emotional responses from which the subjects chose; these were scores to ascertain the degree and the balance between individuation and attachment scores. The test operates on the assumption that a secure attachment base can be supplied by parents, but a child's responsiveness and adaptability to these figures are also factors influencing attachment. Adaptability, in attachment theory, refers to the intrinsic characteristics of the individual which operate as resources to help reduce the potentially destructive effects of separation and loss. The adaptive response fuels individuation. Those who are characterized with Major Attachment Disorder have remained anxiously attached to maintain a closeness to their attachment figures; this can avoid the alienation resulting from their own separateness. Those who become overly detached, labelled Major Detachment Disorder, do so to avoid the potential hurt and anxiety associated with being dependent on an inconsistent attachment figure.

The marginal religious groups had a combined percentage of Major Separation Disorders, including both detached and anxiously attached, of 62.7%. The College comparison group had 29% of this disorder, a significant difference. When adding the amended Visitor group (without affiliates to cult-like organizations) the difference is also significant. The members of the Unification Church (Moonies) had slightly more (5%) of these serious disorders than the Krishnas, but it should be noted that four ISKON (Krishnas) members were unable or unwilling to complete the S.A.T. Three were emotionally upset by the survey, with its emphasis on family background. The assumption is that these individuals would have added to the major separation disorders.

The scores of the Visitors fell in the middle between the cult and the college groups. The Visitor group provided an excellent opportunity to examine a population with high susceptibility needs for membership in a cult but enough affiliative abilities to make joining less internally demanding. The three individuals of this sample who were active in other cult-like organizations were confirmation of the hypothesis that cult participants were more likely to have major separation disturbances. All three exhibited major disorders: two had major attachment disorders and one had a major detachment disorder. Once they were removed from the statistical analysis on the S.A.T., Visitors became more like the College population and the differences between cult and nonjoiner comparison groups were significant. These individuals should have been screened out of the study. Still, the population of those who visited cults (Visitors) pointed to more disturbed attachment patterns, and less ego strength although not in the same high range as the Cult groups. This group also had a fairly high stress level, with more moves, significantly more layoffs or firings, and a higher incidence of increased drug use, (material from questionnaire interview) as compared to the College sample.

These seemed to be important psychological factors explaining attraction to marginal religious organizations. Yet the Visitors did not join (except for three mentioned above). It was surmised that their high frequency of making and maintaining serious romantic relationships, many of them relatively long term, as well as having a reliable group of friends, mitigated against joining.

Observation of the current attachment patterns for the cult sample yielded other interesting findings. The only four cases of Dependent Detachment in this study's sample (total) of 99, occurred for members of the Unification Church (Moonies). When Hansburg originally established his norms, he found this disorder present in only a small percentage of adolescents and adults. It suggests both a very poor resource level and poor personality core strength (Hansburg, 1980). Such a person possesses limited capacity to form a reciprocal attachment relationship and shows a weak exploratory behavioral system. Hansburg writes:

> Because true attachments are so tenuous for such persons, they most readily accept relationships that are of the caretaking variety and for as long as the caretaker provides security . . . the basis for the attachment still remains highly dependent and narcissistic. (pp. 22, 23)

While Dependent detachment protocols comprised only 12.8% of the Unification Church's (Moonies) total, it is significant that it was not found in any of the other groups. It appeared that the most dependent personality types were attracted to organizations with the most structure and demand for conformity.

Major Detachment Disorders were the most frequent patterns for both the U.C. (Moonie) members and the Krishnas. This was highly compatible with other findings, in that members of marginal religious groups are likely to be in a diffused identity state (Lukas, 1982; Gitleson, 1981) and that diffused identity states are correlated with Detached Attachment Patterns (Currie, 1983). The ISKON (Krishnas), in particular, speak of detachment as a life stance, thereby making it easier to do Krishna's bidding. Excessive detachment is also reminiscent of a "false self" discussed by Winnicott (1958). This is a self without autonomy and exists in relation to another object. It is often presented as a grandiose self-structure and used as a defense against anxiety; healthy self-esteem has difficulty emerging when detachment prevails (Horner, 1979).

Major Attachment Disorders were the second most common category for the U.C. (Moonie) members, the Krishnas, and the Visitor group when including current affiliates of cult-like organizations. Approximately 27% of these individuals demonstrated a serious degree of anxious attachment. These results showed, according to Hansburg (1980), severe uncertainty in the capacity to receive loving from an attachment figure. Unrealistic symbiotic needs and low self-esteem are often present, which establishes a yearning for structure, for stability in one's attachment figures, and for the experience of personal acceptance and belonging. Most of all, severe attachment needs allow the self to become absorbed in an all encompassing organization and a chance to merge in an identification with group and leader.

There are three other categories, Secure attachment, Minor detachment and Minor (anxious) Attachment; all are emotionally healthier along the attachment-detachment continuum. Secure attachment, which contained scores within the norms delineated by Hansburg, was present in a minority of cases. The College group contained the highest percent of this category, 20.8%; the U.C. members (Moonies) had the lowest percentage, 3.4%. Minor detachment and attachment disorders were considered less indicative of serious psychopathology; while the attachment-individuation scores may have been slightly elevated or depressed from the norms, the responses for hostility (anger, projection and intrapunitiveness) and painful tension (anxiety, phobic and somatic reactions) were within the norms. Close to 50% of the College sample were categorized with these minor detachment or attachment disorders. And when secure attachments were added to this percentage, over 70% of the College group had emotionally healthier profiles as compared to the cult groups with only 37%.

In summary, hypothesis 2 found that members of marginal religious groups had a significantly greater amount of disturbance in their attachment system as compared to the nonjoiners. Those who visited cults had a much higher percentage of attachment disorders than the college sample. And the visitors who were currently affiliated with some cultlike group had S.A.T. attachment scores similar to the joiners. Thus, attachment disturbance and affiliation with a tight-knit hierarchical marginal religious group have significant correlation. These groups appeal to those young persons who have less adaptive responses and inner resources to cope with separation and loss. The literature previously discussed describes the relationship of attachment theory to separation/individuation. Those who remain anxiously attached seek to maintain a closeness to attachment figures to avoid alienation resulting from their own separateness. The overly detached are trying to avoid potential hurt and anxiety associated with being dependent on an inconsistent attachment figure. Not only do cults provide automatic affiliation and intimacy, but also provide a vehicle for the abrupt separation from family.

Hypothesis 3 affirmed that there was a higher degree of self-love loss and depression among marginal religious group members as compared to the nonjoiner comparison group. The S.A.T. provided an evaluation of both measures. Self-love, as measured by the S.A.T., related to being wanted, loved and cared for by the attachment figure. Such experiences build self-acceptance and healthy self-love. Separation experiences, in infancy and in later life, have been found to strongly affect this system (Hansburg 1980). The S.A.T.'s determination of self-love loss is based on intrapunitive and rejection responses. The members of the marginal religious groups averaged mean scores (9.08) well above the delineated norms (6-8%). Their scores were higher and demonstrated a significant difference when compared to the nonjoiners. Thus, it was concluded that feelings of rejection, of poor self-worth and of being less loveable were more common for cult members.

Depressive syndrome was an added diagnosis on the S.A.T., and it is in evidence when self-love loss percentage is high and exceeds concentration impairment and/or sublimation percentages (self-esteem preoccupation). Close to 50% of both marginal religious groups evidenced depression according to these standards. This contrasted to an average of 28.5% for the comparison groups. The difference was .052 for the chi-square significance level; however, when the Visitors who were currently involved with cult-like groups were dropped from the analysis, the between group difference was clearly significant (p .03). It is of interest that two of those affiliated Visitors were depressed and also exhibited anxious attachment. This further strengthens the thesis of psychological differences between those joining marginal religions and those not.

Hansburg found that depression is often present in severe anxious attachment and usually involves strong self-destructive fantasies and behavior. This has been substantiated in the elderly (Hansburg, 1980) [see Chapter 18 of this book] and in abusive mothers (De Lozier, 1979). [Also see Hansburg, 1976, with regard to early adolescence.] The sources and nature of depression, according to various theories, encompass

> . . . feelings of helplessness, low levels of self-evaluation, disparity between the actual self and the idealized self, severe guilt feelings in relation to parental figures, profound feelings of loneliness, hostile feelings toward an introjected parental figure that is felt to be alien to the self. (Hansburg, 1980, p. 25)

Education was negatively correlated with depression. The higher the educational level, the less likely was the incidence of depression. Many joined the cults at a younger age, interrupting their education and having little opportunity to continue. For others, education can limit the tools needed to be successful in the world and career opportunities suffer. It may prolong identity diffusion, which Lukas (1982) found to be a susceptible period of cult joining.

A high level of depression and self-love loss for cult members was found in previous research (Singer, 1979; Levine, 1976; Galanter, 1978), although it was found to exist prior to joining. This study avoided any depression measure that would assess the period before membership, due to the unreliability of recalling retroactive feeling states. Current belief systems and a new sense of purpose accompanying cult association make direct assessment of past and current emotional states difficult. The indirectness of the projective instrument and its access to preconscious material, proved useful in evaluating depression and made possible the examination of lingering and current depressive tendencies.

Many observers have demonstrated that symptoms of anxiety, confusion and depression were eased by membership in a marginal religious group (Galanter and Buckley, 1978; Galanter et al., 1979; Levine, 1979; Robbins and Anthony, 1972; and Pattison, 1980). This is especially true immediately after joining as illustrated in Galanter's study (1979); 91% of new members reported lower distress scores following conversion. His study is one of the few that contains a comparison group, and reveals that the nonjoiners still have higher general well-being scores. Galanter also reported that the joiners, who, over time, reported a decline in work satisfaction and religious commitment, tended to return to previous levels of distress. Thus, for many members, relief for depression is transitory; this is probably true for the more life-long, chronic cases of depression. The findings of this study document the persistence of depression and self-esteem difficulties [read this as self-love], although this might represent an improvement of the emotional state compared to the precult period.

High depression and low self-esteem [read self-love] have a direct relationship to separation/individuation issues. This may originate with early childhood loss or even adolescent trauma connected to separation or rejection. During adolescence, parental deidealization with the loss of the childhood emotional ties, also creates a sense of mourning. Disengagements from these parental ego supports should be paralleled by ego maturation and the formation of internal regulatory capacities (Blos, 1967). It is postulated that among many of the members of these marginal religious groups, a consolidation of ego and superego has not occurred. This makes emotional separation from parents difficult; a cult is then used as a vehicle for the physical break from home. It also provides a ready-made identity which serves as a support for the fragile ego.

REFERENCES

Ahlstrom, A. *A Religious History of the American People*. New York: Yale University Press, 1972.

Barker, E. "The Ones That Got Away." Conference address at Graduate Theological Union, 1981.

Blatt, S. J., Wein, S. J., Chevron, E., and Quinlan, D. M. "Parental Responsibility and Depression in Normal Young Adults." *Journal of Abnormal Psychology*, 1979, 95(4), 388–397.

Blos, P. *On Adolescence*. New York: Free Press, 1962.

Blos, P. "The Second Individuation Process of Adolescence." *Psychoanalytic Study of the Child*, 1967, 22, 162–186.

Bowlby, J. *Attachment and Loss*, Vol. I: *Attachment* (1969). Vol. II: *Separation*. (1973). New York: Basic Books.

Clark, J. "Manipulation of Madness." Paper presented in Hanover, West Germany, February, 1979.

Currie, P. S. *Current Attachment Patterns, Attachment History and Religiosity as Predictors of Ego-Identity Status in Fundamentalist Christian Adolescents*. Unpublished doctoral dissertation, California School of Professional Psychology, Los Angeles, 1983.

DeLozier, P. P. *An Application of Attachment Theory to the Study of Child Abuse*. Unpublished doctoral dissertation, California School of Professional Psychology, Los Angeles, 1979.

Deutsch, A., and Miller, M. "Conflict, Character and Conversion." *Adolescent Psychiatry*, 1979, 7, 257–268.

Erikson, E. "The Problem of Ego Identity." *Journal of American Psychoanalytic Association*, 1958, 4, 56–121.

Freud, A. "Adolescence." *Psychoanalytic Study of the Child*, 1958, *13*, 255–278.

Galanter, M., Rabkin, R., Rabkin, T., and Deutsch, A. "The 'Moonies': A Psychological Study of Conversion and Membership in a Contemporary Religious Sect." *American Journal of Psychiatry*, 1979, *136*, 165–170.

Galanter, M., and Buckley, P. "Evangelical Religion and Meditation: Psychotherapeutic Effects." *The Journal of Nervous and Mental Disease*, 1978, *166*, 685–691.

Gitelson, I. B., and Reed, E. J. "Identity States of Jewish Youth Pre- and Post-Cult Involvement." *Journal of Jewish Communal Service*, 1981, 57(4), 312–320.

Hansburg, H. G. *Adolescent Separation Anxiety: Vol. I: A Method for the Study of Adolescent Problems*. Springfield, Ill.: Charles C. Thomas, 1972. Reprinted, Melbourne, Fla.: R. E. Krieger, 1980.

Hansburg, H. G. "The Use of the Separation Anxiety Test in the Detection of Self-Destructive Tendencies in Early Adolescence," in D. V. Siva Sankar (ed.), *Mental Health in Children*, Vol. III. Westbury, N.Y.: P. J. D. Publications, 1976.

Hansburg, H. G. *Adolescent Separation Anxiety*, Vol. II: *Separation Disorders*. Melbourne, Fla.: R. E. Krieger, 1980.

Horner, A. *Object Relations and the Developing Ego in Therapy*. New York: Jason Aronson, 1979.

Judah, J. S. *The Unification Church: Conversion or Coercion*, 1982 (in press).

Judah, J. S. "New Religions and Religious Liberty," in J. Needleman and G. Baker (eds.), *Understanding the New Religions*. New York: Seabury, 1978.

Kohut, H. "Forms and Transformations of Narcissism." *Journal of the American Psychoanalytic Association*, 1966, *14*, 243–272.

Kohut, H. *The Analysis of the Self*. New York: International Universities Press, 1971.

Kriegman, D. "A Psychosocial Study of Religious Cults from the Perspective of Self-Psychology."*DissertationAbstractsInternational*,1980,*41*(5)1921,B.

Levine, E. "Rural Communes and Religious Cults: Refuges for Middle Class Youth," in S. Feinstein, et al. (eds.), *Adolescent Psychiatry*. Chicago: University of Chicago Press, 1980, 8, 138–156.

Levine, S., and Scater, N. "Youth and Contemporary Religious Movements: Psycho-Social Findings," *Canadian Psychiatry Association Manual*, 1976, *21*, 411–420.

Levine, S. "Cults and Mental Health: Clinical Conclusions," paper presented at Hebrew University, 1979.

Lukas, 1982 (reference missing from the original bibliography).

Mahler, M., Pine, F., and Bergman, A. *Psychological Birth of the Infant*. New York: Basic Books, 1975.

Marciano, T. D. "Families and Cults," in Kaslow and Sussman (eds.), *Marriage and Family Review*, 1982, *4*, 101–117.

Murphy, E., Bilber, E., Coelho, G., Hamburg, D., and Greenberg, I. "Development of Autonomy and Parent-Child Interaction in Late Adolescence." *American Journal of Orthopsychiatry*, 1963, *33*(4), 643–652.

Nelson, G. "The Spiritualist Movement and the Need for Redefinition of Cult." *Journal of the Scientific Study of Religion*, 1969, *8*(1), 152–160.

Noble, A. *Separation/Individuation Patterns and Participation in Marginal Religious Groups*. Unpublished doctoral dissertation, California School of Professional Psychology, San Francisco, 1984.

Offer, D., and Offer, J. *From Teenage to Young Manhood: A Psychological Study*. New York: Basic Books, 1971.

Offer, D. "Adolescent Turmoil," in Esman (ed.), *Psychology of Adolescence*. New York: International Universities Press, 1975.

Olsson, P. "Adolescent Involvement with the Supernatural and Cults: Some Psychoanalytic Considerations." *Annual of Psychoanalysis*, 1980, *8*, 171–196.

Pattison, E. M. "Religious Youth Cults: Alternative Healing Social Networks." *Journal of Religion and Health*, 1980, *19*(4), 275–286.

Raskin, Boothe, Reatig, Schulterbrant, and Odle, 1971 (reference missing from the original bibliography).

Robbins, T., and Anthony, D. "Getting Straight with Meher Baba: A Study of Drug Rehabilitation, Mysticism and Post-Adolescent Role Conflict." *Journal for the Scientific Study of Religion*, 1972, *11*(2), 122–140.

Schwartz, L. L., and Kaslow, F. W. "Religious Cults, the Individual and the Family." *Journal of Marriage and Family Therapy*, 1979, *5*(2), 15–26.

Simmonds, 1977 (reference missing from the original bibliography).

Singer, M. "Coming out of the Cults." *Psychology Today*, January 1979.

Stierlin, H. *"Separating Parents and Adolescents: A Perspective on Running Away, Schizophrenia, and Waywardness."* New York: Quadrangle Books, 1974.

Ungerleider, T., and Welesch, D. "Coercive Persuasion (Brainwashing): Religious Cults and Deprogramming." *American Journal of Psychiatry*, 1979, *136*, 279–282.

Winnicott, D. W. *Collected Papers*. London: Tavistock, 1958.

STUDIES OF THE ELDERLY

14

Fisk's Study of the Loss of Life Meaning in the Elderly

Aside from my own study (in 1979; see Chapter 18), there has been one other study of the aged with the S.A.T. Entitled "The Effect of Loss of Meaning on the Mental and Physical Well Being of the Aged," it was undertaken by Dr. Peter C. Fisk at the California School of Professional Psychology in Los Angeles and completed in 1979. This study, in contrast to mine, used forty-one elderly people from 65 to 95 who were either widowed or divorced and living in retirement homes. No effort was made to compare them to other elderly people living under other circumstances or having a different marital status. Dr. Fisk was interested solely in studying the loss of life meaning in this group.

Recognizing that the elderly experience the loss of previously held physical and mental powers, places in the community and their sense of identity, Dr. Fisk determined to study what sustains the meaningfulness of existence in the elderly. He began his discussion with two philosophical viewpoints on the meaning of life:

1. Albert Camus, in *The Myth of Sisyphus* (1955), contended:

   . . . what human beings appear to strive towards . . . routine, predictability, order, universal morality and Utopian perfection, all ideals that religion and philosophy have portrayed to man as reachable goals, are, when the natural state of human existence is observed, absurd and ludicrous. Human life is fundamentally objectiveless, meaningless and chaotic.

2. Viktor Frankl, in *Man's Search for Meaning* (1959),
    with whom Fisk obviously agrees, contended:

    . . . if an individual can create a personal meaning, a specific
    purpose for being alive, he will not perceive this absurdity
    and futility that Camus has so vividly described. . . . By
    defining a personal reason for being in this world, all that is
    encountered in one's journey through life becomes valued,
    esteemed and meaningful.

    For Frankl, the will for human beings always to move
    towards meaning is the primary human motivational
    force.

Fisk was concerned with determining to what degree the purpose
or meaning of life to the elderly influenced their physical and mental
well-being. He was impressed with certain types of research which he
felt would be of help in his study of the problem. Rotter (1966) on locus
of control and those who conducted experiments in this area, Phares
(1962), Bellak (1975), Wolk and Ducette (1972), became significant to
him. The concept of internal locus of control and external locus of control impressed Fisk, and he decided to use Rotter's Internal–External
Locus of Control Inventory and thus characterize the elderly as either
IL of C or EL of C. Further, he was interested in the work of Crumbaugh and Maholick (1964), who developed the Purpose-in-Life Test.
He referred to Yarnell's (1975) finding of a negative correlation between the Purpose-in-Life Test and the I-E L of C, suggesting that
people with greater purpose in life view themselves less at the mercy of
luck and more in control of a situation than those individuals with less
meaning, feeling they have no control over their lives (EL of C).

Fisk further considered the significance of attachment and
separation in their relationship to life purposes and meaning in the
elderly. In this area Fisk leans heavily on Bowlby (1975) and Hansburg
(1972, 1979, and 1980). He discusses Bowlby's attachment theory and
concludes from this that "the forced and unwilling loss of an attachment figure must also stimulate a loss of individual meaning." He
presents in detail a summary of Hansburg's study of the elderly (1978)
with the Separation Anxiety Test (which is reported elsewhere in the
current volume) and reports the conclusion that the more aged people
are removed from opportunities both to establish or maintain attachments and to utilize whatever inner resources they possess, the

more pathology will develop. In view of Bowlby's and my theories and studies, Fisk decided to study the effects of separation experiences on the elderly by using the Separation Anxiety Test.

Fisk developed two hypotheses for his study:

1. He hypothesized that there is a relationship between the purpose in life of the elderly and the locus of control orientation (external or internal) during a time when a change of residence has occurred in the lives of elderly subjects of his study. He devised seven subhypotheses for this major one.
2. He hypothesized that there is a relationship that exists between an experienced loss of one's personal life meaning with one's mental and physical well-being (deterioration or stability).

Based on his review of the literature, he began with the concept that those with external locus of control

. . . when they perceive their external environment as altered, to the extent that the creators and re-inforcers of meaning are no longer present, such a person discovers that he does not possess a personal purpose to, or reason for, his life that has been self-created. It is at this point that externalized people feel the events in their lives are beyond their control . . . loss of his outside re-inforcing agents will stimulate a loss of personal meaning, order, control and purpose in his life. Internalized people are not threatened by environmental change and will tend to feel they were the cause of it rather than its effect.

Fisk also considers the significant role of depression as a problem of the elderly. His studies of the theoretical, clinical and research literature (especially Jarvik, 1976 and Epstein, 1976) led him to believe that much of illness and disability in the elderly is psychologically induced, especially when depression is a significant factor. He corroborates this further by discussing the work of Engel and Ader (1967). Fisk addresses himself strongly to the issue of the growth of futility and hopelessness in the elderly as the background for his study and for its implication with regard to the loss of life meaning.

Fisk further discusses three theories of aging which he considered essential to his study: (a) Cumming and Henry (1961) believed in the concept of disengagement—the elderly seek decreased social interaction and welcome relaxation of responsibility and seek detachment from the stresses of society, (b) Dowd (1975) suggested an exchange theory, positing that because the future is shorter, they require greater recognition and acceptance of what they are and what they have contributed to life by having lived, and (c) the activity theory of Kuypers (1973) referring to the maintenance of self-worth and usefulness. The greatest support from the researchers, according to Fisk, has been given to the activity theory.

Using five retirement homes in the Greater Los Angeles area, he selected 47 elderly persons (later reduced to 41) ages 69 to 95 with a mean age of 82.25 years. All were either widowed or divorced. "Though most of the elderly were indigent, they comprised a rather homogeneous sample of lower to upper-middle class, unemployed whites." Fisk selected five self-report questionnaires, including the Internal-External Loss of Control Inventory (I-E L of C), the Purpose-in-Life Test, (PIL) the Semantic Differential (SD), the Hopkins Symptom Checklist (HSCL), and the Cornell Medical Index (CMI). The S.A.T. was the only projective test introduced into the study. No description of these tests will be provided here, and the reader is referred to the original study for such a description (pp. 74–87). The presentation here will deal largely with the results on the S.A.T., and the questionnaires will be referred to tangentially where pertinent.

The Hansburg Separation Anxiety Test was used in this study to provide an added dimension in examining mental well-being as it is compared to loss of meaning. As loss of life meaning was hypothecated to be associated with mental decline, any loss constitutes a separation and possible consequent trauma to one's normal mental functioning. The S.A.T. could tie together both attachment loss and its effect on mental well-being.

Fisk provides the results for 41 elderly persons on the S.A.T. in Table 14.1.

The greatest differences between the strong and mild responses occurred in attachment and painful tension, with nearly a 100% difference in the mean number of responses. This data suggested to Fisk that the need for attachment in these subjects is quite strong and the anguish of separation appears to be most overtly expressed in the category of painful tension (fear–anxiety–pain syndrome).

Another significant table added by Fisk is the comparison of the elderly's percentage of total responses to each of the nine response patterns of the S.A.T. with my criteria for weak, normal, and strong scores. Table 14.2 presents these data.

Fisk emphasized that the greatest effects of loss on the elderly in this study show up in the patterns of attachment need, separation-pain, self-love loss and absurdity. He made comparisons between Hansburg's study of the elderly with the S.A.T. and his own study. He stated that subjects in his study when compared to Hansburg's Group IV consisting of nursing home elderly were not unusually different but subjects in his study displayed a greater need for attachment, more self-deprecation and greater anguish over attachment loss than their counterparts in another retirement home.

Concentrating on the feeling of loss in his group of elderly, Fisk indicated (p. 174): "Depression was observed to be the psychological construct which increased to the greatest extent amongst the subjects over the three month testing period. Loss of meaning was correlated most highly with depression as well." The depressive factor appears far stronger in Fisk's elderly subjects (11.5 compared to 8.5) than in my own somewhat comparable Group IV. The most likely explanation is the difference in marital status. Fisk's group were all widowed or divorced while my group were only partially so. In Hansburg's tables the analysis of elderly subjects by marital status showed the greatest depressive factor among the widowed group. Fisk, apparently, overlooked this factor.

Another significant factor in Fisk's study is the testing of his group on entering the retirement home and again three months later. The re-testing with the Purpose-in-Life Test showed a considerable drop in the subjects' interest and purpose in life. Fisk stated, "Depression was observed to be the psychological construct which increased to the greatest

Table 14.1

MEANS, MEDIANS AND MODES FOR RESPONSES TO "MILD" AND
"STRONG" PICTURES ON THE SEPARATION ANXIETY TEST

Response Pattern	Mild Pictures			Strong Pictures		
	Mean	Median	Mode	Mean	Median	Mode
Attachment	4.90	4.29	3	8.44	8.25	5
Individuation	6.76	6.78	7	4.24	3.39	3
Hostility	2.90	2.43	2	4.95	4.44	4
Pain. Tension	3.43	2.29	0	6.71	5.40	7
Reality Avoid.	3.17	2.25	0	4.10	4.00	4
Conc. Imp.	2.59	2.31	0	2.00	1.36	0
Self-Love Loss	2.44	1.44	0	3.78	3.18	3
Ident. Stress	1.63	1.38	1	2.66	2.56	2
Absurdity	2.46	1.88	0	1.22	1.77	0

extent amongst the subjects over the three month testing period. Loss of meaning was correlated most highly with depression." This combination suggests that there is a relationship between the loss of attachment figures, the diminution of life purpose and depression in elderly widowed persons. I quote further from Fisk:

Depression occurs more frequently in old age than in any other age period (of life). It is more reactive than endogenous in that elderly people are likely to focus on a single traumatic event in their lives, usually a loss, which they believe is responsible for their despair. Life has lost its value and the resulting depression is a display of apathy rather than guilt. Geriatric depression seems to result more from external loss than from intrapsychic conflict. The experienced loss leaves an emptiness and feeling of meaninglessness in life.

This generalization is unnecessary. Individuals differ greatly in their reactions to loss, and in some, guilt may play a larger role. It is also well known that depression in old age is strongly related to loss in personal capabilities and sense of self and therefore should not be ignored as a significant factor.

Table 14.2

PERCENTAGE OF THE TOTAL RESPONSES TO EACH OF THE NINE RESPONSE
PATTERNS ON THE SEPARATION ANXIETY TEST PLUS HANSBURG'S
CRITERIA FOR WEAK, NORMAL, AND STRONG SCORES

Response Pattern	% of Total Response	Hansburg's Criteria			Response Pattern Classification
		Weak	Normal	Strong	
Attachment	26.8	20	20—25	25	S
Individuation	21.6	15	16—28	28	N
Hostility	14.0	12	12—14	14	N
Sep. Pain	17.6	15	15—17	17	S-N
Reality Avoid	12.6	10	10—13	13	N
Conc. Imp.	7.9	Below S.L.L.	Above S.L.L.	Much Above S.L.L.	L
Self-Love Loss	11.5	5	5—8	8	S
Identity Stress	5.7	10	10—14	14	L
Absurdity	5.1	—	0—3	3	S

Fisk was also impressed with the considerable degree of loneliness reported on the S.A.T. by his elderly subjects:

Loneliness was both the predominant response within the "attachment scale" as well as among the sixteen other constructs. Woodward, Gingles and Woodward (1974) defined loneliness as "the most devastating malady of the aged and seems to be their greatest concern" (p. 349). Loneliness is often the result of an inability to unite with another significant object or develop a new purpose in life. Farberow and Moriwaki (1975) found that unresolved loneliness was the major cause of suicides and suicidal attempts among the aged. If loneliness may be viewed as the inability to establish attachment due to some loss, then a deep sense of (self) rejection may arise which may cause one to withdraw and lose self-esteem.

Fisk also noted the frequency of absurd (relatively inappropriate) responses to the S.A.T. in his group of elderly. This coincides with Hansburg's findings, which were quite prevalent with absurd responses in Groups IV and V of the latter study. Having found a direct relationship between responses of absurdity and meaning loss (correlations with the Purpose-in-Life Test), Fisk stated:

As one loses a sense of self and questions the reason for one's existence, he withdraws from reality and from the painful stimuli responsible for such distress. In removing oneself from the aversive conditions, the need to be anxious diminishes and hence, the more one loses meaning and reality awareness, the less one experiences anxiety.

Fisk's data on the various tests, especially the Purpose-in-Life Test and the S.A.T., demonstrated what he believed to be a causative relationship

. . . between meaning loss and depression, anxiety and somatization. . . . The disruptions in one's understanding of meaning in life triggered by significant loss, creates a state in which chaotic confusion prevails. When life events occur to an individual who has suffered a loss of purpose, they (the events) become meaningless. One feels helpless to control them, hopeless in understanding them, fearful of their capacity to do harm and frightened at one's inability to act effectively on the environment. The development of physical ailments serves to protect an individual from interacting and perhaps, experiencing, greater anguish and torment. Hence, depression, anxiety and somatization appear as natural concomitants to meaning loss.

Fisk discussed correlations between the Hopkins Symptom Checklist and responses to the S.A.T. Here it was noted that there was a strong, significant correlation (+ .58 at the .01 level) between depression on the HSCL and self-love loss on the S.A.T. This result is further validation for the interpretation of the self-love loss percentage on the S.A.T. as a measure of the depressive syndrome (see Hansburg, Vol. II, 1980). Strong correlations were also found between absurd responses on the S.A.T. and depression on the HSCL, suggesting a relationship in the elderly between poor reality testing and depression.

The most significant correlation between loss of meaning on the Purpose-in-Life Test and the S.A.T. patterns was with the absurd responses (+ .46 at the .01 level). Loss of meaning seems strongly associated with poor reality testing and fuzzy thinking. Absurd responses had been observed in my study to be quite frequent in those who had been hospitalized for long periods (Group V in that study). Since self-love loss and absurd responses were so significantly associated with diminution in life meaning, the question of cause and effect needs to be raised. If separation from meaningful relationships tends to produce self-rejection, denigration, self-castigation and reality-contact losses, are these the essential ingredients of loss of life purpose and meaning? It would seem that loss of meaningful contacts tends to produce such a result. Fisk also introduced the factor of locus of control indicating that after three months in a retirement home, people who tend to externalize their locus of control (Rotter's test) show a greater loss of meaning although many internalizers will also show an increasing loss of meaning. Externalizers tend to adjust more poorly to a change of environment, but this appears not to be an essential ingredient of loss of life meaning.

In his conclusions Fisk agrees with Mayadas and Hink (1974):

. . . institutions for the elderly dehumanize the environment by collectivizing all activities and social functions in the home (p. 191). It appears that with an abrupt change in residence to a geriatric institution with a loss of meaning for people over 65 . . . the following behavioral effects could be expected. Feelings of hopelessness and lack of personal control over one's life plus a sense of resignation to the fact that, at best, existence will be only marginal, will be experienced. People able to function in their new environment will be motivated by adaptation needs rather than a sense of well being and may gradually withdraw losing some touch with reality. Heightened levels of anxiety, depression and somatization are associated with purpose-in-life decline, with a causal relationship possibly existing. . . . Depression . . . the most prevalent psychological state experienced by the subject population, may be related to a decline in reality orientation and has been associated with somatic discomfort. . . .

If the aged person can sincerely understand the meaning of his life, he may have a minimal amount of psychological and somatic disturbance, whereas an experienced dissolution of purpose is likely to cause great deterioration. . . . Failure to achieve a state of acceptance (life has been meaningful) leads to self-rejection and mental and physical degeneration (Kohlberg, 1973).

Therefore, Fisk recommends that "institutions for the elderly, and any agency serving an elderly population, embark on programs which emphasize individual achievement and satisfaction of the need for personal accomplishment."

REFERENCES

Bowlby, J. "Attachment Theory, Separation Anxiety and Mourning," in S. Arieti (ed.), *The American Handbook of Psychiatry*. New York: Basic Books, 1975.

Bellak, A. "Internal Locus of Control versus External Locus of Control and the Use of Self-Reinforcement." *Psychological Reports*, 1975, *31*, 723–733.

Camus, A. *The Myth of Sisyphus*. New York: Random House, 1955.

Crumbaugh, J., and Maholick, L. "An Experimental Study in Existentialism: The Psychometric Approach to Frankel's Concept of Neogenic Neuroses." *Journal of Clinical Psychology*, 1964, *20*, 200–207.

Cumming, E., and Henry, W. *Growing Old*. New York: Basic Books, 1961.

Dowd, J. "Aging as Exchange: A Preface to Theory." *Journal of Gerontology*, 1975, *30*, 584–594.

Engel, G., and Ader, R. "Psychological Factors in Organic Disease." *Mental Health Program Reports*, 1967, *1*, 1–25.

Epstein, L. "Depression in the Elderly." *Journal of Gerontology*, 1976, *31*, 278–282.

Farberow, N., and Moriwaki, S. "Self-Destructive Crises in the Older Person." *The Gerontologist*, 1975, *15*, 333–337.

Fisk, P. C. *The Effect of Loss of Meaning on the Mental and Physical Well-Being of the Aged*. Unpublished doctoral dissertation, California School of Professional Psychology, Los Angeles, 1979.

Frankl, V. *Man's Search for Meaning*. New York: Simon and Schuster, 1959.

Hansburg, H. G. *Adolescent Separation Anxiety*, Vol. I. Springfield, Ill.: C. C. Thomas, 1972. Reprinted, Melbourne, Fla.: R. E. Krieger, 1980.

Hansburg, H. G. "Separation Disorders of the Elderly," unpublished manuscript, 1979 (published in this book).

Hansburg, H. G. *Adolescent Separation Anxiety*, Vol. II. Melbourne, Fla.: R. E. Krieger, 1980.

Jarvik, L. "Aging and Depression: Some Unanswered Questions." *Journal of Gerontology*, 1976, *31*, 324–326.

Kohlberg, L. "Stages and Aging in Moral Development." *The Gerontologist*, 1973, *13*, 497–501.

Kuypers, J. "Social Breakdown and Competence: A Mode of Normal Aging." *Human Development*, 1973, *16*, 181–201.

Mayadas, N., and Hink, D. "Group Work with the Aged." *The Gerontologist*, 1974, *14*, 440–445.

Phares, E. "Perceptual Threshold Decrements as a Function of Skill and Chance Expectancies." *Journal of Psychology*, 1962, *53*, 399–407.

Rotter, J. "Generalized Expectancies for Internal versus External Locus of Control or Reinforcements." *Psychological Monographs*, 1966, *80*, 1–23.

Woodward, H., Gingles, R., and Woodward, G. "Loneliness and the Elderly as Related to Housing." *The Gerontologist*, 1974, *14*, 349–351.

Wolk, S., and Ducette, J. "Locus of Control and Extreme Behavior." *Journal of Consulting and Clinical Psychology*, 1972, *39*, 129–131.

Yarnell, T. "Purpose-in-Life Test: Further Correlates." *Journal of Individual Psychology*, 1975, *47*, 76–79.

SECTION TWO

Before the reader proceeds to Black's paper on the reliability of the S.A.T., some orientation to significant elements in his paper and to certain unresolved questions is in order. While other studies reported in this volume have indicated the usefulness, reliability, and validity of the S.A.T., Black's study was the most intensive one to date. Not only did the internal consistency coefficients prove to be very close to those obtained in the original study in 1966–1969 (Hansburg, 1972, p. 50), but the test-retest (after six months) reliability also remained generally high for most of the test systems despite some minor problems with the internal consistency and the test-retest reliability of the individuation system. Further, by juxtaposing the Spielberger A-State and A-Trait Tests, Black established that the S.A.T. measures some characteristics which are more profound and more stable and less influenced by temporary states of anxiety or stress.

The problem of the categories described in Volume II of *Adolescent Separation Anxiety* is another matter. Here, there were apparently some misinterpretations of the detailed characteristics of these categories. For example, the anxious attachment category states that the "pain percentage exceeds the normal range" and also indicates that the "hostility percentage exceeds the normal range." Actually, in the original formulation, the pain and hostility percentages were combined and the 30% or higher level for this combination was established as a factor of anxious attachment. Furthermore, the original study included the factor of excessive defensiveness, that is, the combination of withdrawal, evasion, and fantasy, and Black did not include this item. Errors of interpretation of this sort appear in other categories. In addition, the category of anxious attachment was not differentiated into three groups—mild, strong, and severe—as was intended in the original study. These differences in interpretation suggest that a replication study is necessary if we are to retain a strict interpretation of the categories.

What is most interesting, however, is Black's interpretation of what in the original work was entitled the "depressive syndrome." His concept actually almost completely describes the category of anxious attachment if we eliminate item (a). He found this category to be a stable one in the test-retest correlations (.698). In my interpretation it would indicate stability for the anxious attachment category. The depressive syndrome was largely indicated by a higher self-love loss pattern than the self-esteem preoccupation pattern.

Regarding the issue Black raises as to the irrationality of some responses provided for the mild pictures (some of Black's subjects complained about these responses), actually, this manner of presentation was deliberate and was intended to measure the discriminating power and sensitivity to high stressful responsiveness in a mild situation. Obviously, a person who recognizes this absurdity is reacting healthily. Those who respond with such strong reactions in mild situations show evidences of disturbance, usually in the anxious attachment area. Similarly, mild responses to strong pictures indicate the opposite. It is, of course, possible to add some mild anxiety responses that might be considered more appropriate for the mild pictures, but I suspect that this could reduce the effectiveness of the test and its discriminating power.

Black's suggestion with regard to the revision of the individuation pattern raises several questions. Consider the fact that the individuation system did so well in defining differences between numbers of groups in some of the aforementioned studies (Miller, 1980; Kaleita, 1980; Burger, 1981; Levitz, 1982; Brody, 1981; etc.) Further, in my original study *(Adolescent Separation Anxiety,* Vol. I), the individuation pattern was negatively correlated with every other pattern, making it considerably useful as a differentiating factor. Also, in my analysis of separation disorders, the individuation pattern was very helpful in discerning the condition of detachment. Nevertheless, Black has a point here; it could be possible to increase the discriminating power of this pattern by changing the wording of one or two of the items which make up the individuation pattern. This would require a reworking of the statistical and clinical bases for the test. Perhaps such changes could be reserved for a time when the entire test goes through some revision, which might well be undertaken by a doctoral candidate.

It should also be noted that Black accomplished a degree of validation for the S.A.T. by correlating with the Spielberger A-State and A-Trait Tests. The differences appear in the nature of what these tests measure. It seems likely that we can posit that the S.A.T. measures degrees of anxious attachment and detachment and thus the characteristic manner in which individuals handle separation experiences.

15

The Reliability of the Separation Anxiety Test: A Study by Hugh M. Black

The following is a condensed version of a doctoral dissertation entitled "Trait Anxiety and Separation Distress: Analysis of Two Measures in Parents and Their Adolescent Children." This summary of the dissertation was written by Dr. Black and is given here in its entirety at his request. The original dissertation was completed at the California School of Professional Psychology in Los Angeles in 1981.

INTRODUCTION

Observation of children and their relationship with maternal figures led John Bowlby to posit his Attachment Theory, which he presented in his volumes entitled *Attachment and Loss* (1969, 1973, 1980). The need for some instrument to measure variables such as implied by attachment theory for research and clinical predictions had already been recognized by Henry Hansburg (1972). He developed a semi-projective measure of responsiveness to separation stress using his prior clinical insights and adapting some of those of Mahler (1967), Bowlby (1969), Witkin (1965) and White (1963). He theorized that his Separation Anxiety Test would reflect various classes of projected reactions, thus linking patterns of responses. Because of this, the S.A.T. can be scored "objectively" and norms can be established, permitting comparison with other quantitative measures of anxiety.

Hansburg's (1972) pilot research with the S.A.T. using 221

children and adolescents provided strong indications that the S.A.T. generated a relatively comprehensive view of the subject's characterological vulnerability to separation stress. Continued use of the S.A.T. in a clinical setting and only afterwards looking at social histories and psychological and psychiatric evaluations determined the value of the S.A.T. The results of these studies suggested that the S.A.T. was highly predictive of clinical findings. It promised to provide a dimension to evaluations that markedly enhanced their scope. Since that time the S.A.T. has provided data predicted by attachment theory when used with adolescents, younger children and geriatric patients, adults and family systems, thus providing evidence of its additional utility.

However, as of 1980 the S.A.T. had not been sufficiently tested to estimate the degree to which test results are affected by systematic sources of variance. Its recognition as a research or diagnostic tool first required that estimates be obtained of its internal consistency and stability over time when used with both parents and adolescents (APA standards for educational and psychological tests, 1974). Hansburg (1972) had administered an earlier version of his measure to 75 children in residential treatment centers. Split-half reliabilities were obtained for each of the 16 items. The consistency coefficients ranged from .34 to .74, and the consistency of total responses, odd vs. even numbered pictures, was .885. Since in most items a difference in responsiveness is expected on strong vs. mild pictures, and since there are two strong pictures in the odd group and four in the even, these figures were surprisingly high. However, the final version of the S.A.T. had not been tested for internal consistency, and no estimate of temporal stability had been performed.

Hansburg's (1972, 1980) claims for the utility of the S.A.T. imply that it reflects relatively enduring personality characteristics. Projective and semi-projective measures have generally low retest reliability, due in part to the difficulty in standardizing the method of administration, scoring and interpretation. However, the S.A.T. can be thoroughly standardized in these areas.

Retest studies of Rosenzweig's Picture-Frustration Study with intervals of two months and seven and one-half months (Rosenzweig, Ludwig, and Adelman, 1975) produced coefficients between .21 and .71. Studies of the Myers-Briggs Type Indicator (which purports to operationalize Jung's theory of type) with intervals of seven weeks to 14 months (Carskadon, 1977) produced reliability between .48 and .87 for the various scales. Research on the temporal stability of the Family Story Test with a 10-day interval (Kelly and Berg, 1978), which is described as a "structured-projective," provided coefficients ranging from .32 to .7, with total test reliability of .73. Rorschach retest reliability coefficients have been reported on various test factors over a wide range. A well-standardized study of 19 variables, determinants and ratios in the Rorschach over a three-year period (Exner, Armbruster, and Viglione, 1978) yielded correlations of .66 to .9, with a mean of .79. A mean of ratio reliabilities, which resembles more closely the percentages of the S.A.T., was .83. Each of these tests appeared to measure different levels of personality and to produce higher reliability according to the stability and depth of the personality dimensions measured.

If the S.A.T. is to be regarded as a measure of relatively stable dimensions of personality structure, it should yield retest reliabilities that reflect characterological traits rather than ephemeral states. Therefore, in estimating the temporal stability of the S.A.T., [I (Black) decided on] the simultaneous administration of an instrument widely used to measure temporary states of anxiety and the characterological proclivity to experience those states, for comparison. This instrument is known as the State-Trait Anxiety Inventory (STAI).

Spielberger, Gorsuch and Luchene published the STAI, a self-report measure of trait and state anxiety, in 1970. It consists of 20 items, each rated on a four-point scale, describing the present experience of anxiety (A-state), and 20 items similarly rated describing the subject's usual feelings (A-trait). Five years were devoted to developing this instrument, with items carefully selected after numerous testings. By 1980 the scales had been used in more than 1,000 studies (Spielberger, 1980), demonstrating its wide research utility. STAI test-retest reliabilities after one hour of tension-inducing tasks, after 20 days, and after 104 days ranged from .73 to .86 for A-trait and .16 to .54 for A-state. A 10-month interval test-retest study (Newmark, 1972) indicated A-trait reliability of .68 and A-state reliability of .28, as the theory would predict. Three studies done by Joesting (1975, 1976, 1977) in which the STAI was administered before and after examinations revealed significant differences between A-Trait and A-State stabilities as predicted. No sex differences were found in either scale.

The stability over time of the S.A.T. systems should not be less than that of A-trait, as the S.A.T. purports to measure personality dynamics more deeply seated, and thus presumably more stable, than self-report. A test-retest study of the S.A.T., administered concurrently with the STAI, was thought to permit the comparison of variance in the S.A.T. with A-trait and A-state variance, providing an estimate of the stability of the personality factors measured by the S.A.T. in comparison with a well-studied scale.

The S.A.T. purportedly measures personality dynamics that were given their basic formation in childhood, and Hansburg (1980) has stated that it is fundamentally a measure of vulnerability to separation trauma. Furthermore, in administering the S.A.T., subjects are asked if they have ever experienced what is depicted and to imagine what the depicted child would experience. Hansburg stated that subjects who report they have experienced more of the separation events of the S.A.T. are more likely to show traumatization in their protocol. Therefore, the S.A.T. may be relatively sensitive to recent and lifetime traumatic stress experiences. The occurrence of such experiences between testings may interfere with the accurate measure of the S.A.T.'s stability.

Holmes and Rahe (1967) developed a scale for making quantitative judgments about the magnitude of "stressful life events." From past research, a list of 43 items associated with significant change in life patterns was developed and used systematically with more than 5,000 patients. Each patient was asked to rate each event according to the amount of social readjustment required, irrespective of the event's desirability. Marriage was used as the criterion, and other events were rated in comparison to it. Children's ratings of the stressfulness of experience have also been studied (Yamamoto, 1979), indicating that children in Grades 4–6 assess stressfulness in a discriminating manner, often in disagreement with adult assessments of their stress.

Research by Paykel (1974) provided data indicating that events associated with loss over which the subjects had little control were significantly related to the onset of depression within a six-month period. Paykel produced his own list of 61 life events for this study, and asked his subjects to rate them according to "how upsetting the event would be to the average person" (p. 149). In the upper quartile of Paykel's rating, 15 of the 18 events were associated with loss or serious threat of loss. Also on the Social Readjustment Rating Scale (Holmes and Rahe, 1967), 15 of the 21 items with highest mean scores are separation events.

Therefore, a scale constructed on this model using these and other items associated with loss or threat of loss was thought to be the most appropriate measure of intertest stress for the determination of S.A.T. test-retest reliability and sensitivity to separation stress. Rahe (1975) stated that in prospective studies it is more helpful to have subjective estimates of the stressfulness of an event rather than a standardized estimate. The subjects in this study rated each event for stressfulness.

Studies by Paykel (1974) and by Roskies, Iida-Miranda, and Strobel (1977) suggest that events over which the subject has little or no control are responded to with ratings of greatest emotional distress. Thus, for this study, subjects were asked to rate events as occurring against their wishes. Separate scales of separation events were constructed for parents and adolescents. Seventeen of the 32 items used for the parents' form in this study were taken from Holmes and Rahe's scale, while eight were taken from Paykel's list of events associated with depression (1974). The remaining seven were taken from questions used in recent research on separation anxiety (especially DeLozier, 1979, and Miller, 1980). On the adolescents' form, 11 of the 31 items were adapted from Holmes and Rahe, seven from Paykel, four from the questionnaires mentioned above, and nine from the suggestions obtained by the experimenter from teenage consultants who were within the age range of the sample and lived in the same vicinity. Since no previous adaptation of Holmes and Rahe's scale for separation stress has been published, this adaptation was employed.

Tables 15.1 and 15.2 list the test-retest reliabilities of the values with which subjects rated each event in this study. All the correlations are significantly different from zero with the exception of "Loss of a personally valuable article" among adolescents. Overall temporal reliability of the values by which each event was rated was .56 for the adolescent inventory and .79 for the parent inventory. However, further validation is necessary before this adaptation can be regarded as accurately measuring separation stress. In this study, after subjects rated each event for individual degrees of "stressfulness," they were instructed to mark those that had occurred in their lifetime and in the six months prior to the first administration. On the second administration, they rated the same events and were instructed to mark those that occurred between testings.

Table 15.1

STRESS INVENTORY FREQUENCIES, MEANS AND TEST-RETEST CORRELATIONS OF EVENT SELF-EVALUATIONS

(Adolescent Form)

Life Events	Frequencies		Mean Values	Test-Retest Pearson R	
	Lifetime	Between Tests			
Rejected by a group of friends[d] (criterion event)	26	11	50	1.00	
Fired from your job[a]	8	4	52	.41	
Brother or sister hospitalized[a]	28	4	71	.41	
A parent threatens to leave you[c]	11	2	84	.29	
More arguments with your parents[b]	46	29	61	.43	
First day at a new school where you know nobody[a]	47	2	47	.69	
Death of a close friend[a]	11	3	84	.33	
Loss of a personally valuable article (not significant)[b]	37	20	51	.21	$(p > .05)$
A teacher's expression of disappointment in you or your work[b]	46	23	47	.35	
Put on probation for possession of drugs[d]	0	0	71	.34	
Hospitalized for injury or illness[a]	22	3	62	.51	
Change in residence of your family[a]	34	0	50	.37	
Death or loss of a pet[c]	54	15	67	.44	
Eliminated for a team you were trying out for[d]	21	8	49	.37	
Serious illness of parent[a]	15	4	86	.37	
Close friend moving out of state[b]	26	8	63	.42	
Death of a close family member (such as a grandparent)[a]	39	6	82	.39	
Turned down for a date[d]	8	9	54	.40	
Death of a parent[a]	0	0	95	.65	
Leaving home for college or to live in your own apartment[b]	1	0	47	.46	
Flunk a required course[d]	13	5	71	.41	
Having a tooth pulled[c]	37	5	30	.61	
Quarrel with a close friend[c]	55	40	51	.63	
Driver's license revoked for one month or more[d]	0	0	51	.42	
Parental separation or divorce[a]	0	1	83	.63	
One parent away from home for one month or more[b]	12	3	62	.24	

(continued)

(Table 15.1 *continued*)

Life Events	Frequencies		Mean Values	Test-Retest Pearson *R*
	Lifetime	Between Tests		
Rejected when you tried to make a friend[d]	23	9	53	.66
Family financial difficulties[a]	20	7	55	.58
Breaking up with a steady date[b]	27	9	65	.57
A parent's threat to commit suicide[c]	2	0	90	.32
Decision to stop associating with a group of friends[d]	35	16	55	.53
TOTAL INVENTORY				.56

[a]Adapted from Holmes and Rahe's scale.
[b]Adapted from Paykel's scale.
[c]Adapted from recent research on separation.
[d]Provided by adolescent consultants.

Table 15.2

STRESS INVENTORY FREQUENCIES, MEANS AND TEST-RETEST CORRELATIONS OF EVENT SELF-EVALUATIONS

(Parent Form)

Life Events	Frequencies		Mean Values	Test-Retest Pearson *R*
	Lifetime	Between Tests		
Fired from your job[a] (criterion event)	12	2	50	1.00
Serious quarrel with a long-time close friend[c]	28	4	53	.61
Change in residence[a]	55	0	40	.71
Death of a member of your family of origin (parent, etc.)[a]	40	4	79	.46
Son drafted[b]	3	1	62	.72
Trouble with your boss[a]	21	8	41	.58
Sexual difficulties[a]	23	4	53	.75
One of your children injured in a bike or auto accident[a]	33	3	79	.65
Having a tooth pulled[c]	51	1	27	.66
Threat of spouse to commit suicide[c]	3	1	85	.41
Angry quarrels with one of your children[b]	52	31	55	.61
Stillbirth[b]	5	0	65	.77
Serious illness or injury to yourself[a]	22	3	65	.64
Son or daughter leaving home[a]	20	5	55	.62
Jail term[a]	0	0	83	.49
Death of your spouse[a]	1	0	94	.43

(Table 15.2 *continued*)

Life Events	Frequencies		Mean Values	Test-Retest Pearson R
	Lifetime	Between Tests		
Amputation of an arm or leg[c]	1	0	80	.79
Marital separation or divorce[a]	6	1	86	.61
Lawsuit[b]	13	3	59	.63
Son or daughter withdrawing from family life into the drug culture[c]	0	1	86	.62
Loss of a personally valuable article[b]	29	3	37	.53
Death of a close friend[a]	31	4	65	.64
Major financial problems[a]	16	3	64	.57
Infidelity of spouse[b]	6	1	77	.67
Death or loss of a pet[a]	54	9	41	.86
Foreclosure of a mortgage or loan[a]	1	0	62	.70
Increase in number of arguments with spouse[a]	27	8	60	.63
Demotion at work[a]	3	1	52	.55
Intimate friend moving to another state[b]	32	4	37	.62
Unmarried daughter's pregnancy[b]	1	0	65	.71
Threat of your spouse to leave you[c]	13	2	75	.60
Family member hospitalized for illness or injury[a]	51	9	66	.71
TOTAL INVENTORY				.79

[a]Taken from Holmes and Rahe's scale.   [c]Adapted from recent research on separation.

[b]Taken from Paykel's scale.

PROCEDURE

Between August 1980 and April 1981, an internal consistency and test-retest reliability study (with a six-month interval) of the S.A.T. was performed using 69 families residing in and around the San Fernando Valley, Los Angeles. Families were approached through churches and temples of various denominations. Thirty "intact," English-speaking families in which an adolescent age 13–16 lived with both natural parents were obtained in this way. Two families were referred by a personal friend of the experimenter. An additional 37 intact families were subsequently obtained from referral by families who had already consented to participate. Subjects belonged to a wide range of denominations and varied in their church attendance from zero to 100 times during the last year. One hundred twenty-two subjects indicated they were of the white/Anglo group, nine were "Latin," three were American Indian, and four classified themselves "other."

Pairs made up of a child and a parent were selected from each family. Difference in type of pair (mother-son, mother-daughter, father-son, father-daughter) was not a variable in this study; however, at least 15 pairs of each type were selected to provide ample representation. Membership in the same family made the investigation a "family project" and helped ensure each subject's retest availability.

The 30 families obtained from ministers volunteered in different ways. Three ministers volunteered their own families. Four families volunteered as the result of pulpit announcements or bulletin notices, but the majority of minister-referred families were approached personally by the ministers or by letter. Sixteen families were obtained from minister-referred families, and 21 families were obtained from referrals by these families. In obtaining families not minister-referred, preference was given to those families who did not regularly attend church services or belong to a church organization to avoid obtaining a sample biased because of religious orientation. Fifty subjects attended church services 10 times a year or less, and 84 subjects did not claim membership in any church organization. In this way, over-representation by subjects with strong religious affiliation was hopefully avoided. The 69 subject families reflect approximately 50 percent of the families who were referred. Other referral families declined to participate, usually because of lack of time or interest.

While the use of this population is a more straightforward test of theory, it provided data regarding but one segment of the American population. Furthermore, because the subjects were approached individually and requested to participate in the study, an unknown source of possible systematic variance may have been introduced into the selection of subjects to a greater extent than if subjects were obtained on a random basis from the general population. However, this seemed to be a viable selection procedure.

While Hansburg (1972) originally administered the revised S.A.T. to a sample whose age range was 11–14, this study employed a sample of children age 13–16, and their parents. All of the children in this study had reached the onset of sexual maturation by most accepted age-appropriate standards of adolescence. Thus, differences between adolescent and preadolescent children on the measures administered were eliminated. Seniors in high school were not tested because of the uniqueness of the separation threats that many may have imminently faced, such as moving away from home after graduation.

Children who did not live with both natural parents or whose natural parents had been legally separated or divorced from one another during the child's lifetime were eliminated. A particular trauma of the kind caused by departure or death of a natural parent might have introduced variables beyond the scope of the study. This investigation focused on "non-clinical" families as preliminary to any investigations on the effects of various kinds of treatments in S.A.T. scores. "Non-clinical" as defined for the purpose of this study meant the absence in the immediate family of anyone who in the year previous to the beginning of data collection had been in treatment for psychiatric or behavior disorders or received psychotropic medication. The term implied no judgment about the mental health of the subjects. It was felt that subjects currently undergoing some form of psychotherapy or psychiatric treatment may respond differently from test to retest due to the effect of the treatment.

After the family had agreed to participate in the study, the experimenter visited the family home to explain the purposes and requirements of the research. The experimenter described the research, and the parents made the decision as to which one would participate. All subjects were then instructed to answer all the questions on a screening questionnaire. While no attempt was made to assess reading ability in terms of grade level, any potential subject who could not complete the questionnaire would have been dropped from the study. (No subject complained of difficulties in completing those measures or in understanding the directions.)

Each questionnaire was separately scanned when finished to see whether each subject understood the questions and whether all questions were answered. By means of this screening procedure, two families were dropped from the original sample of 71 families, one because a family member was receiving psychotropic medication and one because the adolescent had been adopted. Eligible families were told that an administrator would contact them in the near future. Four administrators, including the experimenter, were used to administer the measures. All 69 families were retested within plus or minus 30 days of the six-month anniversary of the first administration. Both administrations were done in each family's home to avoid possible effects introduced by another location.

At the end of the second administration, subjects were asked to fill out a debriefing form. Included in this form was a straightforward questionnaire to make some assessment of memory effects. While the procedure is admittedly less accurate than asking each subject what pictures and responses he/she remembered from the first administration before the second administration, it also does not contaminate responses or introduce unknown variance.

RESULTS

Test data were analyzed by ANOVA tests for possible systematic variance emanating from sample characteristics or administrative procedures. The variables tested included family role (adolescent or parent), age of adolescent, income of parent, sex, religion (Jewish, Catholic, or Protestant), church attendance in the past year, membership in a church organization, ethnicity (Caucasian vs. all others), order of administration (S.A.T. first or STAI first), and administrator. Some significant relationships were discovered. Adolescents reported significantly higher A-trait scores than did parents. Due to this finding, adolescent and parent A-trait scores were not combined but were tested separately on subsequent analyses involving A-Trait. Females had significantly higher scores on the S.A.T. pain system at both administrations than males. Therefore, males' and females' S.A.T. pain system sores were analyzed separately on subsequent analyses involving this variable.

Furthermore, a positive correlation significantly different from zero was found between parent income and parents' scores on the S.A.T. individuation system. However, the correlation coefficients were low (Administration I: r = .28; Administration II: r = .27) and accounted for less than 8% of the variability in parents' scores on that system. Since only half of the sample was so influenced, and since the correlations were low, it was thought unnecessary to statistically control this relationship. No correlations significantly different from zero were obtained between scores on the measure used to test the effect of memory on S.A.T. responses and test-retest differences in S.A.T. systems or scales.

Two subjects gave a total of less than 15 responses to the S.A.T. Scores derived from such a total are thought to be only tentatively interpretable (Hansburg, 1980). Since this study was designed in terms of adolescent-parent pairs, all the scores of both members of each of the two families were eliminated from the study.

The internal reliability of total S.A.T. responses was .86, which is similar to the figure of .885 obtained in a split-half reliability test of the unrevised S.A.T. done by Hansburg (1972). This study provided a "modified split-half" analysis, as Schafer and Jones (1977) suggested in measuring the internal consistency of instruments composed of heterogeneous factors and items. "Well-chosen" splits, or comparisons of equivalent items, is the appropriate method for testing the internal reliability of the S.A.T. The 12 S.A.T. pictures were divided into two groups to perform a matched-half analysis of internal consistency. Each of the two groups had three strong and three mild pictures. The agreement of a clinical psychologist skilled in the scoring of the S.A.T. and the experimenter was obtained for the matched halves (see Table 15.3).

Internal reliability coefficients of total responses to mild and strong pictures and to systems, subsystems and scales are presented in

Table 15.3

S.A.T. PICTURE TITLES: MATCHED-HALVES

Group I	Group 2
MILD PICTURES	
IV The child is leaving his/her mother to go to school	II The boy/girl is being transferred to a new class
V The child is leaving his/her parents to go to camp	III The family is moving to a new neighborhood
VII The boy/girl's older brother is a sailor leaving on a voyage	IX The mother has just put this child to bed
STRONG PICTURES	
I The boy/girl will live permanently with his/her grandmother and without his/her parents	VIII The judge is placing the child in an institution
VI After an argument with the mother, the father is leaving	XII The boy/girl is running away from home
X The boy/girl's mother is being taken to the hospital	XI The boy/girl and his/her father are standing at the mother's coffin

Table 15.4. Matched-half reliability correlations for S.A.T. systems, except for the individuation system, exceeded .70. Scale reliability correlations, excluding empathy, well-being, sublimation, anger and anxiety, exceeded .50. Internal consistency for the pain system and its scales was also calculated for each sex separately, since a significant difference on this dimension had been noted (see above). However, noticeable differences in internal consistency between males and females was noted only on the anxiety scale, with both scores below .50.

A further matched-half reliability analysis was performed for the responses to mild and strong pictures for each S.A.T. scale to determine

Table 15.4

S.A.T. MATCHED-HALF RELIABILITY (Pearson R)

Total Separation Anxiety Test	r = .86
Total Mild Pictures	r = .78
Total Strong Pictures	r = .76
Attachment System	r = .73
Loneliness Scale	r = .63
Empathy Scale	r = .41
Rejection Scale	r = .67
Individuation System	r = .67
Adaptation Scale	r = .62
Well-Being Scale	r = .40
Sublimation Scale	r = .34
Hostility System	r = .73
Anger Scale	r = .47
Projection Scale	r = .56
Intrapunitiveness Scale	r = .61
Pain System	r = .71
Anxiety Scale	r = .37
(Males)	r = .43
(Females)	r = .33
Phobic Reaction Scale	r = .52
Somatic Pain Scale	r = .75
Defensiveness System	r = .73
Withholding Scale	r = .57
Evasion Scale	r = .63
Fantasy Scale	r = .69
Self-Evaluation System	r = .77
Self-Esteem Subsystem	r = .62
Self-Love Loss Subsystem	r = .74
Identity Scale	r = .52
Impaired Concentration Scale	r = .67

which parts of any scale might be most fruitfully reviewed for possible revision. Frequencies were tested in chi square contingency tables, and all were found to be significantly related except for anxiety responses on mild pictures. Given the extremely limited range of responses (0 to 3) possible on the mild or strong pictures of each scale, this degree of internal consistency appears substantially high.

Test-retest differences in S.A.T. systems and scales were first compared with the "stress difference score." The stress difference score was obtained by calculating the difference between the stress scores reported for the six months preceding the first administration and the stress scores reported between administrations of the S.A.T., in order to control the systematic variance expected from this source. However, no correlations significantly different from zero were found. Subjects used one separation event as a standard for determining the degree of stress for each other event. This standard event may have had a different meaning for each person, which might call into question the comparability of stress scores across subjects. Therefore, the mean scores across subjects for each event were calculated. However, stress difference scores obtained from individual scores calculated from the mean values also provided no evidence of any correlation significantly different from zero between stress differences and S.A.T. systems differences from test to retest.

Table 15.5 presents test-retest correlations on all S.A.T. systems, sub-systems and scales. Temporal stability for the pain system and its scales was also calculated for each sex separately, since a significant difference on this variable had been noted (see above). Noticeable differences between the sexes were detected only on the pain system as a whole and on the somatic pain scale. Test-retest correlations for A-state and A-trait of the STAI and for Mental Set scores (the number of pictured events subjects reported that had happened in their lives) are also indicated for comparison. All of the S.A.T. systems except for the individuation system have test-retest correlations higher than that of A-trait.

In developing the use of the S.A.T., Hansburg (1979) identified six separation disorders from his experience with patients and their protocols. They are derived from criteria which in most cases involve Hansburg's quartile norms (see Tables 15.6 and 15.7). The criteria for diagnostic syndromes as defined in this study were taken directly from his description of the syndromes.

Hansburg's diagnostic categories proved considerably less stable than the S.A.T. systems for this sample (see Table 15.8). Using Hansburg's criteria, 30 subjects were classified in two categories. Each of the two categories of all 30 subjects was analyzed for stability over time. Therefore, each of these 30 subjects was analyzed twice for temporal stability of diagnostic category. All but two of these subjects were

Table 15.5

TEST-RETEST RELIABILITY (Pearson R)

Total Separation Anxiety Test	$r = .84$
Total Mild Pictures	$r = .82$
Total Strong Pictures	$r = .70$
Mental Set Responses	$r = .65$
STAI/A-State	$r = .47$
STAI/A-Trait	$r = .73$
Attachment System	$r = .77$
Loneliness Scale	$r = .68$
Empathy Scale	$r = .62$
Rejection Scale	$r = .69$
Individuation System	$r = .61$
Adaptation Scale	$r = .56$
Well-Being Scale	$r = .70$
Sublimation Scale	$r = .48$
Hostility System	$r = .81$
Anger Scale	$r = .69$
Projection Scale	$r = .70$
Intrapunitiveness Scale	$r = .73$
Pain System	$r = .76$
(Males)	$r = .67$
(Females)	$r = .80$
Anxiety Scale	$r = .66$
Phobic Reaction Scale	$r = .67$
Somatic Pain Scale	$r = .73$
(Males)	$r = .36$
(Females)	$r = .82$
Defensiveness System	$r = .78$
Withholding Scale	$r = .66$
Evasion Scale	$r = .70$
Fantasy Scale	$r = .64$
Self-Evaluation System	$r = .80$
Self-Esteem Subsystem	$r = .61$
Self-Love Loss Subsystem	$r = .79$
Identity Scale	$r = .69$
Impaired Concentration Scale	$r = .67$

Table 15.6

"NORMAL RANGE" FOR S.A.T. SYSTEMS

Systems	Normal Range
Scales	
Attachment System	20-25%
Loneliness	
Empathy	
Rejection[a]	
Individuation System	16-28%
Adaptation	
Well-Being	
Sublimation[a]	
Hostility System	12-24%
Anger	
Projection	
Intrapunitiveness[a]	
Pain System	15-17%
Anxiety	
Phobic reaction	
Somatic pain	
Defensiveness	10-13%
Withdrawal	
Evasion	
Fantasy	
Self-Evaluative System	
(a) Identity Subsystem	10-14%
Identity Stress	(age 13 and older)
(b) Self-Esteem Subsystem	percentage higher
Impaired concentration	than self-love loss
Sublimation[a]	
(c) Self-love Loss Subsystem	5-8%
Rejection[a]	
Intrapunitiveness[a]	

[a]Scale used more than once

Table 15.7

DIAGNOSTIC CATEGORIES

I. Anxious attachment

  1. attachment percentage exceeds the normal range[a]

  2. pain percentage exceeds the normal range[a]
  3. plus one of the following:

      a. More attachment than individuation responses on mild pictures[a]
      b. hostility percentage exceeds the normal range

      c. more self-love loss than self-esteem responses[a]
      d. identity stress percentage above or below the normal range

II. Hostile attachment

  1. attachment percentage exceeds the normal range[a]

  2. pain percentage exceeds the normal range[a]
  3. more hostility than pain responses

III. Hostile detachment

  1. individuation percentage above the normal range
  2. defensiveness percentage above the normal range
  3. more hostility than attachment responses

IV. Dependent detachment

  1. attachment percentage below the normal range

  2. individuation percentage below the normal range[a]

V. Excessive self-sufficiency

  1. more individuation than attachment responses over the entire test
  2. more individuation than attachment responses on strong pictures

VI. Depression

  1. the presence of at least four of the following:[b]
      a. self-love loss exceeds the normal range

      b. self-love loss exceeds self-esteem[a]

      c. individuation percentage below the normal range[a]

      d. more attachment than individuation responses on mild pictures[a]
      e. hostility plus pain percentages exceed 30% of the total
      f. defensiveness percentage exceeds normal range
      g. identity stress percentage exceeds normal range

---

[a]Criteria used more than once.

[b]This standard was adopted by the experimenter because Hansburg was not
explicit regarding the number of criteria necessary to place subjects in
the depressed category.

diagnosed both "anxiously attached" and "depressed." Forty percent (n = 12) of those who had double diagnoses on the first administration had double diagnoses on the second. The "depressed" diagnosis appeared to be the most stable and the most frequent: 46% (n = 63) of the sample had a diagnosis of "depressed" at the first administration, and 70% (n = 44) of that group were "depressed" at the second administration.

Only two subjects, from different families, scored within Hansburg's criteria for "normal" on all S.A.T. systems at first administration, and neither subject did so at the second administration. Fifty subjects (37% of the sample) did not meet the criteria for any diagnostic category at the first administration and also did not score within the norms. Of these, 29 (58%) fit no diagnostic category at the second administration. Of the 34 subjects who were diagnosed "anxious attached" at the first administration, 38% (n = 13) were so diagnosed at the second administration, and of the nine subjects diagnosed "dependent detached" at the first administration, 22% (n = 2) were so diagnosed at the second.

Table 15.8

TEST-RETEST STABILITY: DIAGNOSTIC CATEGORIES

Category	Administration I	Administration II	Proportion in the Same Category
Anxious Attached	34	13	.382
Hostile Attached	2	1	.50
Hostile Detached	0	empty cell	
Dependent Detached	9	2	.222
Excessively Self-Sufficient	4	0	.00
Depressed	63	44	.698
Healthy	2	0	.00
Two Diagnoses	30	12	.40
No Category ("Other")	50	29	.58

DISCUSSION

Data from the S.A.T. systems obtained at the first administration generally demonstrate a degree of internal consistency indicating that they pull from the same separation reaction across differences in pictures. Only the individuation system has a reliability coefficient (r = .67) that falls short of .70. The self-esteem sub-system of the self-evaluation system also has a lower consistency (r = .62); this is probably due to the fact that one of the scales included is sublimation, which is also part of the individuation system and exhibits the lowest internal reliability of all the scales (r = .34).

Hansburg (1972) conceived of the individuation system as reflecting the subject's capacity to deal with separation on the basis of his/her own resources. An examination of the content of the individuation system responses in the S.A.T. suggests that at one time it may reflect that self-resourcefulness, but at other times may reflect a defensive, withdrawn self-isolation. Hansburg recognized the latter aspects of the individuation system, especially when individuation system responses exceeded attachment system responses, as reflected in the results of his first use of the S.A.T. He stated that "on the whole, better-adjusted children showed lower individuation than attachment indexes" (p. 60). In subsequently constructing his diagnostic categories (1979) he regarded excessive individuation responses as reflecting defensive detachment. This study suggests that the rational basis for the individuation system needs to be rethought and clarified, though the consistency is admittedly only slightly less than that of other systems. Two distinct systems may be necessary to make the distinction between healthy and compulsive self-reliance. However, if the responses of the sublimation scale alone were revised to remove their ambiguity, the individuation system might provide sufficient internal reliability.

When the items were further analyzed according to consistency of responsiveness to mild or strong pictures, they revealed a surprisingly high degree of internal consistency. This analysis allowed for a frequency range of only four (0 to 3) because there are but three strong and three mild pictures in each of the matched halves of the S.A.T. Of the total of 17 scales, only four yielded contingency coefficients below .4 on either strong or mild pictures, i.e., empathy, sublimation, anger and anxiety. With this minimal range, any coefficient significantly different from zero is noteworthy. Thus, at this basic level of analysis the

S.A.T. demonstrates a general internal consistency and the test and its components indicate an adequacy for research or diagnostic purposes.

The only finding reflecting sex-related differences was a significantly higher mean number of responses to S.A.T. pain system scales by females than males. These scales include anxiety, phobic reaction and somatic pain. This finding may be related to some empirical findings from other studies which indicate that even in early childhood girls exhibit lower pain thresholds than boys (Hoffman, 1975). In connection with this finding, mothers reported responses to baby girls' cries that were more linked to their perception of girls' need for their mothers' interventions than were their responses to boys' cries. The mothers perceived the boys as "sturdier" and therefore crying for attention rather than physical needs. If this differential treatment by mothers and female caretakers is present throughout childhood, males in our culture may be socialized to deny their own painful tension, while females may be socialized to express pain and seek relief from an outside source. If so, the differential responsiveness of females and males to this aspect of the S.A.T. would be expected.

The pain system and its scales were separately analyzed for each sex. There are three component scales for this pain system, i.e., anxiety, phobic reaction and somatic pain. The consistency of anxiety responses to mild pictures were not significantly different from zero for either males or females. The "anxiety" scale provides individual responses to pictures such as "the child feels that something terrible is going to happen to him/her now," or "the child is afraid to leave." Responses to mild pictures, so expressed, may appear irrational to many subjects. Several subjects in this sample made comments to this effect. Responses to the mild pictures by the "normal" subjects in this study were consequently very infrequent (only 31 subjects made one or more responses). Responses reflecting less severe anxiety to mild pictures might be used in any revision of the S.A.T., and anxiety responses to strong pictures might be rethought and revised in the context of each pictured event to increase internal consistency.

A positive relationship between A-trait and lifetime separation stress as reported on the Stress Inventory was obtained ($r = .35$), indicating that 12% of the variance in A-trait is accounted for by this variable. The actual variance accounted for by life separation stress may be greater than these findings indicate, given the fact that this study made first use of this adaptation of Holmes and Rahe's scale and relied solely upon face validity.

Adolescents also showed significantly higher life stress scores than parents when self-evaluated, not mean, values were used. The reason for this is the greater frequency adolescents reported having experienced events unique to their form of the Stress Inventory than the frequency parents reported having experienced events unique to their form (see Tables 15.1 and 15.2). On the adolescent form, there were more of the commonly experienced separation events than on the parent form. Examples of such frequently reported events unique to the adolescent form are "first day at a new school where you know nobody" and "a teacher's expression of disappointment in you or in your work." On particular similar items of the Stress Inventory, parents and adolescents had nearly identical mean evaluations. The totals of mean evaluations, when adjusted for difference in number of items, were also nearly identical.

The total test reliability of evaluations of the stressfulness of events from test to retest (adolescents: $r = .56$; parents: $r = .79$) compares favorably with the test-retest reliability obtained by Sarason, deMonchaux and Hunt (1975) on the Holmes and Rahe scale ($r = .55$). With the exception of one item on the adolescent of the Stress Inventory ("Loss of a personally valuable article"), the cognitive structures of meaning through which the other items are measured show moderate to high reliability coefficients (see Tables 15.1 and 15.2). Reliability coefficients were generally higher among parents than adolescents. This lower reliability, combined with item differences, may partially account for the higher adolescent stress scores.

Adolescents were found to have significantly higher A-trait scores than parents. Compared with undergraduate college students, high school students also had significantly higher mean scores (Spielberger et al., 1970). The findings of this study are consistent with a progression of age and of developmental differences. As a person matures he may become more confident and less vulnerable to threats to his self-esteem. Elevated A-trait scales are associated with such vulnerability. Adolescents' higher A-trait scores may be associated with their higher stress scores and lower retest reliability of evaluation of stressful events.

It may be speculated that a person may become less vulnerable and more confident in the face of separation and other events through the greater stability of the cognitive structures which process the event. Elevated self-evaluation stress scores and A-trait scores in adolescents are consistent with other findings of heightened anxiety among adolescents who are struggling with the conflicts of individuation and independence characteristic of that period and have not yet acquired the stability of cognitive structures eventually to be acquired with maturity. No such differences were found on the S.A.T. scores. This result suggests that the S.A.T. reflects a dimension of personality less sensitive to current conscious experience of stress than does A-trait.

Generally strong stability over time for each of the S.A.T. systems except individuation was demonstrated. Within the individuation system, the scales "adaptation" and "sublimation" are the least stable, suggesting that these scales may be less reflective of enduring personality characteristics than of transient states of responsiveness. The stabilities of the other S.A.T. systems exceeded A-trait stability, thus providing further evidence that the S.A.T. systems generally reflect aspects of personality more deeply seated or more stable than does self-reported subjective anxiety measured by A-trait. The retest reliability coefficient (r = .65) for the S.A.T. self-report, memory-based item (Mental Set Responses) also reflects this fact. The lower stability of the individuation system probably reflects the problems with its component scales based upon qualities noted above.

Since males and females differed in their responsiveness to the pain system, this system was analyzed for test-retest reliability for each sex separately. In general, females reported various forms of painful tension more reliably than males. A notable sex-related difference in stability of responsiveness to the scale "somatic pain" (females: r = .82; males: r = .36) is indicated. This item provides such responses as "getting a stomach ache" or "dizzy and faint." Explanation for such a difference between sexes in stability of somatic pain responses is lacking. This item provided good internal consistency for both sexes at the first administration of the S.A.T.

A positive relationship was predicted in this study between S.A.T. attachment and pain systems test-retest differences and separation stress difference scores. The stress difference score is the difference on the Stress Inventory for separation events six months previous to the first administration and those reported between administrations. It was thought that such sensitivity to current separation stress might be similar to the degree of sensitivity in the STAI and thus suggest some relationship between the measures. Predicted evidence for such a relationship was not obtained.

However, low but significantly post hoc correlations were obtained between separation stress difference scores and the S.A.T. individuation (r = .18) and hostility system (r = .17) test-retest differences. As noted above, Hansburg (1972) found that increased individuation and hostile responsiveness in reaction to separation stress is associated with a defensive, detached and self-isolatory pattern of response. This study suggests that at least at the level of separation stress experienced by this sample between testings, a number of subjects may have responded in the above fashion. This study further suggests that detached responsiveness to current separation stress may be related to increased scores on A-trait and A-state. However, the correlations obtained were all of low magnitude, presenting the strong possibility that they emanate from other mutually independent sources of variability in separation stress difference scores.

In general, however, the principal implication of this study regarding the S.A.T. and the STAI is that they measure personality variables at different levels. Wagner's (1976) paradigm for conceptualizing personality structures posits a "Facade Self" with which one interacts socially and an "Introspective Self" which encompasses self-feelings and intentions. According to his analysis, self-reports such as the STAI and the Stress Inventory reveal aspects of the Facade Self, while semi-projective measures such as the S.A.T. reveal aspects of the Introspective Self. The generally greater test-retest stability of the S.A.T. than the STAI and its imperviousness to recent separation stress provide evidence that the S.A.T. may measure "deeper" and more enduring aspects of personality. If the distinction outlined by Wagner's paradigm reflects the relationship between the S.A.T. and STAI, any connection between them must be inferred, not directly investigated.

Hansburg (1979, pp. 16–33) elicited pathological syndromes from his clinical experience with juveniles, associated with differences in their S.A.T. protocols (see Table 15.7). They are derived from criteria which in most cases involve Hansburg's norms (see Table 15.6), which he derived by deviating one quartile in either direction from the median of 250 children ages 11–14 in child care and at public schools in New York. Generally, this classification system for separation disorders does not appear to provide an unambiguous or dependable determination of response patterns to separation stress for this population. An exception is the category "depressed," into which 47% (n = 63) of the sample fell. Seventy percent (n = 44) of the subjects were also classified "depressed" at the second testing.

This sample, which was taken from a population coping with life's stresses without psychological/psychiatric help, provided an extremely small percentage (1.5%, $n = 2$) of "healthy" subjects and a large percentage (64%, $n = 82$) classifiable within at least one of Hansburg's categories. If the second administration is taken into consideration, only 23% ($n = 31$) did not qualify for one of the diagnostic categories in either administration. All the other subjects were classifiable, following Hansburg's criteria, in at least one separation disorder on either the first or second S.A.T. administration or both. Thirty subjects (22%) qualified for more than one category. If accurate, these diagnostic categories indicate that a high proportion of this "nonclinical" population shows effects to some degree from one or more separation disorder.

The source of the categories' instability are unknown and may be multiple. They were derived from Hansburg's clinical use of the S.A.T. and not from systematically gathered empirical findings. Hansburg (1979) has indicated that the diagnoses are not mutually exclusive. Moreover, the norms employed as principal criteria of the categories were derived nonparametrically. The general lack of stability found in the diagnostic categories may result in part from the difference in population, especially from the adult part of the sample. However, those 82 subjects who met the criteria for one or more classes of separation disorders were compared by a chi square analysis with the 52 subjects who did not meet criteria for one or more disorders by using the variable family role (parent or adolescent). Significant differences were not found. Adolescents in this subject were older (ages 13–16) than Hansburg's normative sample (11–14), making strict comparability between samples impossible.

One probable major source of category instability is Hansburg's "normal range" for proportions of total S.A.T. responses in each system (see Table 15.6). Since the systems have been demonstrated to present adequate test-retest reliability, such response pattern instability is unexpected and undesirable. Hansburg's use of median quartiles to determine norms may have been appropriate as a first step, given his small sample, but the norms thus derived must be regarded as only approximate. Norms derived from a larger sample and a more diversified population by means of standard scores may provide criteria that will determine response patterns which have greater stability over time. In addition, empirical studies might gather self-reports, reports of others, and structured clinical observations of the patterns of response of subjects to separation stress. Phenomenologically organized syndromes could then be compared with the S.A.T. protocols of the same subjects. In light of these findings the categories might be restructured. Also, empirical study may provide the basis for establishing formulae to weigh differentially certain scales to correct for the number of responses and other psychometric faults.

In summary, this study has investigated Hansburg's S.A.T. and found evidence that its internal consistency and stability over time are generally sufficient for use in research or for diagnostic purposes. The data indicate that the aspects of personality it measures are relatively enduring. Suggestions for its improvement as a clinical and research tool have been made. Its semi-projective structure allows refinement and standardization, which can make it a valuable supplement to self-reported, memory-retrieved data regarding attachment and separation issues.

REFERENCES

APA. *Standards for Educational and Psychological Tests.* Washington, D.C.: APA, 1974.

Black, H. M. *Trait Anxiety and Separation Distress: Analysis of Two Measures in Parents and Their Adolescent Children.* Unpublished doctoral dissertation, California School of Professional Psychology, Los Angeles, 1981.

Bowlby, J. *Attachment and Loss*, Vol. I: *Attachment.* New York: Basic Books, 1969.

Bowlby, J. *Attachment and Loss*, Vol. II: *Separation.* New York: Basic Books, 1973.

Bowlby, J. *Attachment and Loss*, Vol. III: *Loss.* New York: Basic Books, 1980.

Carskadon, T. G. "Test-Retest Reliabilities of Continuous Scores on the Myers-Briggs Type Indicator." *Psychological Reports*, 1977, *41*, 1011–1012.

DeLozier, P. P. *An Application of Attachment Theory to the Study of Child Abuse.* Unpublished doctoral dissertation, California School of Professional Psychology, Los Angeles, 1979.

Exner, J. E., Jr., Armbruster, G. L., and Viglione, D. "The Temporal Stability of Some Rorschach Features." *Journal of Personality Assessment*, 1978, *42*, 474–482.

Hansburg, H. G. *Adolescent Separation Anxiety*, Vol. I. Springfield, Ill.: Charles C. Thomas, 1972.

Hansburg, H. G. "Psychological Systems and Separation Disorders." Paper read at the meetings of the APA in New York City, September 1979.

Hansburg, H. G. *Adolescent Separation Anxiety*, Vol. II. Melbourne, Fla.: R. E. Krieger, 1980.

Hoffman, L. W. "Early Childhood Experiences and Women's Achievement Motivations," in M. T. S. Mednick, S. S. Tangri, and L. W. Hoffman (eds.), *Women and Achievement*. New York: John Wiley and Sons, 1975.

Holmes, T. H., and Rahe, R. H. "The Social Readjustment Rating Scale." *Journal of Psychosomatic Research*, 1967, *2*, 213–218.

Joesting, J. "Test-Retest Reliabilities of the State-Trait Anxiety Inventory in an Academic Setting." *Psychological Reports*, 1975, *37*, 270.

Joesting, J. "Test-Retest Reliabilities of the State-Trait Anxiety Inventory in an Academic Setting: Replication." *Psychological Reports*, 1976, *38*, 318.

Joesting, J. "Test-Retest Correlations for the State-Trait Anxiety Inventory." *Psychological Reports*, 1977, *40*, 671–672.

Kelly, R., and Berg, B. "Measuring Children's Reactions to Divorce." *Journal of Clinical Psychology*, 1978, *34*, 215–221.

Mahler, M. S. "A Study of How the Child Separates from the Mother." *Mental Health Program Reports*, N. I. M. H., 1967, *1*, 113–124.

Miller, J. B. *The Effects of Separation on Latency Age Children as a Consequence of Separation/Divorce*. Unpublished doctoral dissertation, California School of Professional Psychology, Los Angeles, 1980.

Newmark, C. S. "Stability of State and Trait Anxiety." *Psychological Reports*, 1972, *30*, 196–198.

Paykel, E. S. "Recent Life Events and Clinical Depression," in E. K. E. Gunderson and R. H. Rahe (eds.), *Life Stress and Illness*. Springfield, Ill.: Charles C. Thomas, 1974.

Rahe, R. H. "Epidemiological Studies of Life Change and Illness." *International Journal of Psychiatry in Medicine*, 1975, *6*, 133–146.

Rosenzweig, S., Ludwig, D. L., and Adelman, S. "Retest Reliability of the Rosenzweig Picture-Frustration Study and Similar Semi-Projective Techniques." *Journal of Personality Assessment*, 1975, *39*, 3–11.

Roskies, E., Iida-Miranda, M., and Strobel, M. G. "Life Changes as Predictors of Illness in Immigrants," in C. D. Spielberger and I. G. Sarason (eds.), *Stress and Anxiety*, Vol. IV. New York: John Wiley and Sons, 1977.

Sarason, I. G., de Monchaux, C., and Hunt, T. "Methodological Issues in the Assessment of Life Stress," in L. Levi (ed.), *Emotions: Their Parameters and Measurement*. New York: Raven Press, 1975.

Schafer, R. *Aspects of Internalization*. New York: International Universities Press, 1968.

Schafer, W. D., and Jones, J. R. "A Modified Split-Half Approach to Internal Consistency Estimates for the Personal Orientation Inventory." *Psychological Reports*, 1977, *41*, 1020–1022.

Spielberger, C. D. Personal Communication, July 30, 1980.

Spielberger, C. D., Gorsuch, R. L., and Lushene, R. *The State-Trait Anxiety Inventory*. Palo Alto, Cal.: Consulting Psychologists Press, 1970.

White, R. *Ego and Reality in Psychoanalytic Theory*. New York: International Universities Press, 1963.

Witkin, H. A. "Psychological Differentiation and Forms of Pathology." *Journal of Abnormal Psychology*, 1965, *70*, 317–336.

Wagner, E. E. "Personality Dimensions Measured by Projective Techniques: A Formulation Based on Structural Analysis." *Perceptual and Motor Skills*, 1976, *43*, 247–253.

Yamamoto, K. "Children's Ratings of the Stressfulness of Experiences." *Developmental Psychology*, 1979, *15*, 581–582.

SECTION THREE

This section provides an opportunity for those using the S.A.T. to examine a number of papers I have produced over the years—some published before and some published here for the first time.

The first was written for the staff of the Psychiatric Clinic of the Jewish Child Care Association. Entitled "Studies of Families with the Separation Anxiety Test," it was read to the clinic staff in October, 1975. It is presented here to provide some ideas with regard to the test's use with entire families, and it should be read in the light of later attempts to use the method with adults as well as the elderly.

The second paper, entitled "Detection of Self-Destructive Tendencies in Early Adolescence," appeared in Volume III of *Mental Health in Children*, edited by D. V. Siva Sankar (1976). It is reprinted here in its entirety with the permission of the publisher (P.J.D. Publications Limited, Westbury, N.Y.). The purpose of this paper was to suggest certain patterns of attachment and related problems of separation which tended to be characteristic of persons with severe anxious attachment disorders, often propelling youngsters toward suicide or other self-destructive reactions.

The third paper, originally intended for the *Journal of Gerontology* but never revised for that periodical, is entitled "Separation Disorders of the Elderly." It was written in 1979 and presented to the American Orthopsychiatric Association meeting in Washington, D. C., in 1979. This research was performed by one research assistant, one clinical psychologist, and me in a number of centers for elderly persons, as well as on individuals selected at random in Brooklyn. It was the first attempt to use the same test on elderly persons, but altering the directions somewhat.

The fourth paper is entitled "Extended Family Availability and Maternal Reactions to Separation." It was written in 1981 and read at a meeting of the New York State Psychological Association in May 1982. A study of thirty-one mothers of a group of 5-year-olds in the kindergarten classes at the East Midwood Day School in Brooklyn, it was meant to gather more data on maternal reactions to the S.A.T. and, at the same time, to test certain patterned relationships between extended family availability and separation reactions. The data presented in this latter paper were of both theoretical and research significance and indicated some aspects of attachment and separation not adequately noted in other presentations of mine.

This section represents a further elaboration of some of my ideas in the field of attachment and separation and should help to clarify my own conceptual framework and my efforts to accumulate more information on the meaning of the separation anxiety patterns and their use in understanding human behavior.

16

Studies of Families with the Separation Anxiety Test (1975)

INTRODUCTION

In an effort to deal with the family dynamics relating to separation problems, I have given the S.A.T. to four families. Two were intact families, and two had separated or divorced parents. The procedure has been experimental in nature with the hope of revision at later dates. The theoretical formulation in relation to this procedure has been that parents will identify the separation problems of children by projecting their own separation difficulties. I also expected a degree of confusion between the parents' childhood reminiscences and the current child placement reaction. It was anticipated that, in some cases, over-identification would be common in symbiotic problems and confused identifications would occur in more ambivalent individuals. What was felt to be significant was a revelation of the intrafamilial dynamics related to separation. It was recognized that, no matter how disturbed a situation and no matter how much hostility existed, there were long-term attachments that held the family together. The question was how significant the need was to investigate parental reactions to separation from the child, especially if the parent had initiated the separation.

It was expected that social workers would refer those families in which strong attachments existed, in which there was a considerable amount of overt anxiety either in the children or the parents or both, and in which, although placement seemed to be the treatment of choice, serious questions existed as to whether child or parent(s) could withstand the separation without serious consequences. For this reason, I would have expected symbiotic conditions to dominate this group of cases. The fact that strong attachment problems existed is, of course, no necessary cause for eschewing or for discontinuing placement. I am well aware that, in some cases, progress in personality development is often seriously hindered by excessive or seriously ambivalent attachments. On the other hand, pathological attachment-disorders may be of such a nature as to result in aborted placement, or sudden breaks in placement, due to a child's or parent's need to disrupt the placement.

The S.A.T. seemed particularly adapted to the study of separation dynamics in these families. The situations and the pictures provide significant comparisons between the youngster and his family members and how he handles the ties to them, as well as how they may handle the attachments and separations to and from him. Leaving the family for placement produces parental reactions that are sometimes very disturbing. It arouses parental attachment and separation problems dating back to their own childhood, disturbs the emotional equilibrium that existed up to that point, produces a threat to the mechanisms of behavior and to the defenses that have been adopted in the family, and thus precipitates rearrangements in family behavior. It seems likely that the test would indicate the extent of the distress, the types of defenses which are set in motion, and the ability to handle the problems created.

The possibility of asking the parent to indicate how the parent in the picture feels was, of course, the most obvious and reasonable question. However, contaminating intellectual and reasoning factors were considered most likely to become involved. An adult is more likely to respond with what he thinks is expected of him rather than what he feels. On the other hand, if the parent is asked to identify with the child, he is more likely to project. This is based on the assumption that, when a person is asked how someone else would feel, he is more likely to project deeper concerns than if asked how he himself feels.

It is, of course, a significant question as to whether or not placement, for most children, is a necessary expedient; therefore, the parental feelings are of importance. Such a thought has become more tenable in child-care practice as it has become increasingly evident that the attitudes of natural parents towards separation from their children is of considerable significance. In fact, the trend is in the direction of maintaining the family if at all possible. Thus, the attitudes and the actions of parents who are being separated from their children become of prime importance.

Obviously, this research into the use of the S.A.T. in families can be justified only if we consider the following to be significant:

1. All children who are referred for placement do not necessarily need placement as a treatment of choice. Many families are so constituted that separation of any member is a serious trauma.

2. Knowledge of family dynamics is valuable for family treatment purposes, both in those cases of children who are placed and those in which the decision is to retain the child in the family.

3. The S.A.T., because it is a more objective instrument than interviews—but not a substitute for them—may reveal the kind of dynamism in families that is required for treatment. In addition, as a clinical instrument, it may very well help in deciding whether the family can tolerate separation, with or without treatment, and whether the child can potentially be handled by the agency. Further, it may aid in resolving uncertain or doubtful clinical and placement issues in the evaluation of the family and to corroborate interview impressions or present a new view of the separation problems involved.

A further question relates to whether or not the S.A.T. has any validity with parents or, for that matter, with adults. There is no objective evidence for this—the cases included in this evaluation represent only an exploratory clinical effort. However, thus far, the material obtained has been so revealing and so corroborative of other impressions obtained from both clinical staff members and agency staff social workers that it is worthwhile reporting in order to stimulate further investigation.

FAMILY SUMMARIES

Case I: Son, Mother, and Daughter

In this study, a 40-year-old mother of five children, separated from a psychopathic father, sought to place one of the children, a 14-

year-old boy, from a temporary shelter arrangement to a more long-term facility in the JCCA. The boy had a history of running away from another facility, and the question was raised as to whether it would be possible for this boy to remain away from his mother. Living in the mother's home at the time was a 12-year-old sister. The remainder of the children were already living in other facilities.

The S.A.T. was given to mother, son, and daughter. The most impressive result of this study was the extent of the expressed need for individuation or self-reliance at the expense of more normal separation reactions. This enforced necessity for adaptation versus emotional outlets or even normal areas of denial was seen as an indication of the mother's neglect of the children's normal attachment needs. The boy and the girl both showed highly constricted pictures. The girl showed far more affect than the boy, which indicated that she could be more responsive to therapeutic intervention. The boy demonstrated more severe concentration disturbance than the girl, but the girl showed a developing character disorder similar in some respects to the boy's. The excessive affect (37%), the low attachment level, the high self-sufficiency index, and the extent of evasion indicated that soon the girl would develop serious adjustment problems and would act out.

On the other hand, the mother demonstrated a strong attachment need, but at the same time, a very strong adaptation reaction. The extent of her separation anxiety was quite strong and similar to that of the daughter. The indications were that she was a narcissistic, dependent, needful person who, although recognizing the need to adapt, could not handle her own separation experiences. The result was an inability on her part to deal with the children's needs. Further, there was evidence that the mother was unrealistic as well as ambivalent in her handling of separation experiences. (The latter is documented by her excessive inappropriate responses.)

Based on these protocols, the following statement was made in my report:

My general impression is that of a rather unrealistic mother who has been emotionally neglectful of her children and has made it difficult for them to reach out to her in any situation. Thus, these children have been left emotionally to their own devices. I doubt whether anything worthwhile could be accomplished if the boy were returned to his mother. It seems likely that, despite what has happened in the past, the boy needs to be cared for in a residential setting.

In the year that followed, the boy made a good adjustment to a group residence, and the girl was later similarly placed. She was recommended for treatment, and at this writing, the child is still attending therapy sessions regularly and making some progress despite evidence of mild intellectual slowness and a skin disorder. The major intrapsychic dynamic is that of a narcissistically dependent and neglectful mother and the resultant acting-out youngsters with serious problems in object relations, demonstrated obviously on the S.A.T. and corroborated by preceding and subsequent developments. It has been learned that the mother has gratified her own dependent needs by becoming a paramour and a kept woman of a wealthy married man. All five children of her marriage are now in placement.

Case II: Son, Daughter, Father, and Mother

In this family, the patient was a 13-year-old boy who came to Joint Planning Service and who, despite a number of years of psychotherapeutic treatment efforts, had not responded. He was abusive and violent, especially toward his mother and his 11½-year-old sister. Generally, he was considered unmanageable and strong-willed, with occasional school truanting, stealing, and other behavioral problems. The essential focus in this case was related to the boy's intense concern about separation from the mother and the mother's ambivalence. In the course of the study by Joint Planning Service, the father, who was divorced from the mother, appeared as a stumbling block, despite the very destructive quality of the boy's behavior in the family. (This case has been written up in great detail and is referred to in the references at the end of this paper.)

Several interesting dynamics were revealed by the S.A.T. in this case. One of the most significant was the intense attachment need displayed by all members of the family, ranging from 26% to 29%, which are considered much higher than average. This appears strange, considering the extent of the hostility existing in the family and the final divorce taking place between the parents. It is not strange, however, if one considers the hostility as an important affect relating to separation and as a measure of the intensity of attachment. (See paper on "Separation Hostility: A Prelude to Violence" in references.) As part of this problem, the family members, with the exception of the boy's sister, displayed intense feelings of rejection in the face of separation, and the similarity was quite striking. Separation denial (reality avoidance) appeared to be a shared trait. Another striking resemblance was the unusually high attachment individuation balance, an indication of serious distortion of the capacity for object relations and its comparison to the individual sense of self-reliance and of self. Especially strong hostility reactions were shown mostly in the records of the mother and the boy, a suggestion that affect expression in both individuals was more readily elicited in the defensive hostility areas.

The record patterning revealed further that the father was the least resourceful and, basically, the most dependent individual in the family. Therefore, he had the greatest need to hold the family together; the divorce, which had separated him from the family, was completely against his expressed wishes. On the other hand, the mother's record demonstrated more serious disturbances, with strong evidence for self-destructive and suicidal patterning, although she seemed more capable of functioning in work.

The sister maintained herself in the family by means of a character deviation in which complaints were used to avoid responsibility. Her S.A.T. results were constricted; but, similarly to her brother, she demonstrated a responsiveness to the strength of the stimulus—a good prognostic sign. Generally, she showed strong drives for sublimation, a considerably better capacity to express separation pain, and fewer feelings of self-love loss. Dynamically, it seemed that this girl had adopted defenses that would continue the protection of the mother and would avoid open confrontation in the style of her brother.

The mother's interaction with the children showed many atypical phenomena involving exaggerated affect reactions, hostility with powerful denial, a deep intrapsychic evasiveness, and a high level of self-love loss. The suicidal pattern obtained suggests that she transmitted intense fears of abandonment to the children—a very serious problem in light of the father's separation from the family.

The conclusion that a strong symbiotic system pervaded this family was inevitable. Psychologically, the family was not really able to separate, but maintained their relationships in a highly destructive manner.

It was soon after this study that the father, with the assistance of the paternal aunt, was able to convince the mother that placement would not be desirable. This effectively caused a withdrawal of the case from the agency. The case is an excellent example not only of how the S.A.T. can reveal a family pattern but also how a symbiotic system, organized and led by one individual, can prevent adequate treatment for a family member.

Case III: Daughter, Mother, and Father

This family group was referred for S.A.T. study at the insistence of a Joint Planning Service social worker, with the expressed intention of determining whether or not placement of the daughter would be possible. The girl (16½ years old) had referred herself to the agency, indicating a wish for placement away from the family. She had already moved out, living with an older sister or with a friend.

The major factor demonstrated in this case was the girl's own separation pattern of obvious need for relief from the overwhelming attachment needs of the parents. She showed a constricted (31 responses) pattern, with minimal attachment need and limited sensitivity to the separation stimuli; but, at the same time, she showed a high level of separation pain and separation denial. There was definite evidence that the girl wished to withdraw from the separation problems, and the anxiety seemed less related to attachment and more related to the need to break away. Evidence for strong narcissistic reactions was demonstrated and there was very little indication of self-love loss. These patterns strongly suggested that placement would be tolerated by the girl and was essential to her well-being at this time.

The mother's pattern was a highly neurotic one with a strong attachment level (33%). She showed less acceptance of separation in the mild than in the strong pictures, showing an excessive sensitivity to separation stimuli. There was evidence of an unsuccessful attempt at stoicism, suggesting a woman carrying a tremendous emotional burden. Anger remained relatively underexpressed, whereas strong feelings of self-love loss, depression, and rejection were evident. This pattern is found in individuals with degrees of self-destructiveness in their personality. There was no doubt that this pattern indicated an overbearingness that the girl's pattern obviously could not tolerate.

The father showed an entirely different pattern, manifesting a highly dependent, attachment-oriented, needful person, limited in personality but impulsive and explosive (affect levels reached 47% — 20% anger and 27% pain). Such a high degree of emotional reaction to separation accompanied by this degree of attachment indicated the strong protest against separation. Thus, from his point of view, he needed the daughter as an additional attachment figure, which, obviously from her pattern, she did not want to gratify. The father's reality testing was not always good, and it was likely that he had limited tolerance for attachment-need frustrations. It was obvious that the father's needfulness extended to many areas of his life, and, in this area, he would be driven to many forms of primitive gratification.

The areas of confirmation for the above family constellation were obtained from historical materials derived from social work contacts. The father was retired for disability when he was only 45 years old. He did no useful work and was quite dependent on family contacts. He overate and sat around a good deal. The mother made demands on and pushed all members of the family. Yet, in an effort to maintain the girl in the home, they appealed to Jewish Family Service, which, apparently in an effort to save the family from disintegrating, wanted to keep the girl with the parents. However, when the report of the S.A.T. study was made available to Jewish Family Service, they then relented and the girl was placed in a residential treatment center with salutary results. Perhaps subsequent events, while unfortunate, proved to be fortuitously valuable: the mother developed terminal cancer that would no doubt have seriously added to the girl's adjustment problems. This family study appeared to have been of considerable practical assistance in effecting placement when conflict had arisen between two agencies with differing motivations with regard to the desirability of such placement.

Case IV: Son, Father, and Mother

This young man, nearly 19 years old was living at the Youth Residence and was referred by a social worker for a family study to determine whether degrees of family attachment were negatively affecting his adjustment to the residential treatment center.

The S.A.T. pattern on the boy showed an intense attachment need and high levels of separation pain. Both of these varied, representing 50% of his responses. Evidence for a basically symbiotic core was manifest and was at times quite intense and indiscriminate. The indications were that any suggestion of change or shift in environment, especially when momentary or more extended, would give rise to powerful feelings of loneliness, fear, anxiety, physical pain, and a need to resolve the intensity of these feelings. The relative strength of the feelings of rejection suggested that he might, at times, be overwhelmed by suicidal or self-destructive feelings. The intensity of separation pain seemed to lead to violent and possibly irrational efforts at self-assertion. He had an intense need to sublimate and in some form to adapt, but the real problems seemed to be a powerful ambivalence between an anxious attachment and a need for self-reliance. Caught up in this disturbance, he appeared to resolve the problem at times in favor of any one of these. Thus, one would expect that he could alternate between intense attachment need (such as trying to reach his parents), intense self-destructive feelings, and a desire to handle everything on his own. The resultant instability would be very debilitating.

The mother proved to be an important key to the boy's difficulty. Despite her surface appearance and manner of intellectual and emotional suavity, she demonstrated considerable disturbance on the S.A.T. She had difficulty determining with whom to identify in the pictures, especially when she was asked to refer the problems involved to her own childhood relationships. She demonstrated very poor discrimination between the mild and the strong stimuli, a characteristic noted in her son's record and additional evidence of her own deep-seated symbiotic problems. Further, she selected many inappropriate responses, an indication of poor reality testing in separation situations. Her high attachment-need level and insufficient self-reliance pattern belied her surface self-sufficiency. In addition, there was a high degree of self-love loss, indicating a powerful sense of guilt. Strong over-identification with the boy was demonstrated with resulting intense hostility toward the separation process. It seemed likely that the mother's ineffectuality in dealing with separation without strong emotional stress was continuously reinforcing the boy's difficulty in working through his own separation from her.

The father, too, showed impairment of judgment with regard to mild and strong separation stimuli—a picture indicating further why the boy found it so difficult to discriminate mild from strong forms of separation from the support of environmental figures. The father, too, demonstrated excessive attachment need, even on mild pictures. The father's patterns were generally confused, with many inappropriate reactions, but his disturbance was not as blatant as the mother's. The father did not feel as emotionally overwhelmed as the mother and the boy, and seemed more preoccupied with ego-functioning effects of separation. His disturbance between himself and the boy appears to refer largely to why the boy does not adapt or why he is not more successful, rather than to the boy's emotional problems. The father seemed more confused and less understanding of both the boy's and the mother's problems and showed a lack of clarity in his capacity to feel about his wife and his son.

It was strongly recommended that the boy remain at the Youth Residence and avoid living with the parents. Stability of environment was considered essential in order to maintain this boy, and treatment of parental needs would be highly useful in dealing with their confusions and over-identifications. The family demonstrated intense guilt, feelings of needfulness and confusion, and could not be helpful to the boy in a daily living situation.

Despite efforts to maintain this boy at YRC, he rashly insisted on leaving to attend an out-of-town college. Prognosis for success in such a situation without treatment was poor with regard to the avoidance of eventual breakdown. It was felt that he would be likely to constantly appeal to the parents for their emotional support, and they, because of their own confusions, would not be able to supply this support. His own instability could lead to serious impulsive, possibly self-destructive, acts. At this writing, no facts are available about his present status.

SUMMARY AND CONCLUSIONS

Recognizing that this exploratory study of four families represents only a small and, as yet, unchartered approach to separation dynamics, what can we derive from the study that can be useful?

First, I believe it provides a stimulus toward further objective ways of studying the forces that seem to move parents and children in their efforts at attachment on the one hand, and their attempts at self-realization and nonpathological disentanglement on the other hand. The study recognizes that parents bring to family life a history of their own separation problems and that these problems are projected and displaced on the children—often in such a way as to create pathological needs with their attendant symptomatology and defenses. At times, parental separation pathology is not so clearly discerned in interviews, even when these interviews are quite penetrating.

Second, the S.A.T. seems to penetrate parental separation problems in a number of ways, although there are a number of technical problems that must be investigated. For example, would it be more helpful to devise a similar test, using the parent as the focal figure and utilizing phrases which would apply to adult feelings? Does the conflict over self-projection and identification with the child obfuscate the basic separation patterns of the parents? How significant are intellectual as well as sociocultural parental expectations in the nature of obtained responses? These, and similar technical questions, have heuristic value for researchers that can help us deal with further objectification in this area.

Third, what we often noted in these summaries was the extent to which one or both parents were focal figures in the orbital family dynamics when it came to separation phenomena. This is an important factor in considering not only which parent, if any, may be unconsciously sabotaging placement or treatment, but also which parent may be most useful in enabling the family to go forward. At the same time, we can detect similarities as well as differences in the separating capacity, as well as the separation patterns of various family members. These similarities and differences sharpen our clinical insights. Thus, in Case I, both children showed serious impairment of attachment capacity with excessive self-sufficiency, resulting in serious pathology of the character structure. At the same time, the mother was seen as a needful person who eventually abandoned all of her children in favor of taking on a childlike, dependent position for herself. In Case II, the opposite situation obtained—intense attachment needs pervading the entire family but maintained in a hostile, destructive manner. In that case, the father's severe symbiotic need was the focal point for preventing placement. In Case III, the focal problem centered around a neurotic mother and a highly needful father, both blocking placement. Finally, in Case IV, we saw an unstable youth in a strongly attached family—guilt-ridden, confused, over-identified, and ambivalent. The struggle for autonomy was constantly put forth, but violated by the unstable and unpredictable directions of their personality factors. In all of these cases, we saw how the S.A.T. patterns penetrated the external defenses. Further, in all cases, the follow-up of the families demonstrated that the original directions projected by the S.A.T. proved generally accurate.

REFERENCES

Bowlby, J., Address to JCCA Staff (March 27, 1974). On file in JCCA Library.

Bowlby, J., "Attachment Theory, Separation Anxiety and Mourning," in *American Handbook of Psychiatry*, Vol. VI (2nd ed.): New Psychiatric Frontiers. Ed. D. A. Hamburg and H. K. Brodie. New York: Basic Books, 1975.

Hansburg, H. G., *Adolescent Separation Anxiety: A Method for the Study of Adolescent Separation Problems*. Springfield, Ill.: C. C. Thomas, 1972. Reprinted: Melbourne, Fla.: R. E. Krieger, 1980.

Hansburg, H. G., "Separation Hostility: A Prelude to Violence." Proceedings of the 20th International Congress of Psychology, August 1972, Tokyo.

Hansburg, H. G., "Relationship between Specific Relationship Experiences and the Reactions to the Separation Anxiety Test." Unpublished, 1971.

Hansburg, H. G., "A Study of Caseworker's Appraisal of the Separation Anxiety Test." Unpublished, 1971.

Hansburg, H. G., "The Use of the Separation Anxiety Test in the Detection of Self-Destructive Tendencies in Early Adolescents," in *Mental Health in Children*, Vol. III, Ed. D. V. Siva Sankar. Westbury, N. Y.: P. J. D. Publications (in press).

Hansburg, H. G., "The Use of the Separation Anxiety Test in the Study of an Entire Family." Unpublished, 1975.

Hansburg, H. G., "Separation Problems of Displaced Children," in *Emotional Problems in Peace and War*, Ed. Roland Parker. Pittsburgh, Pa.: Stanwyx Press, 1972.

Hansburg, H. G., "A Study of Adolescent Separation Stress." *American Journal of Orthopsychiatry*, 1972.

Orgun, I. N., "Adolescent Separation Anxiety (A Review)." *Medical Insight*, Vol. 5 (3), March 1973.

17

Detection of Self-Destructive Tendencies
in Early Adolescence
(1976)

INTRODUCTION

Self-destructive feelings and behavior have long been linked with unfortunate, seriously disturbing or tragic separation experiences. The suicide of young frustrated and rejected lovers has been memorialized in many stories and plays, the most famous being Romeo and Juliet. The self-destructive behavior of many youngsters who are abandoned by their parents is a common occurrence. More devastating is the slow erosion of the inner security by the constant inaccessibility of parental figures, who, although physically available, are either emotionally insensitive or unresponsive or constantly misunderstanding of the child's needs. At the same time, it is a truism that the capacity to separate from parental or other closely significant persons for necessary periods and for personal explorations of the social and physical environment is essential for individuation and ego development.

Bowlby's concept known as attachment theory (Bowlby, 1974) provides us with a significant base of operations for understanding the pathology of self-destructiveness. Psychoanalytic concepts more traditionally employed the attack on the introjected love object. Bowlby, instead, gives more attention to attachment frustration with its accompanying emotional turmoil that intrudes on the capacity to cope with environmental demands. Actual or threatened abandonment is seen as an experience which disrupts functioning capacity. Bowlby states, "there is extensive support for the view that anxious attachment is a common consequence of a child having experienced actual

separation, threats of abandonment or combinations of the two"
(Bowlby, 1974). Additionally, anger is conceived as a normal, healthy
component of attachment deprivation and as an effort toward
regaining the association with the love object (Bowlby, 1973, 1974;
Hansburg, 1972). The fact that anger can become pathological is then
pointed out as a serious consequence of continued frustration of attachment need. Although Bowlby does not deal with the potential self-
destructiveness derived from this, there is a considerable body of
evidence supporting this.

Thus, the failure to achieve dependability from an attachment
figure may lead to attacks against the self under certain conditions.
These conditions have been described by many workers who have
studied suicide or suicidal equivalents in children and adolescents. It is
the thesis of this paper that youngsters who experience the intense conflict of strong attachment need, and equally strong frustration and instability in the gratification of this need, suffer from severe separation
ambivalence. Further, this ambivalence is coupled with severe
emotional turmoil, which, even if temporarily assuaged, continues as a
subsurface phenomenon which will reappear, sometimes without warning, if abandonment or threats of abandonment develop or are anticipated. This will be accompanied by a great sense of helplessness,
pain, hostility, intense denial, difficulties in maintaining self-love
(feelings of rejection and intrapunitiveness), and inability to face the
normal identity stresses of adolescence. This pattern is likely to lead to
self-destructive reactivity or to a psychotic break during the increasing
demands of adolescent adjustment. The derivation of this thesis comes
from the literature on child and adolescent suicide and from my own
studies in the use of the S.A.T. (Hansburg, 1972).

Mahler's (1968) theory of three stages of object relations—autistic,
symbiotic, and separation-individuation—despite differences in terminology, closely resembles Bowlby (1973, 1979) and Ainsworth's
(1969) concept of the development of proximity-seeking as contrasted
with exploratory behavior with the awareness of accessibility of an attachment figure. The gradual development of self-reliance as confidence in the accessibility of the attachment figure increases is similar
in both theories, based upon their varied observations with different
populations. The anxiety and other attendant emotional reactions such
as anger, aggression, and loss of concentration on activities are
described in both theoretical formulations. The differences relate to

the intrapsychic tactics that are adapted to deal with separation. Mahler prefers the concepts of the introjection of love objects and object constancy, whereas Bowlby is partial to the feeling of self-reliance (see also White's concept of competence and effectance) and the ability to find needed attachment figures in the environment when dependency needs require it. Bowlby (1973) eschews the use of the term "symbiosis," which is considered phase-specific (see also N. Friedman, 1967), but psychoanalysts like Mahler consider the symbiotic quality as a phenomenon that attains internalized psychological significance. Regardless of the difference, it seems likely that we can use the term "symbiotic" as representing more severe degrees of attachment need, even when the symbiotic object no longer derives either unconscious or conscious gratification from the relationship.

In our cases in this study, it is conceivable that failures in the gratification of the symbiotic needs at early stages of development (before 18 months) made it difficult for the child to negotiate the separation-individuation phase with any confidence. Thus, an intensified state of vulnerability to emotional turmoil during separation experiences in later life becomes a relatively fixed characteristic of separation behavior. Defensive character maneuvers must then ensue in order to protect against the internally felt stress.

The incidence of suicide and suicide attempts among children and adolescents has increased markedly in recent years according to United States' Vital Statistics (1970). This increase has been largely in the 15- to 19-year-old group, although there have been some increases in the ages from infancy to 14 years. Males generally show a larger percentage of such acts than females. I am told that, during 1972, 22 cases of children 4 to 12 years old were hospitalized at Mt. Sinai Hospital in New York for attempted suicide. Actually, the incidence of self-destructive behavior is difficult to measure and is far greater than suicide attempts (Whitehead, 1973), depending on the population studied and the methods and interpretations utilized in the studies.

At the Jewish Child Care Association, there have been many reports from group residences concerning self-destructive behavior and threats of suicide. Recent literature on suicide attempts (see reference list) have proliferated in an attempt to locate the risk population and to develop methods of prevention and treatment. It has become especially urgent to develop prediction techniques that would be of value in determining the degree of childhood and adolescent potential self-destructive risks. In the course of work in diagnosing separation problems in early adolescence, I have developed the S.A.T. method. Using this method, I have been able to identify a pattern of response that shows a marked similarity to the description of the child who is vulnerable to self-destructive and/or suicidal tendencies (Hansburg, 1972A-D). The descriptions of such children have appeared in the literature with increasing frequency.

Tobbachnick and Farberow (1961) stated the following:

The important dynamics (suicide) are as follows: depression, particularly when accompanied by anxiety, tension and agitation, hostility and guilt (these seem to lead to acting out motor impulses that may be directed upon the self), and dependency needs, particularly if they have been frustrated or threatened to any considerable degree.

In my study, I have used the word *attachment* rather than *dependency*, as I believe with Bowlby that this concept is more appropriately differentiated from generalized dependency by its more specific and demanding nature in children.

Schecter, in a work by Schneidman and Farberow (1957), indicated:

Dynamics of depression have been well described. In general, in adults, these descriptions have stated that, when an individual's hostility cannot be expressed outwardly, it is turned against the introjected objects which, because they are part of the self, results in the attempted or actual destruction of the self. Depressions in children have also been described clinically. While the same dynamics of hostility directed against the formerly loved, but now hated, introjected objects we hypothesized, these descriptions have also stressed the factor of the extreme dependence of the child on the parents, his love object. Thus, whenever children feel the threat of the loss of a love object, they not only develop feelings of rage towards the frustrating object, but feelings of helplessness and of worthlessness as well. This results in, and is equivalent to, a depression. . . . it is when the degree of tension is extremely high and the defense mechanisms break down or become ineffective that suicide or suicidal equivalents may appear.

The author felt that children, rather than attempting suicide, simply expressed their self-destructive feelings in other ways. These may be called "suicidal equivalents," that is:

an attenuated attack on the introjected object which results in depressions, accidental injuries, anti-social acts and the like, all of which have the potentiality for ending in the destruction of the individual. They are desperate efforts at regaining contact with the lost gratifying object.

Wolff (1972) described the pattern of suicide among adolescents as:

those associated with depression, with social withdrawal, loss of initiative and self-esteem, sadness, crying spells, and sleep disturbances being major manifestations of depression. . . . the pattern usually emerging in the adolescent attempting suicide is that of an unhappy, lonely, often sensitive person. . . . the syndrome which has high rates of suicide share a common feature, reduced ego capacity. Persons with lower thresholds for tension might habitually use chemical agents to reduce the tension load and inadvertently program themselves to use suicidal means to control continued overloads of anxiety.

In the same edited work, Cantor (1972) urged the following:

I am certain that serious research can be conducted to determine whether a suicidal personality exists. It should also be possible to someday predict who in a group of individuals would more likely commit suicide.

Studies of animals, particularly nonhuman primates, have also demonstrated how self-destructive they can be if separation experiences are prolonged or tragic. An interesting example of the latter was provided by Jane Goodall in her work with chimpanzees in an African setting. The following example is drawn from her book, *In the Shadow of Man*, and quoted elsewhere (Begers, 1973). The incident is derived from a family of chimpanzees in which the mother is Flo, the daughter is Fifi, and the son is Flint. Goodall states:

I would strongly suspect that the kind of affection between a chimp mother and her offspring and a human mother and her children is very, very similar. The motivation to protect, to nurture and to suckle is very close in both species. Flint's grief at his mother's (Flo) death, for example, underscores this point. Flint had been with his mother when she died while crossing a stream. For three days after her death, Flint returned to her body and tried to extricate maggots from the corpse. Within a week following the death of his mother, Flint became so lethargic and depressed that he lost a third of his weight. He exhibited all the signs associated with severe depression; he refused to eat and would sit huddled up in a ball. On the fifth day, Flint met his sister, Fifi, and it seemed as if her presence helped him relax. When she moved away, we were sure that Flint would follow. Although Fifi waited patiently, Flint lay down under a bush. During the last two weeks of his life, he hardly moved at all. The day before he died, he returned to the place in the stream where his mother had been. He spent a long time looking at the rock on which she had been before he moved away.

Such severe attachment and its tragic consequences when death separates a child from its mother strongly suggest the possibility of a pathological condition in which a sense of helplessness (Seligman, 1973) related to a severe separation results in obvious self-destruction.

It appears logical, therefore, that we should be concerned with the identification and treatment of human children who show such pathological attachment without adequate attendant defenses. The S.A.T. seems particularly adapted for such identification. Working together in the Psychiatric Clinic of the JCCA, Christine Duplak and I have tentatively been able to elicit patterns of response easily diagnosable as the suicidal equivalent or self-destructive reactivity. These patterns have been examined in an empirical, clinical manner and collated later with psychosocial histories obtained from the records in five cases. While there are no two patterns exactly alike, there are certain similarities that suggest a diagnosis of weakened ego strength, strong ungratified attachment need, depressive and withdrawal defenses and considerable losses of self-love and self-esteem. In addition, powerful pain reactions are often evoked without the necessary defenses to deal with the pain. In all of these cases, the suspicion of self-destructive reactions to separation is strongly justified.

For those who have some familiarity with the S.A.T. Method, I present below the specific patterns which are diagnosable as self-destructive:

1. A strong attachment need in the presence of a low separation-individuation level.

2. A strong attachment and a weak separation-individuation level on mild pictures, a reversal of the normative condition and an almost ambi-equal individuation on mild and strong pictures—a representation of a serious deficiency in the attachment-individuation relationship.

3. The presence of intense separation pain, intense separation hostility, or both, with pain generally somewhat stronger, but the total of these representing a form of separation turmoil of more than one-third of the total responses.

4. Evidence that self-love loss is stronger than self-esteem loss in every case, with the self-love loss being espe-

cially strong in relation to the normative picture obtained in other cases.

5. An abnormal denial pattern with a definitely heightened denial percentage.

6. A weak identity stress reaction, a phenomenon suggesting a general lag in the maturation level, especially
in the psychosexual area.

CASE REPORTS OF SELF-DESTRUCTIVE PATTERNS

The cases described below were encountered during the normal
course of clinical practice in the Psychiatric Clinic at JCCA. I began to
recognize the patterns involved after the first rather dramatic case
came to my attention. The delineation of this pattern became clearer
with each new case and with startling clarity. I did not believe that this
was the only pattern to be found in cases of self-destructive intentions
or acts, but, up to this time, I have failed to find any other pattern
associated with this behavior, although I am certain that it will emerge
with increasing contact with such patients.

Case 1: N.G., Age 12 years, 8 months

N.G. was referred by the Far Rockaway Group Residence and
given the S.A.T. on November 22, 1971 by Christine Duplak. Duplak
consulted me with the resultant protocol, and I was told nothing of the
circumstances of the referral. The resultant protocol of 94 responses appears in the Appendix exactly as it was produced, and it is accompanied by the summary chart obtained from it.

In addition to the patterns revealed, there were a number of interesting reactions to the pictures. For example, on the mild separation
picture which shows a child sleeping and a mother leaving the room,
he selected the following responses: rejection, loneliness, withdrawal,
and empathy—a combination indicating an unusual reaction to such a
mild stimulus, especially when one considers his age. The picture of the
child leaving the mother to go to school produced six responses: impaired concentration, phobic feeling, generalized anxiety, withdrawal, somatic reaction, and anger—obviously a strong emotional
disturbance to a mild separation stimulus. There were other mild pic-

tures producing strong reactions. Reality testing was poor (eight absurd responses). In addition, there were five projection responses—an indication that separation stress was producing a paranoid reaction, which could certainly be interpreted as an ominous development.

While the patterns of response indicated a normal total attachment percentage, an overly strong attachment reaction appeared on mild pictures. The most significant item was an extreme drop in the individuation level—that is, the acceptance of separation experiences (3%). This must be considered a serious development, an indication that he felt completely helpless in the face of such experiences. The separation pain level was so strong as to exceed the attachment level, a pathognomic indicator of the danger of decompensation in the presence of intolerable pain. Strong affect hunger, with attendant inner turmoil, was indicated. The hostility level was also overpowering (19%), suggesting that he was being inundated by severe, unalleviated separation disturbance. Separation denial approached high levels (17%), and since the fantasy level was low and withdrawal and evasion strong, the probability of acting out was strengthened. In line with this, the self-love loss was very high (14%) and overshadowed self-esteem loss—demonstrating deep feelings of rejection. The attachment-individuation balance had moved to the unstable side, a manifestation of unstable reactions to separation.

It seemed likely from this protocol that N.G. was in a serious condition and was ready to act out in the direction of self-destruction. No other sensible interpretation was possible. All of the attributes previously discussed were present—a strong, ungratified attachment need, a very low separation acceptance (individuation), strong separation hostility and separation pain, very high self-love loss involving deep feelings of rejection, intense separation denial, weak identity stress and serious weakness of the attachment-individuation relationship. In addition, there were two serious indicators of illness—a large number of absurd responses (poor reality testing) and a paranoid reaction to separation.

The prediction that this boy would do something to destroy himself was partially fulfilled within two weeks on December 7, 1971. Precipitating factors included a break-up with a girlfriend and an argument with students on a school bus. He had been complaining of a desire to leave the residence and to live with a brother. He began to talk seriously of suicide, "by jumping off the roof, putting his head through the window, or taking pills." He was then hospitalized at Elmhurst General for a period of six weeks. He was discharged with a diagnosis of schizophrenic reaction, schizoid affective type, was placed on medication, and was recommended for long-term placement and residential treatment. Subsequently, he was placed at the Pleasantville Cottage School. Many difficulties appeared, and in July 1972, he ran away, but was later returned. At this writing, he is still at Pleasantville.

The history indicated that N.G. was the youngest of three brothers and had always been considered to be the most sensitive. He was very tall and heavy, so he appeared far older than his years. His relationship with his parents had always been poor, and he apparently did not miss his mother when she died. (N.G. was 4 years old at the time.) When the boy was 11 years old, the father was hospitalized for acute depression and suicidal thinking, and subsequently died of a heart attack in the hospital. In May 1970, the caseworker had described N.G. as a "verbal, sensitive, preadolescent who presented a superficially well functioning picture. However, he has a tremendous craving for emotional and financial security and maternal attention." Apparently, it was the placement and separation from the family and the father's death that precipitated the serious depression and paranoid ideation. Despite this, he was intelligent and quite successful in school. A fluctuating adjustment appeared in the group residence during the year and a half prior to the onset of serious disturbance.

It is interesting to note that, in earlier psychiatric and psychological studies, this boy had simply been described as an intelligent, sensitive boy who was showing an "adjustment reaction of childhood." It is obvious that the true nature of his disorder went unrecognized because of a failure to study his reactions to separation experiences. The evidence in this case suggested a strong correlation between the patterns of the S.A.T. and the progression of events in this boy's life. The test indicated that self-destructive potential was very strong and likely to ensue. It seems likely that the hospitalization and subsequent placement in a residential treatment center was essential to save him from self-destruction. There is also a suggestion that this boy is highly vulnerable to intense disturbance when his attachment needs are not met or when even mild separations occur. Surveillance is essential to prevent future breakdowns of this kind.

Case 2: M.G., Age 12½ years

This boy first came to my attention in February 1972. He had been seen for psychological examination by Patricia Horn, and during the course of this, was given the S.A.T. Horn brought this material to me in consultation, and I was not apprised of any details, nor did I see the boy. The test protocol appears in the Appendix.

He gave a total of 62 responses—19 to the mild pictures and 43 to the strong pictures. The percentage difference between these two figures was excessive (38%)—an abnormal sign. He showed very strong qualitative, as well as quantitative, reactions to the strong pictures—especially to the grandmother, judge, and runaway pictures—and strong enough reactions to the hospitalization and death of the mother pictures. There were also strong reactions to a few mild pictures—school and camp—indicating intense emotional feelings with regard to separation from the maternal figure.

The pattern of responses indicated, without doubt, a serious emotional disturbance, especially strong in the area of self-destructiveness. His attachment percentage was quite strong (29%) and, when compared to the very low (8%) individuation, represented a serious failure in the separation-individuation process. It was also observable that there were practically no individuation responses on the strong pictures—a very unusual result—whereas the difference between the individuation on the mild and strong pictures was negligible. This highly sensitive separation index was accompanied by severe self-love loss (4 rejection and 4 intrapunitive responses), all on the strong pictures. Such severe self-deprecation, in addition to the failure in the separation-individuation process, is an ominous sign.

Accompanying the above were strong pain and hostility, an index of considerable separation turmoil. Also present were intense separation denial involving 7 withdrawal, 3 fantasy, and 3 evasion responses—a 21% level. This intensive denial must be considered as both delusional and asocial. Lastly, the identity stress level was below the norm. All of these factors were theoretically and clinically pathognomic of a self-destructive personality. In this case, the evidence suggested that he was capable of reality breaks, even though the number of absurd responses was within normal limits.

The pattern in this case strongly resembled that of N.G. Subsequently, what I learned about M.G. confirmed the depth of the attachment need and his self-destructive tendencies. The psychologist was impressed by the corroboration of other interpretive material obtained from drawings, Rorschach, and T.A.T. She said in her report:

because of his anticipation of being rejected and/or hurt in interpersonal relations, M.G. often tries to withdraw from and/or avoid becoming involved with others. . . . there are indications of M.G.'s concern about his own sanity. The depth of his despair and his inability to control his life in conjunction with the possibility of impulsive outbursts, the relative ineffectuality of his defenses and his turning anger against himself, indicate the possibility of serious self-destructive tendencies.

It was later reported to me that M.G. was seen wandering around in a daze, both at the residence and at school. On several occasions, it was observed by the teacher that he was attempting to injure himself by jabbing the point of a pencil compass into his arms several times. A camp report (summer 1970) indicated the boy's disturbed social relationships and his tendency to depressed states. In a checklist, destructiveness was checked in the "very much" column, as were attention-seeking, head-banging, temper outbursts, and withdrawal. His overall self-confidence was double-checked as "very poor," as was his ability to develop friendships. His school report (1970) also checked "withdrawn" and "depressed," and it was recorded that he habitually ripped up his own papers in class. A camp report in 1972 stated that he was "moody, withdrawn and involved with self and family problems. Very negative about himself and the world at large."

M.G. had improved a good deal after removal from the home and placement at the Mt. Vernon group residence. Several diagnoses had indicated a very intelligent youngster of variable functioning; probably basically schizophrenic. His worker at the residence indicated that, although he has improved a great deal:

Life is a daily struggle for him and it is only within an accepting, understanding and supportive atmosphere that . . . M.G. has a chance. . . . He still occasionally lapses into bizarre behavior. . . . it is only through continued living in a therapeutic milieu that M.G. may develop a coping mechanism to make it possible for him to withstand the demands of a society which seems too difficult for him to bear at present.

The corroboration of historical and diagnostic material from other sources with the pattern of the S.A.T. is striking. On the basis of the test, it was recommended that treatment be initiated immediately. It was later learned that M.G. was put into more intensive casework therapy, individually and in group, and has done much better since. Nevertheless, he is a highly vulnerable youngster, who, under stress of any significant separation, has strong potential for self-destructive acting out.

Case 3: J.C., Age 11½ years

This boy was given the S.A.T. at the request of the psychiatrist. It was administered by Christine Duplak, who also saw his twin sister, M.C. Of the five cases described in this report, J.C.'s record showed the greatest strength and the mildest self-destructive patterning.

He gave a normal number of responses (62%), with some lowering of the percent difference between the mild and strong pictures. There was some suggestion of overreaction to the mild pictures, which included such reactions as phobic feelings, generalized anxiety, loneliness, fantasy, and anger, a sure sign of acute emotional distress at that time. The complete lack of well-being responses was noteworthy and was pathognomic of serious difficulty in accepting separation. It was interesting that the sleep picture caused an intrapunitive reaction—the mother was leaving the room because the boy had not been good.

The most important factors in the patterns obtained included a general lowering of the individuation pattern to 11%, a severe intensification of reality avoidance (21%), intense separation pain (19%), higher than normal hostility and a self-love loss stronger than self-esteem loss. Identity stress was weak (7%). This pattern was consistent with the self-destructive potential described previously. Yet this patterning must be considered as mild in comparison to the two more serious cases described above.

The psychologist's remarks referred largely to the intense distress and vulnerability to anxiety generated by separation. It was her feeling that the resultant disturbance due to separation would be neurotic rather than psychotic in nature. Further discussion with the psychologist indicated that an acute state, rather than a symbiotic condition, was present and that a current situation had stimulated the present pattern on the test.

Both J.C. and his twin sister M.C. had resided in a foster home for at least 10 years. They had been quite happy there and did not want to return to live with their psychotic mother. After a weekend home visit, the natural mother suddenly decided not to permit them to return to the foster home. This decision threw them into a panic. Shortly thereafter, they were seen by a staff psychiatrist who felt that serious damage to the mental health of both children would result from retention by their natural mother. It was after a case conference that recommendation was made for referral for an S.A.T.

J.C.'s behavioral, emotional and intellectual history had generally been satisfactory. Several examinations, given at earlier ages, and psychosocial evaluations had shown him to be a healthy, happy youngster, although with some tendency toward constriction and withdrawal in critical situations. In early childhood, he was considered to be more dependent than his sister. After two years in one foster home, the children were replaced in their more recent one. At that time, social work notes indicated that J.C. was more sensitive than M.C. There were also indications of compulsivity and perfectionism, which eased somewhat with latency. He was highly sensitive to slight criticism, a pattern correlating highly with the sensitivity and vulnerability seen in the S.A.T.

Since May 1972, both J.C. and M.C. have been back in their mother's home with all their other siblings. They went through some stormy periods, and then, in October 1972, the mother began to have more trouble managing the children. By November 1972, J.C. was having continual behavior problems at home. He became more defiant and more involved in angry altercations with the mother, and he had severe temper tantrums. The mother's psychotic need to use the oldest male child in the home as a scapegoat soon became apparent, and the boy's struggle for acceptance and love from the mother was constantly frustrated. As a result of a conference with the caseworker, J.C. was referred for psychiatric evaluation. The psychiatrist reported that he was both "depressed and impulsive." On March 23, 1973, I received a note from the social worker that, subsequent to the psychiatric examination, J.C. had become very angry in an argument with his mother, gone to his room and, on the way, kicked a hole in the wall with his tennis shoes. During the argument, he said, "I want to kill myself, I am no damn good." It was later learned that, at one time, one of J.C.'s older brothers had attempted suicide through excessive drug intake and had been hospitalized.

Recommendations for psychotherapeutic treatment on an outpatient basis were made by the psychiatrist and by myself in con-

sultation with the caseworker. There is evidence in the case that an increasing intrapsychic stress was developing between the boy and his
mother. It appeared to be based in large part on an intense need for
maternal approval and contact. It strongly suggested that an intrapsychic disturbance was developing as this boy moved into
adolescence and that the separation-individuation process was beginning to give him more serious trouble. It is likely that this trouble was
being exacerbated by the psychotic reactivity of the mother.

Case 4: L.W., Age 13 Years

This early-adolescent black girl was referred to me for an S.A.T. in
October 1972 by an intake social worker from the Joint Planning
Division of JCCA. At the time, the only information available to me
was that the Angel Guardian Home in Brooklyn, a Catholic foster care
agency, was seeking placement for the girl in one of JCCA's facilities.
The protocol of 54 responses and the summary chart are presented in
the Appendix beginning on page 253.

She had 24 responses on mild pictures and 30 on strong pictures.
Loneliness was the most frequently recorded response (10), a result that
indicated intense inner emptiness under even mild separation conditions, and secondary phobic, anxiety and withdrawal responses of
strong intensity. This indicated the extent of intense pain. Intense
feelings of considerable frequency were stirred by the mild pictures,
resulting in only a 12% differential between mild and strong pictures.
Thus, on the class transfer picture, responses included feelings of rejection, impaired concentration, phobic feeling, anxiety, loneliness, and
withdrawal. Anxiety and loneliness were reported on the sleep picture
as well.

Important pattern disturbances were demonstrated. Attachment
responses were 30% of the total, indicating a strong symbiotic un-
dercurrent. This was emphasized by the 15% separation-individuation
reactions, which represents a severe disturbance of the balance.
Significant aspects of the balance were shown by the excess of attachment to individuation reactions on mild pictures—which was
unusual and is typically found in basic symbiotic problems. Further,
the separation-individuation reactions to the mild pictures were equal
to those on the strong pictures—a phenomenon indicating the serious
problem of the earlier separation-individuation process. Severe inner

separation pain was demonstrated (31%), a finding of considerable significance. At the same time, there was an unusual suppression of separation hostility reactions (5.6%). When the latter was coupled with the high-level pain and the severe symbiotic and poor separation-individuation reactions, we are left with evidence of severe unconscious super-ego problems. The 13% withdrawal response suggested a strong tendency to a loner status and a sullen withdrawal accompanied by panic. It was also noted that self-love loss was stronger than self-esteem loss, a phenomenon which, when accompanied by the above patterns, indicates that she falls back on narcissistic involvement.

We would therefore expect that threats of geographic or intrapsychic separation from significant attachments would lead to alternation between withdrawal, inhibition, and depression or outbursts of panic. Such a condition could, no doubt, lead to self-destructive reactions. It is further noted that the identity stress level is low—a poor prognosticator for self-image development in adolescence and, at the least, the likelihood of immature psychosexual development. In my report on this girl, I stated: "She had deep, ungratified attachment needs and her immaturity and emotional development made it difficult for her to express these needs in a normal way." It was recommended that residential treatment be avoided for a time and efforts made to treat the foster family.

Subsequent to the examination, I consulted the case worker on the history and read the record. The life experiences of this girl provided considerable reasons for the condition noted above, but there were some differences between what the test showed and psychiatric opinion. She had been referred for treatment to a child guidance clinic because, in the past year, she had become sullen, resentful and withdrawn. She refused to eat and often complained of being "picked on" by the foster mother. Her behavior and her words became quite threatening, and the foster mother became fearful that L.W. would do something quite drastic. She began talking about killing herself and the foster mother; as a result, the entire family came under great strain.

L.W., a second child, was born prematurely to a mother who had been a delinquent girl, a runaway, incorrigible and sexually permissive. She had been in institutions and had lived alternately with her maternal grandmother and mother. The mother abandoned L.W. as a baby in the hospital, and her whereabouts was unknown until October 1966 when L.W. was 7 years old. Seen for a short time, the mother disappeared again in December 1966 and was never seen or heard from again. The father was unknown. L.W. lived in a nursery as an infant and was then placed in the present foster home in November 1961 at the age of two. She had many ups and downs in this home, being obedient, polite and well-behaved for periods of time and, at times, bursting out with hostility and defiance. Some of this was related to the discovery of the existence of her own mother.

In May 1970, she was reported by the school to be inattentive and indifferent, but shy and polite. A counselor noted that L.W. seemed to have a depressed personality and described her as a loner. She appeared to relate to her peers, but tended to be withdrawn and unresponsive. Previous to this report, in February 1970, the school telephoned the case worker stating that L.W. had informed the teacher that she wished to die and might kill herself. She also complained that no one loved her. Various physical complaints, including stomach and knee pains, were made, but physical findings were negative. She was then referred (May 1970) for study at a mental hygiene clinic. Psychological testing at the time revealed that she was of slow intelligence, bland and overtly unemotional. Jealousy and hostility toward a foster sibling were reported. Projective tests at the time yielded little of value because of constriction.

After a school change and some medication, L.W. did better, but periods of quiet were at times interrupted by severe outbursts of stubbornness, manipulativeness and hostility toward her foster mother and foster sibling. In March 1971, she refused to attend school. In addition, whenever her foster mother denied her anything, she went into a rage. Ambivalence by foster parents with regard to handling and placement continued while the psychiatrist and case worker made efforts at residential placement. Shortly thereafter, her foster parents appeared to have alleviated the problems and decided to keep her home.

Things ran smoothly with no recurrence of disturbance, and sessions at the agency's clinic were discontinued. Then, by the summer of 1972, a resurgence took place. L.W. was felt to be threatening to the happiness of the entire family, and placement was again requested. The agency worker said: "It is felt that the foster family never incorporated this child as a true member of its household." However, and despite this, on September 25, 1972, her foster mother decided that the placement request was precipitant and based mainly on the father's impulsiveness. The family again wanted to keep her. The psychiatrist then found L.W. to be almost mute, unresponsive and with an intense distaste for the foster home. She was referred back for further psychotherapy, but in October 1972, another disturbance with further study and referral occurred. The ambivalent home status continued with increasing disturbance and resentment in L.W. By February 1973, she was beginning to request placement out of the home, and the Angel Guardian psychiatrist referred her for further psychological testing.

The Ferer Structured Completion Test was administered, and on this test, marked suicidal as well as homicidal reactions were laid bare. The psychiatrist said: "In my opinion, L.W. will not make a suicidal attempt of any severity so long as she believes that there are people interested in her and attempting to plan meaningfully and constructively for her. However, should she be forced to remain in a living situation she perceives as inimical to her interest and one in which she is subjected to constant, unwarranted criticism, it is my feeling that her capacity for acting out in this fashion would be increased."

At this writing, the Joint Planning Division is recommending hospitalization prior to consideration of residential treatment. The one interesting difference between the S.A.T. protocol and the background material is the suppressed hostility on the former and the overt hostility on the latter. It appears that the turmoil in this girl was expressed largely through attachment need (30%) and separation pain (31%), a total of 61% of the responses. Since the test material reported reactions to separation, whether mild or severe, it seems likely that this girl was emphasizing her attachment need and severe pain at separation and the lack of restitution, whereas, in the environment, this girl was overtly clamoring for restitution of the lost love object. The latter appeared to have been stimulated by the short appearance of the natural mother, although it became obvious that the ambivalence of the foster parents in the handling of this girl was a serious contributing factor. Constant threats of abandonment were seriously exacerbating her condition. The inability of this girl to psychologically gratify her attachment need in this family setting, and the extraordinary emotional pain she was experiencing in the process, resulted in an intense clamoring for maternal attention which was not forthcoming in a meaningful way.

Since the time of the above events, L.W. attempted suicide by slashing her wrists when the foster father attempted to take her back to the agency for placement. This dramatic occurrence is a startling corroboration of the significance of the self-destructive pattern being discussed here.

Case 5: E.B., Age 15

This girl was given the S.A.T. on November 10, 1972. She resided at the Pleasantville Cottage School and was tested by Dr. George Sackheim, who had had no previous experience with the test. Dr. Sackheim brought the test protocol to a seminar meeting of the Psychologist Division of the Psychiatric Clinic of JCCA for evaluation. Nothing in this girl's background was known to me at the time of presentation, but was known to one member of the seminar group. The obtained protocol is presented in the appendix.

It should be pointed out that, during the administration of the S.A.T., there are mental set questions which precede the request for responses to the pictures. E.B. reported an unusual number of separation experiences (10 out of 12 pictures). Such severe disruption of life relationships represents an abnormal experience when compared to the average number of "yeses" obtained on the mental set questions. There were a total of 62 responses, with 26 on the mild and 36 on the strong pictures. This gave a percentage difference of 16%, which is somewhat low and indicates an increased sensitivity to the mild pictures. This was especially noteworthy on the school transfer picture in which she had 7 responses—rejection, fear, loneliness, withdrawal, projection, intrapunitiveness and identity stress—an unusual patterning for a girl of this age. Of further significance was the selection of the loneliness response on each of the 12 pictures. Additionally, there were strong emphases on the phobic and withdrawal responses. There was no evidence of inadequate reality testing.

Nevertheless, a very serious patterning of disturbance was revealed. As noted on the pattern chart, 29% of the responses were in the attachment area. Such strong need for closeness was accompanied by only 3 responses (5%) on the separation-individuation pattern. There was a strong attachment need pattern on the mild pictures, exceeding the individuation pattern, while the individuation patterns on both mild and strong pictures were practically equal. This serious weakness was accompanied by intense separation hostility—largely intrapunitive—a turning inward of strong hostile feeling. Separation pain was very severe, reaching 22% of the total. The evidence of severe emotional turmoil in the presence of separation phenomena was obvious. Strong self-love loss (13%) greatly exceeded self-esteem loss, indicating a serious breakdown in self-confidence and a regression to narcissism. Separation denial was strong (16%) with considerable emphasis on withdrawal and fantasy.

The above pattern describes a deeply needful individual beset by serious weaknesses in the separation-individuation process, resulting in severe emotional turmoil and self-destructive potential. She is, thus, a highly sensitive and vulnerable girl constantly open to serious emotional disturbance at the slightest threat of separation from the source of love and security. The resulting instability indicates the need for a carefully protected environment in which care is taken to avoid precipitant ego frustrations or deprivations of supportive relationships.

The history of this girl is tragic in many respects as attested by the long case record of the JCCA. Born in Greece, she was abandoned by her mother when the father died and placed in the care of an older woman. Very little is known of her early development. At age 4 and along with another Greek orphan girl, she was adopted by an elderly couple who had lost all of their three children in adolescence by tragic illness and accident. These adoptive parents were, themselves, very shaky in their physical and emotional well-being, the mother being a depressed and bitter woman. As it turned out, E.B. was disliked by the adoptive mother and favored by the adoptive father. When she was 9 years old, E.B. was placed in a foster home, due to the serious illness of her adoptive mother. The adoptive mother died shortly thereafter, and E.B. was blamed for this by the adoptive father. In the foster home, she was very difficult and unable to relate adequately and was replaced in another home where she remained until age 12. During this three-year period, she related better but was difficult and destructive. The foster father became seriously ill when E.B. was approaching adolescence, and she was transferred to the JCCA's Mt. Vernon Group Residence. The foster father then died suddenly of a heart attack.

When E.B.'s adjustment at Mt. Vernon proved very precarious, she was placed at Grasslands Hospital for a short time and then returned to JCCA and placed at Pleasantville Cottage School. She was now 13 years old. Earlier, when she was 11, she had been described by a psychiatrist as deeply troubled, depressed and anxiety-ridden, with feelings of loneliness and insecurity, and embittered, suspicious and lacking in basic trust of people. Her dependence on parental assurance for feelings of worth and significance was still very strong. Her sense of self and her ego development were very shaky. Two years later, the psychiatrist said that she was not psychotic but that she easily regressed in a crisis. She was considered impulsive, with a low frustration tolerance, prone to depressive episodes because of her extreme sensitivity, feelings of rejection and deep-seated guilt feelings.

During the past several years, she had shown wide mood swings between hysteria and depression during psychotherapeutic treatment. It was most interesting that, with her beautiful singing voice, she sang melancholy songs and talked about needing someone to love her (note the high attachment need on the S.A.T.). Recent psychiatric and psychological studies of this girl have emphasized her problems in object relations, her unconscious need for reunion with her lost mother, her inability to form really close and satisfying human relations because of the intense need for the basic maternal figure. Her present psychiatrist suggested that: "It is probably not farfetched to assume that this girl will avoid at all costs the possibility of another disappointment or rejection as has occurred in her short lifetime." Another psychiatrist and her recent examining psychologist characterized her as having "a Marilyn Monroe syndrome." The psychologist found evidence of suicidal potential in the TAT, and, in addition, he noted that heterosexual relationships would be likely to be casual, superficial and unsatisfactory. The psychologist found further that this girl suffered from severe unconscious guilt and that her acting out and defiance were in response to great inner emotional suffering. E.B. was considered to be of bright normal intelligence, with considerable variability in functioning.

The corroborative material in this case is quite extensive and especially noteworthy in a number of areas. The S.A.T. indicated the intensity of the loneliness and affect hunger which was described in various terms by the case worker, psychiatrist and psychologist. The depressive trend, as well as inner emotional turmoil, was emphasized by both psychiatrist and psychologist. Weak identity formation was seen by the psychologist in the Rorschach and her identity stress index in the S.A.T. Especially significant is the corroboration of self-destructive potential in the TAT material and in the implications of the history of the frequency of illness and death in adoptive and foster families, resulting in strong inner depression. While all those who have had contact with her describe her as a very personable, intelligent and capable adolescent with positive potential and a strong drive to prove herself, there lurks within her a trend from which, if permitted to surface as a result of a keen disappointment and a separation experience, a suicide attempt could result.

The five cases presented above are summarized in Table 17.1. The similarity of patterns is unmistakable and should be considered as a basis for further research on self-destructive vulnerability to separation experiences.

Table 17.1

SEPARATION ANXIETY TEST PROTOCOL SUMMARIES OF FIVE CASES OF YOUNGSTERS WITH SELF DESTRUCTIVE TENDENCIES

FACTOR PATTERN	CASES AND AGES						
	I-12½	II-12½	III-11½	IV-13	V-15	Median	Comp. Norms
1 A. Attachment	21%	29%	22%	30%	29%	29%	Very High
B. Individuation	3%	5%	11%	15%	5%	5%	Very Low
2 A. Attach-Ind.	Mild	Mild	Mild A-I	Mild A-I	Mild A-I	Mild A-I	Serious
B. Balance Deficits	A-I	A-I	Ind. Bal	Ind. Bal	Ind. Bal	Ind. Bal	Weakness
3 A. Separation Hostility	19%	16%	13%	5½%	16%	16%	Strong
B. Separation Pain	22%	17½%	19%	31%	21%	21%	Very Strong
4 A. Conc.-Sub. Ratio	5%	6%	8%	5½%	1½%	5½%	A weaker than
B. Self-Love Loss	14%	13%	9%	7½%	13%	13%	B
5 Separation Denial	17%	21%	21%	13%	16%	17%	Very High
6 Separation Identity Stress	6%	4½%	7%	3½%	10%	6%	Weak
Attach.-Indiv. Balance	47%	82%	40%	22%	34%	40%	Strong but not diff.
Absurd Responses	8	2	1	1	3	2	Generally Normal
Mild-Strong Diff.	20%	38%	22%	12%	18%	20%	Generally Normal

A COMPARATIVE STATISTICAL STUDY OF THREE GROUPS OF CASES RELATIVE TO SEPARATION-DETERMINED SELF-DESTRUCTIVE VULNERABILITY

In this section of the report, I shall make comparisons between the group of five cases presented above and two other groups of cases. These latter two groups consist of one group of fourteen unselected clinic cases and thirty cases selected from the records of unselected populations from my original study of adolescent separation stress. The purpose of this comparison is to note the relative presence of the self-destructive patterns in these groups which were diagnosed in the group of five cases. This also provides an opportunity to rate the extent of self-destructive vulnerability in other cases. In order to make this comparison, I should like to reiterate and then elaborate on the six factors which appear in the records of the five cases with self-destructive tendencies and which are summarized in Table 17.1.

Factor 1: This deals with attachment in relation to separation and individuation. There is a normal or very strong attachment percentage which is based upon the responses of loneliness, feelings of rejection and empathy, which is the index adopted originally for the test. At the same time, there is a severe lowering of the separation acceptance or individuation index. This percentage is based upon the responses of adaptation, well-being and sublimation. The comparison of these two indices indicates such a severe lowering of the individuation percentage in relation to the attachment percentage based on the original norms for the test as to suggest a serious disorder of the separation-individuation process.

Factor 2: This refers to the relationship between the attachment individuation construction and the strength of the separation stimulus. On the six mild pictures, the five children referred to above showed a stronger attachment reaction than individuation reaction, a serious reversal of a normal reaction. This suggested an overly strong reaction and a severe sensitivity to slight separation experiences, a phenomenon suggesting an anxious attachment as defined by Bowlby. Such a sensitivity would have to be considered as a strong vulnerability to separation experiences and environmental changes from familiar to unfamiliar settings. Included in this factor was a general equality between the individuation reactions on the mild and strong pictures. Both of these conditions indicated an abnormal deficit in the reactions to the separation stimulus.

Factor 3: We deal here with the strength of the reported emotional turmoil which results from the separation experiences. These affect reactions include six responses grouped under separation hostility and separation pain, the former including anger, projection and intrapunitiveness and the latter fear, anxiety and somatic reactions. In our five cases, the combination of these affect areas was very high, encompassing between one-third and two-fifths of the responses (Table 17.1, Appendix II). In all five cases, separation pain exceeded separation hostility, and in four out of the five cases, hostility was quite strong. This indicates that, in combination with the disturbance in the separation-individuation process, there is a considerable affect upheaval of great inner significance.

Factor 4: This aspect is concerned with the strength of separation denial, an index consisting of withdrawal, evasion and fantasy. When this is strong, especially if fantasy dominates, it signifies a delusional trend. In our five cases, it can be seen from the data that this factor was definitely stronger than the norm (17%). Such a factor would represent a danger to the self when it is combined with the other indexes and could add to the danger of suicidal reactions in the presence of separation.

Factor 5: This factor refers to the severe loss of self-love in relationship to the self-esteem pattern. The self-love loss index consists of rejection and intrapunitive responses. A higher than normal percentage here is an indicator of an abnormal self-rejection; the normative population generally shows a higher self-esteem loss than self-love loss. Our five cases showed Factor 5 present in each case.

Factor 6: Here we are concerned with the identity stress response. In each of the five cases, the identity stress percentage was low or very low. This suggested difficulty in handling the normal regressive tendency of early adolescence; therefore, a hindrance to psychosexual maturation. This difficulty strongly indicates a fear of going to pieces during a separation experience and, therefore, an unwillingness to accept any personality change at this stage of life.

The data in these five cases, which are summarized in Table 17.1, suggest that, when all six factors are present, the combination has lethal or destructive potential toward the self. This theoretical formulation coincides with the clinical data as well as with material drawn from the literature. We see a severe, almost unquenchable, affect hunger for being wanted and loved by an attachment figure, a tremendous difficulty in accepting even mild separation, a severe inner emotional turmoil which is unneutralized, a trend toward withdrawal and possibly delusional reactions, a severe sense of self-castigation and denigration and a lack of ability to handle identity stress. Lacking an adequate defense in the face of these weaknesses, these children may be prone to depressions and/or delusional episodes.

Now, let us consider a random sampling of 14 cases drawn from our clinic records of youngsters who were given the S.A.T. These cases showed a median age of 12½, which is the same as our five cases listed above. From Table 17.2, we will note that each of the 14 cases has been checked for each of the six factors. The presence of a factor in a given case is noted by a / sign, while the absence is noted by an X. We will note that no case showed all six factors; one case showed five fac-

Table 17.2

DEGREE OF SELF DESTRUCTIVE SEPARATION
ANXIETY TEST PATTERNS ON FOURTEEN
UNSELECTED CLINIC CASES

Case	Age	Pattern Significant Factors						Total	Index
		1	2	3	4	5	6		
1	10	X	X	X	X	X	/	1	17%
2	12	X	X	X	X	X	/	1	17%
3	13½	X	X	X	X	X	X	0	0%
4	14½	X	X	/	X	X	X	1	17%
5	14	/	/	/	/	/	X	5	83%
6	14½	X	/	/	X	/	/	4	67%
7	12½	/	X	/	X	X	/	3	50%
8	13	/	/	/	X	X	X	3	50%
9	12	X	X	/	/	X	/	3	50%
10	12½	X	X	/	X	X	X	1	17%
11	12	X	X	/	X	X	/	2	33%
12	11	X	X	X	/	/	/	3	50%
13	12	X	X	X	/	X	/	2	33%
14	13	X	X	X	X	X	X	0	0%

Median 12½ Range of Points 0-5 Median 2 Median Index % 33% Number of Cases Showing Significant % (above or at 50) 6 43% Points of strong significance 3 (emotional turmoil) and 6 (identity stress)

Factors most differentiating between self-destructives and the unselected clinic cases: 1, 2, 4, 5.

tors and one case four factors. Eight cases showed zero to two factors, and four cases showed three factors. The median percentage of factors was 33%. The last column would suggest the potential for self-destructive behavior; six cases show a 50% potential or more.

An examination was made of the records of these 14 children, and, in the six cases noted above, there was much stronger evidence than in the other eight cases of considerable sensitivity to separation. These children seemed more threatened by object loss, and their defenses were strongly masochistic. It is also important to note that we are dealing with gradations of capacity for defense against self-destructiveness. In Table 17.2, it may be seen that Factors 3 and 6 were not as differentiating as Factors 1, 2, 4 and 5. From these data, it seemed that attachment need with poor balance between this and individuation, as well as separation denial and identity responses, were most differentiating between our five cases and the unselected clinic cases.

Table 17.3 presents an evaluation of self-destructive patterns (referrable to the five cases) in an unselected group of 30 cases from a school population of non-placed children. Striking differences appear. Only 20% of this group showed indexes from the six factors of 50% or more. Only one child showed a really strong potential for self-destructiveness as measured by this scale. Factors 1, 2 and 6 differentiated most between this population and our five cases.

Table 17.4 indicates that the more we move from the strongly self-destructive population through clinic cases and then the more normative population, we see a gradual decrease in the degree of the presence of the six factors. Noteworthy is the finding that Factors 1 and 2 were least present in both the clinic and normative population. Such a finding suggests that the attachment level, in relation to the individuation level on both mild and strong pictures, is a very sensitive indicator for self-destructive potential. While these two factors are the most sensitive, it seems obvious that, when the other four factors are combined with these two, the potential is far greater. For example, intense emotional reactions, as seen in Factor 3 (separation hostility and separation pain), occurred in our five cases (Table 17.1) while in our unselected clinic cases, 57% of the children showed this intensity, and in our unselected normative population, only 13% showed this. There is some suggestion from this material, if one is permitted a bit of theorizing, that many children may have counteracting defenses which

Table 17.3

DEGREE OF SELF DESTRUCTIVE SEPARATION
ANXIETY TEST PATTERNS OF THIRTY NON-PLACED
CHILDREN IN A RANDOM POPULATION SAMPLING

Case	Age	Pattern Significant Factors						Total	Index
		1	2	3	4	5	6		
1	12½	X	X	X	X	X	X	0	0%
2	13	/	X	/	/	/	/	5	83%
3	13	X	/	/	X	/	X	3	50%
4	12½	X	X	X	X	/	/	2	33%
5	13	X	X	/	/	X	X	2	33%
6	13	/	X	/	/	X	X	3	50%
7	13	X	X	X	X	X	X	0	0%
8	13½	X	X	/	X	/	/	3	50%
9	13	/	X	/	X	X	X	2	33%
10	12½	X	X	/	X	/	X	2	33%
11	12½	X	X	X	X	X	X	0	0%
12	13	X	X	X	X	/	X	1	17%
13	12½	X	X	X	/	/	X	2	33%
14	14	X	X	X	X	X	X	0	0%
15	14	/	X	X	X	/	X	2	33%
16	13½	X	X	/	/	X	X	2	33%
17	12½	X	X	X	/	/	/	3	50%
18	14½	X	X	/	/	X	X	2	33%
19	14	X	X	X	/	X	X	1	17%
20	14½	X	X	X	/	X	X	1	17%
21	12	X	X	/	/	X	X	2	33%
22	14	X	X	X	/	X	X	1	17%
23	14½	X	X	X	/	X	X	1	17%
24	13	X	X	X	/	X	X	1	17%
25	13½	X	X	X	/	X	X	1	17%
26	13	X	X	X	X	/	X	1	17%
27	13½	X	X	X	/	X	X	1	17%
28	15½	X	X	X	/	/	X	2	33%
29	12½	X	X	X	X	X	X	0	0%
30	12	/	X	/	/	X	X	3	50%

Median 13½ Range of Points 0-5 Median 2 Median Index %
33% Number of Cases Showing Significant % (above
or at 50) 6 20% Points of Strong Significance 3
(emotional turmoil), 4 intensity of self love
loss, and 5, separation denial
Factors most differentiating between self-
destructiveness and the unselected normal population, 1, 2 and 6.

prevent separation turmoil from disrupting the ego—a kind of im-
munization probably related to a stronger separation-individuation
achievement.

Table 17.4

SUMMARY OF SELF-DESTRUCTIVE TENDENCIES FOR THREE GROUPS DEPICTED IN
TABLES 17.1, 17.2 and 17.3

Group	No. of Cases	Age Range	Median Age	% Cases at 50% or Above Self-Dest.	Differentiating Factors
A. Self-destructive Cases	5	11½-15	12½	100%	1,2,3,4,5,6
B. Unselected Clinic Cases	14	10-14½	12½	43%	1,2,4,5
C. Unselected Normal Population	30	12-15½	13	20%	1,2,6

Factors which are most differentiating are 1 (severe lowering of total individuation in relation to attachment need) and 2 (attachment-individuation balance deficits
-high level of attachment response to mild stimuli and fairly equivalent individuation
response to mild and strong stimuli).

SUMMARY AND CONCLUSIONS

This paper has been concerned with the relationship between self-
destructive potential in early adolescence and a specific pattern of
responses on the S.A.T. Theoretical and clinical material from the
literature indicated that there is a strong relationship between intense
separation experiences from significant love objects and self-destructive
or suicidal trends in humans as well as in animals. At least, there is
evidence that fears of abandonment, as well as actual loss of love objects, can be precipitating factors in suicidal behavior. Locating children whose sensitivity and vulnerability to separation are intense and
whose patterns are self-destructively responsive to actual or threatened
separation from significant attachment figures has been considered an
important task for mental health workers.

The S.A.T. is so designed as to reveal internal feeling reaction to intensity gradations of separation experiences. During the course of my
work with this instrument at the JCCA, I have uncovered what appears to be a special group of highly sensitive youngsters who are prone
to self-destructive reactions under separation stress, whether

threatened or actual. The five youngsters described in this report are certainly not diagnostically similar; they range from psychotic propensities to neurotic problems and character difficulties. Yet, they all show a S.A.T. pattern markedly similar and with evidence from other data of self-destructive trends.

The milieus in which these children have lived varied from foster homes to group residences to institutional settings. Their histories are considerably different in many respects but, in all cases, fears of abandonment and actual abandonment had been experienced with great intensity. While patterns of defense and ego potential vary, their sensitivity to attachment deprivation appears to be expressed in severe overt distress of a magnitude likely to result in a self-destructive or suicidal attempt.

The evolvement of the recognition of this test pattern came to me slowly as each case was presented. It certainly cannot be considered as final in any sense. Further, it is likely that other patterns exist in which a trend toward self-harm will be discerned. To uncover such patterns might necessitate several types of studies; some might be post hoc (subsequent to suicide or self-destructive efforts) and others follow-up studies of large populations over long periods of time to determine the degree and extent of such behavior among test-determined potential cases as differentiated from controls.

In the present study, it was possible to make comparisons of three groups of youngsters for the presence and extent of the six factors (described on pages 246–247). It was seen that unselected clinic cases showed a considerably lessened number of cases with the six-factor pattern and unselected normative populations still far less. These data provide some, but not by any means final, confirmation of the significance and prevalence of the pattern.

I should not like to leave this paper without considering the clinical significance of these data. The material suggests that, in the presence of strong attachment need, some children are unable to accept even mild separation experiences and show a definite disturbance in the separation-individuation process. This results in severe emotional turmoil—an effort to retrieve the lost love object—but, at the same time, a severe lowering of self-love. This corroborates Bowlby's concept of protest and despair. The strong feeling of abandonment which ensues and the inability to handle the normal identity stress and regressive pulls of early adolescence produce an unusual combination of depression and impulsiveness which endangers the welfare of the child. When this is combined with a pull toward denial, temporary delusional reaction is possible.

From this material, it follows that these children require special care by child care agencies. The most significant safeguard is likely to lie in the provision of long-term attachment figures. In addition, it seems likely that these youngsters will need to be carried in psychotherapeutic treatment as a bulwark against suicide attempts. From the experience with these five cases reported herein, there is some suggestion that, when active intervention by mental health workers is made available, there is a likelihood that successful suicide attempts will not ensue.

APPENDIX: THE FIVE CASE PROTOCOLS

A summary of the five protocols is presented below. The original text may be referred to for additional details.

Case 1: N.G., Age 12-8 (12 years, 8 months)

Rejection—8 (Mild 2, Strong 6), Imp. Conc.—4 (M 2, S 2), Phobic—8 (3, 5), Anxiety—9 (5, 4), Loneliness—10 (4, 6), Withdrawal—9 (5, 4), Somatic—4 (1, 3), Adaptive—1 (1, 0), Anger—8 (4, 4), Projection—5 (1, 4), Empathy—8 (3, 5), Evasion—6 (2, 4), Fantasy—1 (0, 1), Well-being—1 (1, 0), Sublimation—1 (1, 0), Intrapunitive—5 (0, 5) and Identity Stress—6 (2, 4). Total: 94 (Mild 37, Strong 57).

Patterns: Attachment—26 (Mild 9, Strong 17), 21%; Individuation—3 (M 3, S 0), 3%, Hostility—18 (5, 13), 19%; Painful Tension—21 (9, 12), 22%; Reality Avoidance—16 (7, 9), 17%; Conc. Imp. vs. Sub.—3:2, 5%; Self-Love Loss—13 (2, 11), 14%; Identity Stress—6 (2, 4), 6%; Absurd Responses—8 (2, 6).

Case 2: M.G., Age 12-5

Rejection—4 (Mild 0, Strong 4), Imp. Conc.—2 (M 1, S 1), Phobic—3 (2, 1), Anxiety—5 (3, 2), Loneliness—8 (2, 6), Withdrawal—7 (2, 5), Somatic—3 (1, 2), Adaptive—1 (1, 0), Anger—5 (1,

4), Projection—1 (0, 1), Empathy—6 (1, 5), Evasion—3 (1, 2), Fantasy—3 (0, 3), Well-Being—2 (1, 1), Sublimation—2 (2, 0), Intrapunitive—4 (0, 4), and Identity Stress—3 (1, 2). Total: 62, (Mild 19, Strong 43).

Patterns: Attachment—18 (Mild 3, Strong 15), 29%; Individuation—5 (M 4, S 1), 8%; Hostility—10 (1, 9), 16%; Painful Tension—11 (6, 5), 17½%; Reality Avoidance—13 (3, 10), 21%; Imp. vs. Sub. 2:2, 6%; Self-Love Loss—8 (0, 8), 13%; Identity Stress—3 (2, 1), 5%; Absurd Responses—2 (0, 2).

Case 3: J.C., Age 11-8

Rejection—2 (Mild 0, Strong 2), Imp. Conc.—4 (M 1, S 3), Phobic—6 (5, 1), Anxiety—6 (2, 4), Loneliness—8 (3, 5), Withdrawal—7 (3, 4), Somatic—0 (0, 0), Adaptive—6 (3, 3), Anger—4 (2, 2), Projection—0 (0, 0), Empathy—4 (0, 4), Evasion—0 (0, 0), Fantasy—6 (2, 4), Well-Being—0 (0, 0), Sublimation—1 (1, 0), Intrapunitive—4 (1, 3), and Identity Stress—4 (1, 3). Total: 62, (Mild 24, Strong 38).

Patterns: Attachment—14 (Mild 3, Strong 11), 22%; Individuation—7 (M 4, S 3), 11%; Hostility—8 (3, 5), 13%; Painful Tension—12 (7, 5), 19%; Reality Avoidance—13 (5, 8), 21%; Imp. vs. Sub. 4:1, 8%; Self-Love Loss—6 (1, 5), 9%; Identity Stress—4 (1, 3), 7%; Absurd Responses—1 (0, 1).

Case 4: L.W., Age 12-11

Rejection—3 (Mild 1, Strong 2), Imp. Conc.—1 (1, 0), Phobic—7 (4, 3), Anxiety—7 (3, 4), Loneliness—10 (5, 5), Withdrawal—7 (4, 3), Somatic—3 (0, 3), Adaptive—4 (1, 3), Anger—2 (1, 1), Projection—0 (0, 0), Empathy—3 (1, 2), Evasion—0 (0, 0), Fantasy—0 (0, 0), Well-Being—2 (1, 1), Sublimation—2 (2, 0), Intrapunitive—1 (0, 1), and Identity Stress—2 (0, 2). Total: 54, (Mild 24, Strong 30).

Patterns: Attachment—16 (Mild 7, Strong 9), 30%; Individuation—8 (4, 4), 15%; Hostility—3 (1, 2), 5½%; Painful Tension—17 (7, 10), 31%; Reality Avoidance—7 (4, 3), 13%; Imp. vs. Sub. 1:2, 5½%; Self-Love Loss—4 (1, 3), 7½%; Identity Stress—2 (0, 2), 3½%; Absurd Responses—1 (1, 0).

Case 5: E.B., Age 15-3

Rejection—3 (Mild 1, Strong 2), Imp. Conc.—1 (M 1, S 0), Phobic—7 (3, 4), Anxiety—6 (2, 4), Loneliness—12 (6, 6), Withdrawal—7 (5, 2), Somatic—1 (0, 1), Adaptive—3 (1, 2), Anger—4 (1, 3), Projection—1 (1, 0), Empathy—3 (0, 3), Evasion—0 (0, 0), Fantasy—3 (0, 3), Well-Being—0 (0, 0), Sublimation—0 (0, 0), Intrapunitive—5 (2, 3), Identity Stress—6 (3, 3). Total: 62 (Mild 26, Strong 36).

Patterns: Attachment—18 (Mild 7, Strong 11), 29%; Individuation—3 (M 1, S 2), 5%; Hostility—10 (4, 6), 16%; Painful Tension—14 (5, 9), 22%; Reality Avoidance—10 (5, 5), 16%; Conc. Imp. vs. Sub.—1:0, 1½%; Self-Love Loss—8 (3, 5), 13%; Identity Stress—6 (3, 3), 10%; Absurd Responses— (0, 3).

REFERENCES

Ainsworth, M. D. S., and Wittig, B. A. "Attachment and Exploratory Behavior of One Year Olds in a Strange Situation." In *Determinants of Infant Behavior*, Vol. 4. Ed. B. M. Foss, London: Methuen, 1969.

Begers, C. "Beauty and Her Beasts." *Saturday Review: The Sciences*, Vol. 1, No. 1 (Jan. 27, 1973). Interview with Jane Goodall at Stanford University, pp. 34–37.

Bowlby, J., *Separation: Anxiety and Anger*, Vol. 2: *Attachment and Loss*. London: Hogarth Press, 1973.

Bowlby, J., "Attachment Theory, Separation Anxiety and Mourning," in Hamburg, D. A. and Brodie, H. K. (eds.), *American Handbook of Psychiatry*, Vol. VI: *New Psychiatric Frontiers*, 1974.

Farberow, N. L., and Schneidman, E. S. *Clues to Suicide.* New York: McGraw-Hill, 1957.

Farberow, N. L. *Cry for Help.* New York: McGraw Hill, 1961.

Friedman, N. *Varieties of Symbiotic Manifestations.* New York: Institute for Psychoanalytic Research Training, 1967.

Hansburg, H. G., *Adolescent Separation Anxiety.* Springfield, Ill.: C. C. Thomas, 1972. Reprinted: Melbourne, Fla.: R. E. Krieger, 1980.

Hansburg, H. G., "Separation Problems of Displaced Children." in *The Emotional Stress of War, Violence and Peace.* Ed. R. Parker, Pittsburgh: Stanwyx House, 1972.

Hansburg, H. G., "Adolescent Separation Hostility: A Prelude to Violence." Tokyo, Japan: Proceedings, XX International Congress of Psychology, 1972, p. 599.

Hansburg, H. G., *Clinical Issues in Psychology*, 4 (30), 1972.

Hansburg, H. G., *American Journal of Orthopsychiatry*, 42 (330), 1972.

Mahler, M. D., *On Human Symbiosis and the Vicissitudes of Individuation*, Vol. I., *Infantile Psychosis*. New York: N.Y. International Universities Press, 1968.

May, Rollo, *Power and Innocence*. New York: W. W. Norton and Co., 1972.

Seligman, M., *Psychology Today*, 7 (43), 1973.

Vital Statistics of the United States, Vol. II, *Mortality*. U.S. Health and Education Welfare Services, 1970.

Whitehead, P.C., Johnson, F. G., and Ferrence, R. *American Journal of Orthopsychiatry*, 43 (1), 1973. "Measuring the Incidence of Self-Injury," p. 142.

Wolff, K. *Patterns of Self-Destruction*. Springfield, Ill.: C. C. Thomas, 1972.

18

Separation Disorders of the Elderly
(1979)

THEORETICAL CONSIDERATIONS

If we conceive of separation experiences as a constant life-stress factor (Bowlby, 1969), then it is certain that, as humans move into age levels of 65 and beyond, this experience will become as continuously demanding (if not more so) as ever. There is good reason to believe that, in old age, because of the greater reduction in activity and limitations of power and because of past separation experiences with family members, the stress of separation from loved ones, especially as death approaches, would produce disturbances in emotional life and, therefore, in behavior. This was verified indirectly by the highly significant affirmative responses to the question, "Do you worry that persons most close to you won't be with you when you are dying?" (one of the three most significant questions discriminating levels of death anxiety in a questionnaire for the elderly developed by Conte, Weiner, Plutchik & Bennett, 1975).

Bowlby (1969) has pointed out that attachment is a significant factor from the cradle to the grave and has important survival value. For this reason, separation from significant attachment figures or from important life endeavors must also be considered as a threatening phenomenon, not only of early life but also of middle as well as old age. So important is this in the elderly that the frequent isolation that accompanies old age, because of debility and problems of the self-image, often enforces unwitting and/or unwilling separations. This would suggest that specific emotional disturbances may well arise, not only

257

because of the physical disorders of old age but also because of either self-imposed or externally induced deprivations of attachment need. It would seem likely that individuals who are capable of gratifying the need for attachment to others are more likely to survive the emotional ravages of old age than those who, for various reasons, are unable to do so.

It follows from the above that those among the elderly who are most needful of attachments (especially those who are most seriously handicapped by physical disability) would be most vulnerable to threats of, or actual, abandonment by close persons or caretakers. On the other hand, those who are least needful and most able to utilize their personal resources in dealing either with handicaps or approaching death will be least vulnerable to emotional disturbance. It is obvious that much would depend upon the individual's personality traits and past life experiences. It also seems likely that much will depend upon the current life-style or life conditions which characterize the elderly.

Further, as age increases, the individual experiences diminution of some functions, which may well simulate the process of loss, that is, the loss of part of the self. This loss may well affect the sense of identity and influence integrative capacities. The fear of loss of one's integrity or integrative powers is a constant problem in the elderly. This vulnerability to the loss of part of the self is likely to induce inner emotional turmoil unless supportive attachment figures provide both reassurance and opportunities for constructive channels of self-expression.

Individuals who have survived to old age and who have succeeded with a pattern of excessive self-sufficiency and merely surface relationships, or who have been characterized by a "false self," are faced with the possibility of decompensation. If such takes place, then they are more likely to experience serious emotional disorders in old age because the only level they can experience attachments is at the pre-Oedipal period.

In line with the above theoretical considerations, it seems that the manner and techniques of human object relations is an area of human experience that is symptomatically useful in understanding the problems of old age. For this reason, methods which can measure, qualify and describe attachment needs, capacity for the use of personal resources, separation affect and defenses of denial, loss of self-esteem, etc., should be useful in diagnosing problems of the elderly.

METHODS FOR STUDYING THE ELDERLY

The literature on the elderly, describing observational, retrospective, clinical interviews, tests, etc., has been quite extensive in recent years. Aside from dealing with the physical problems and their psychological effects, the areas of emphasis have been on such subjects as attitudes toward death (Kubler-Ross, 1969), suicide (Schneidman, 1961), intellectual, motor and sensory disabilities (Rapaport, 1946), body image concerns (Plutchik et al., 1976), depression and grief (Parkes, 1972), separation from children (Goldfarb, 1955), etc. Specific discussions and studies of attachment, separation, and loss problems of the elderly have been sparse. The literature is replete with clinical, hospital, senior citizen club group interviews and tests dealing with the problems manifested by the elderly at home and in the community. In these studies, there has been marked emphasis on the need for a variety of forms of psychological, social and financial assistance, as well as medical care. There have been many implications suggesting that the need for relatedness experiences among the elderly are considerable, but little has been done to explore Bowlby's theoretical formulation of the lifelong need for attachments, the dangers of threats of abandonment and the theory of loss.

In the present study, I have adapted a method which I had originally devised for the study of adolescents (Hansburg, 1972). Although this method was standardized for adolescent youngsters, it was found to be very useful in clinical evaluations of parents and other adults, who found the test easy to take and relatively simple to respond to. The clinical insights into the dynamics between members of the family were of considerable value when used in the study of families (1975; see Chapter 16). An adult is asked to identify with the youngster in the pictures, which presents a rather interesting task for the subject. Since there is no standardization for this procedure with adults, the analysis of the case was accomplished by comparative study of the data within the structure of the test alone but with occasional references to other clinical cases. The result of this procedure has been rewarding in clinical case studies. I was fully aware of the hazards of adapting an instrument of this sort to elderly persons, but, reacting to the proverb, "Nothing ventured, nothing gained," I decided to make the effort to see whether the results would be meaningful. If worthwhile results were obtained, consideration could then be given to the development of an instrument measuring similar feelings and reactions, especially designed for the elderly.

PROBLEMS FOR STUDY

In applying the above instrument to the elderly, a number of significant problems seemed pertinent to study. Do the elderly show disorders of the attachment and separation processes and, if so, are they similar in many ways to those of youngsters and other adults? Are these separation disorders more prevalent among those elderly who are more limited in their life space and in their social, intellectual and physical functioning? Are the normative patterns of attachment and separation similar to those seen in young people or are the patterns generally different? In considering the age levels of 65 to 90, is there any relationship between age and the various factors in the S.A.T.? Are there differences between those still married and those widowed or never married? Do the physically handicapped and those confined by illness show any pattern differences in relation to other elderly? These and other related problems are interesting as they may shed further light on the emotional problems of the elderly.

PROCEDURE AND POPULATION

The procedure consisted mainly of the administration of the S.A.T. to approximately 100 elderly persons ranging in age from 65 to 90, Of these persons, 53 were tested by a student, Mrs. Hazel Schnurr, 21 by a psychologist at the Kingsbrook Medical Center and, later, 26 by myself. Individuals were tested in a number of different environments:

1. employed individuals, largely self-employed
2. retired, unemployed, living at home and not affiliated with any active group
3. a senior citizens' group active in a club in a local Jewish community center
4. individual elderly residing in the Metropolitan Jewish Geriatric Center (a large nursing home), and
5. elderly confined at the Kingsbrook Medical Center for physically handicapped and terminally ill patients.

Among these 62 females and 38 males were many widowers and widows and a few who had never been married. Three records were, for various reasons, excluded from the data, leaving 97 records. The median age of all those tested was approximately 75 years. Individuals in the first two groups were tested either at their place of employment or in their own homes. The third group was tested at the Ocean Parkway Jewish Center, the fourth group at the Maimonides Hospital Far Rockaway Nursing Home (the Metropolitan Jewish Geriatric Center) and the fifth group was examined by Stephanie Warshall (psychologist) at the Kingsbrook Medical Center. The groups were nearly equal in total number, although the median ages were not quite the same. As might be anticipated, the first three groups were, on the whole, slightly younger than the last two.

Testing was done individually, and the responses recorded at that time. Each individual was told that he or she (a separate form of the test was used for the men and women) should try to identify with the child in the picture and, if possible, to recall how he or she would have reacted as a child. Only a few of the elderly reported having problems in following this procedure.

RESULTS

It was originally intended to study the results of this research primarily through a comparison of the patterns (basic to the S.A.T.) for the five groups of the elderly. It was posited that these groups would vary from each other because of the differences in the life circumstances in which they lived. However, as further indicated under "Problems for Study," many interesting questions were thought to provide an area of study. Therefore, I have accordingly divided the results into various areas.

Area A: Results According to Life Situation

Aside from the eight patterns noted above, I shall indicate the median for inappropriate (absurd) reactions, differences between mild and strong stimuli responses, total responses, percent of those showing strong symbiotic[1] patterns, percent of those showing strong personality core reactions, number of self-destructive or suicidal factors present and the percent of those showing acting-out tendencies. In Table 18.1, the data for this area are presented in summary form without the statistics representing the analyses of variance and the reliabilities of differences. In so doing, it is possible to note the trends which characterize the relationship between the various groups. In order to understand this material fully, it would be useful to be familiar to some extent with the SAT and the patterns which help us to understand the dynamics to which the various items refer. However, I shall attempt to

---

[1] The term "symbiotic" is used here to refer to intense attachment need as well as limited feelings of self-reliance. Bowlby ("Attachment Theory, Separation Anxiety and Mourning" (1974), *American Handbook of Psychiatry*, Vol. VI: New Psychiatric Frontiers, Ed. D. A. Hamburg and H. K. Brody) believes that this term is "not happily chosen" because it is a phase-specific phenomenon denoting an adaptive partnership between two organisms and borrowed from biology; each organism contributes to the other's survival. However, I believe that this term may be used when there is evidence for *an intense wish on the part of an individual for this kind of relationship and in which he(she) feels that such a relationship is essential to survival.* This intense wish borders on a desire for fusion with an attachment figure and is demonstrated on the S.A.T. by strong attachment, very low self-reliance (individuation), strong affect (hostility and anxiety), strong separation denial and low identity stress, as well as intense separation self-love loss.

Table 18.1

MEDIAN RESPONSES ON THE SEPARATION ANXIETY TEST FOR FIVE DIFFERENT GROUPS OF THE ELDERLY

Grp	A Atc	B Ind	C Hst	D Pain	E Den	F S-E Pre	G Lve Los	H Idn Str	J A-I Bal	K % C Str	L % Symb	M M-S Dif	N S-D Fcts	P Abs	Q Total R	R Act Out
I	25	24	19.5	16.5	5.5	11	8	9	30	50	14	25	1.5	2.8	46	0
II	19	19	16	13.5	14.5	11.5	9	7	2	40	35	20.5	2	3.9	60.5	20
III	22.5	22	14	14	16	15	8	8	19.5	17	42	18	1.5	6.4	68	28
IV	20.5	21	14.5	14	13	9.5	8.5	5	18	25	55	16.5	2	7.1	73.5	30
V	23	14	16	22	14.5	8	11.5	9	20	17	75	11.5	5	10.7	85	33

Abbreviations: A, Attachment; B, Individuation; C, Hostility; D, Pain; E, Denial; F, Self-Esteem Preoccupation; G, Self-Love Loss; H, Identity Stress; J, Attachment-Individuation Balance; K, % of Elderly with good core strength; L, % Elderly with symbiotic trends; M, Mild-Strong differences; N, Self-Destructive factors; P, Absurd responses; Q, Total R; R, % Acting out; Group I - Employed, Group II - Non-Employed, Home, Group III - Senior Citizens Club, Group IV - Metropolitan Geriatric Center, Group V - Kingsbrook Medical Center

Note: Standard deviations of the differences between medians were used on all of the data to obtain reliabilities and degrees of variance. We include here only the results without the extensive variability statistics.

describe the results in language that is generally utilized by the mental health professional.

If we study Column B in the table, we will note that the most severe separation distresses in terms of resourcefulness are noted in Group V, in which the percentage drops to 14, while the strongest group is Group I (employed). Yet, the median attachment level is nearly the same for these two groups. Checking Column D, we see a sizable jump to 22 in the pain level for Group V, while all the other groups are fairly close. We also note in Column E that the employed group shows a considerable diminution in denial in comparison to the others. The weakness in the self-esteem preoccupation area in Group V is countered by considerable strength in this area in the senior club group (III). What is important is the evidence of weakness shown by Group V when we compare Column F to Column G, the latter dealing with the loss of self-love. Group V is the only one in which Column F is exceeded by Column G. This indicator has been found in previous studies with both adolescents and adults to represent vulnerability to depression and self-immolation.

As we continue to study this Table, we become aware that the style of life which is most actively involved in outside activities produces the best profiles, and those least involved produce the worst. This is most readily demonstrated by an analysis of Columns K through R. Here we will note that the core personality strength (a combination of attachment and individuation levels for each individual) begins highest with the employed and drops off considerably as we proceed down Column K. The separation weaknesses increase as we proceed (Column L) from the employed to the Kingsbrook Medical—thus, symbiotic indicators appear lowest among the employed, somewhat stronger in the non-employed at home, still somewhat stronger in the club group, increasingly stronger in the nursing home and finally reaching a point in the Kingsbrook Medical Center, representing 75% of the 21 patients tested in that group.[2] This indicator is of considerable usefulness in understanding vulnerability to separation experiences.

The reaction to the strength of the separation stimulus is an important factor in understanding personality. Good discrimination demonstrated by more responses to the strong pictures than to the mild ones is more characteristic of the balanced and strong personality. We

[2] An explanation of this indicator and its significance appears in the S.A.T. Manual (*Adolescent Separation Anxiety*, Vol. II).

will note in Column M that the median difference (norm for adolescents is 20%) starts at 25% for the employed and gradually decreases
to 11.5 in the Kingsbrook group. This suggests a gradual decrease in
discriminative judgment and greater vulnerability to milder stimuli,
with increasing loss of contact with the activities of outside life. In
Column N, we see an interesting and perhaps not so startling result.
Here, we note that the Kingsbrook group is high in self-destructive factors (1976; see Chapter 17, where is provided an explanation for this
column). There are 6 such factors in the test, and, while the other
groups hover between 1.5 and 2, Kingsbrook shows 5. In Column P,
we note the gradual increase of inappropriate reactions (absurd reactions) moving from 2.8 for the employed, 3.9 for the unemployed home
group, 6.4 for the senior club group, 7.1 for the nursing home and 10.7
for Kingsbrook. This reality testing measure indicates decreasing
reality contacts with increasing confinement. In addition, Column R
demonstrates that more acting out takes place among the elderly as we
proceed from the greatest life involvement to the least. Finally, we will
also note the gradual increase in responsiveness to separation (Column
Q) in the same direction as the above.

A recapitulation of these results shows that eleven out of sixteen
items are differentiating of the five groups of elderly. This is a strong
indication that the style of life, no doubt representing a combination of
personality and life circumstances, is a significant predictor of reactions to separation experiences. The increasing needfulness, vulnerability, depression and self-destructiveness which characterize the
elderly when they are gradually moved out of the mainstream of life
becomes obvious from these results.

As if to emphasize the results, an interesting occurrence at the
Kingsbrook Medical Center is worth noting at this point. During the
course of this study (1976), a new building had been completed for the
hospital, and it was planned to move many of the patients to this
building. When the psychologist noted the vulnerability to separation
and the high number of self-destructive factors present in the records of
many of the patients, she discussed the matter with the administrative
staff but was reassured that all necessary precautions had been taken
for the welfare of the patients. Within a short period after the move,
eight of the ten most vulnerable patients (as measured by the S.A.T.)
died. One of these practically destroyed himself by standing out in the
rain insufficiently clad. This incident suggested that vulnerability to

separation is an important phenomenon in the elderly and should not be taken lightly.

Another incident is of interest at this point. Shortly after the testing at the senior citizen's club was completed, one of their members died suddenly. His wife, who was among the twenty individuals tested, showed the six factors of vulnerability to depression and self-destructiveness. At the time of the sudden death, the shock wave was considerable and she was prostrated. Knowing the pattern observed on the test, I informed members of the club group that she should be watched carefully and that it would be advisable that she not be left to live alone under any circumstances. Heeding this warning, a married son, living in another state, came to stay with her and then took her to reside at his home with his family. Whether it was this action that hastened her recovery will never be known, but, after a period of mourning and a gradual accommodation to her new surroundings, she was able to become involved with a new senior group and take her place in the community. It is possible that this mental health intervention, based on the use of the S.A.T., saved this 66-year-old woman from a deep depression and/or suicide. The pattern described in this woman was strongly symbiotic (in the sense used in the test) and indicated that she would, under the circumstances, be impelled toward living with others and would be unable to manage on her own. (It will be noted that the unemployed home Group II had the lowest median attachment and the lowest pain levels of all five groups.)

Area B: Results According to Age

It was noted previously (p.261) that the ages of the nursing home and hospital groups were somewhat higher than in the other three groups and that this was obviously expected because increasing frailty and illness are part of the aging process and are more likely to result in some form of placement where medical care and social experiences are more available. For this reason, the question was raised as to whether it is the age factor which is largely responsible for the results obtained in Area A.

The data were then arranged by age groups of all of the 97 individuals in the study regardless of style of life or physical or mental condition. These data are presented in Table 18.2. A careful study of this table suggests, in general, that there is no relationship between age and the most significant elements of the S.A.T. Here and there are some minor indications of a significant element, such as the total number of responses in which there appears to be a gradual increase in responsiveness with age. The rise in the ages 70 to 90 does not seem too considerable, although there is a trend. One-fourth of the group were in the 65 to 69 year range, and this group showed a median responsiveness considerably below the other age groups. Whether older elderly are more sensitive to the test may be so, but the general data do not bear this out.

There is some indication that the age group between 75 and 79 tested somewhat differently from the other age groups. This group showed the highest attachment level, the lowest hostility, the lowest denial, a greater self-love loss than self-esteem preoccupation, the weakest identity stress reaction, the highest percentage of individuals with strong symbiotic indicators, the highest number of absurd responses and the lowest number of individuals who tended to act out. This result appears to suggest the possibility that this is the weakest age group. The percentage of this age group was lowest in the weakest environmental group (Kingsbrook—12%) while the highest percentages of this age group were at the nursing home (55%) and at the unemployed home group (43%). This would therefore suggest that the problem of this age group was not due to its relationship to the environmental factor.

Table 18.2

MEDIAN RESPONSES TO THE SEPARATION ANXIETY TEST FOR FIVE DIFFERENT AGE GROUPS OF THE ELDERLY

Age Grp	A Atc	B Ind	C Hst	D Pain	E Den	F S-E Pre	G Lve Los	H Idn Str	J A-I Bal	K % C Str	L % Symb	M M-S Dif	N S-D Fcts	P Abs	Q Total R	R Act Out
65–69	20.4	19.2	17.4	16.5	15.5	13	9.5	8.4	21.3	11	33	20	2	3.5	47½	22%
70–74	20.8	19.5	16.5	16.2	15.5	13	9.6	7.2	14.4	40	20	16½	1.5	3.5	60½	30%
75–79	24.5	21.8	14	16	12.1	9.5	10.8	5.3	15.8	22	44	15	2	7.5	66½	11%
80–84	19.9	24	16.5	14.2	14.5	13	8.7	7	17	16½	22	15	2	4	69	42%
85–89	19.5	19	16.7	12	19	9.5	8.7	9	22	40	0	21	1.3	4	69	20%

See Table 18.1 for abbreviations.

The current data, therefore, seem to suggest that age among the elderly is not a primary determinant of the reactions to the S.A.T. There does seem to be a possibility that the ages between 75 to 80 are crucial in some respects, but it would require replication of this data with other subjects to confirm this. If this suggestion would be proven valid, it would be of interest to determine what factors are responsible.

Area C: Results According to Marital Status

An examination was made of the records with regard to marital status, and four groups were found: (1) married, (2) widowed, (3) never married and (4) divorced. What was most interesting was that only two of the entire group were divorced while 40 were married, 45 widowed and 10 never married. It was our intention to check out this data to determine whether any of the factors in the S.A.T. were related to marital status. This factor seemed pertinent since living with someone, or having someone as close as a spouse visit if one was confined, might be a significant factor in the way in which an individual coped with separation experiences. It was not our intention to undertake a correlative study with the history of marital relations since that would have entailed research that was beyond the study's scope. Table 18.3 presents the data on marital status. The material on the

Table 18.3

MEDIAN RESPONSES TO THE SEPARATION ANXIETY TEST FOR THREE MARITAL STATUS GROUPS OF THE ELDERLY

Mtl Grp	A Atc	B Ind	C Hst	D Pain	E Den	F S-E Pre	G Lve Los	H Idn Str	J A-I Bal	K % C Str	L % Symb	M M-S Dif	N S-D Fcts	P Abs	Q Total R	R Act Out
Mar	21	24	19	13	13	12	8	7	21	25%	10%	14	2	5	53	15%
Wid	22	21	15	15	14	10	10	5	19	13%	22%	22	2	4	75	15%
Nev Mar	21	19	12	14	16	14	6	3	6	20%	10%	6	2	4	58	20%

See Table 18.1 for abbreviations.

Mtl - Marital status

Mar - Married

Wid - Widowed

Nev Mar - Never Married

divorced members has been eliminated since the number was too small to be meaningful.

Most of the differences between the three groups are not significant. However, there is some general evidence that the widowed elderly are much more sensitive to separation experiences than either of the other two groups. This sensitivity is demonstrated in their definitely increased responsiveness and in the increased percentage of individuals with symbiotic indicators in comparison to the married persons. Those who had never married proved to be the least sensitive to separation. Married persons demonstrated greater core personality strength than the widowed and more than those never married. The never married group showed a number of interesting weaknesses in areas of significance, i.e., identity stress, attachment-individuation balance and mild-strong differences. These areas, when poor, indicate immaturity and poor discriminative judgment. These characteristics are associated with limitations in personality development, at least insofar as object relations are concerned and the ability to regress without decompensating. The never married showed a definite diminution of affect in the face of separation experiences in comparison to the married and widowed. It would appear that they show less distress, either pain or hostility. This suggests the possibility that, under social conditions, being unmarried has greater survival value than being married or having been widowed. It may dull emotional reactions to contact need, but, in the process, it may result in personality limitations in object relations.

Area D: Results According to Sex

Male-female differences in the elderly on the S.A.T. were thought to be an interesting problem to evaluate. There were 36 males and 61 females in the group. This was not an intentional selection but turned out this way because the original study did not anticipate looking into this problem. Nevertheless, a comparative study was attempted in all areas of the test, and Table 18.4 is the result. It can be seen from this table that females are far more sensitive to the separation experiences depicted than males. They select far more responses, show greater self-love loss, a greater tendency to loss of appropriateness, poorer discriminative judgment with regard to mild and strong stimuli, more self-destructive factors and poorer balance between attachment and individuation. These results would suggest that elderly women are more dependent upon object relations than males and, for this reason, would feel greater need for attachments and therefore show more disturbances in one form or another when separations occur.

Table 18.4

MEDIAN RESPONSES TO THE SEPARATION ANXIETY TEST FOR MALE AND FEMALE GROUPS OF ELDERLY

Sex	A Atc	B Ind	C Hst	D Pain	E Den	F S-E Pre	G Lve Los	H Idn Str	J A-I Bal	K % C Str	L % Symb	M M-S Dif	N S-D Fcts	P Abs	Q Total R	R Act Out
Male	23½	23½	18	13	11½	10½	7	7½	20½	45%	17	21½	1	1½	53	48%
Fem	21	21	14	14	14	13	11	6	15	13%	42	16	2	5	76	27%

See Table 18.1 for abbreviations.

The male-female differences become even more marked if one examines Columns K, L and R, which depict the percentages of individuals who are either symbiotic (excessively attachment-oriented), tend to act out separation reactions and/or have strong personality core reactions to the separation stimuli. These figures leave no doubt that the elderly male tends to be emotionally stronger but is far more likely to act out his feelings, while the females are more intensely needful and much less able to withstand the emotional impact of separation. Nevertheless, females show considerably less tendency to act out their separation problems.

Area E: Comparison of Elderly and Adolescent Separation Problems

Any professional familiar with the psychological problems of youngsters would seriously hesitate in making comparisons to individuals who are close to the end of life. The processes of internal separation from attachments to parental figures and displacement to others (peers, as well as adult surrogate figures) in order to individuate at a level of adult behavior in a community would appear to be a far cry from those processes affecting the elderly. The latter are struggling to maintain their individuation in the face of changes moving in the opposite direction. In spite of these considerable differences, there appear to be some fundamental characteristics in the manner of handling separation (whether psychological or geographical) which may remain similar throughout the life span.

I have made a comparison of the responses to the S.A.T. between populations of relatively typical adolescents and the elderly in this study who were typically involved in life activities. The resemblance in the data is quite striking. Approximately 60 of the first three groups of elderly were compared with approximately 100 early adolescents, who were tested in five different school settings in my original study, published in 1972. A few areas showed very small differences, and most of them were unreliable.

It is interesting to note that the elderly (and, from my experience, other adult age groups) tend to show slightly higher levels of attachment responses, partly, no doubt, because, in identifying with the youngsters, they may tend to exaggerate needfulness. At the same time, individuation levels are also higher but total affect levels are the same. Hostile feelings appear to be somewhat stronger in the elderly, and pain levels are much stronger in the youngsters. The latter suggests that the psychological separation pains (fear, anxiety and somatic reactions) are somewhat stronger in adolescence than in the elderly, if the S.A.T. is valid for the latter.

The elderly are generally somewhat more responsive to the test, giving more responses, but the medians do not vary too significantly. What was interesting was the considerable similarity in the percentages of youngsters and elderly who show symbiotic, as well as acting out, tendencies. No doubt, the differences in the manner of expressing these tendencies would be interesting to examine through observational techniques.

CLINICAL EVALUATION OF SEPARATION DISORDERS OF THE ELDERLY

I have previously mentioned (p. 264) how the S.A.T. was used to note extreme vulnerability to separation experiences in the elderly. We saw how attachment needfulness with attendant disturbances of fear, anxiety, bodily pain, weakness in handling regressive pull, separation denial through withdrawal and fantasy and increasing feelings of rejection and intrapunitiveness (depression) were increasingly evident in elderly persons confined to a hospital for the chronically disabled and terminally ill. The test was noted to be very useful in detecting such patterns which, in adolescence, I had described with the phrase "self-destructive" (Hansburg, 1976). This type of disorder has also been noted in other younger adults (Hansburg, 1976) in their thirties and forties.

In the above cases, Bowlby's term "anxious attachment" is applicable, but the patterns in these cases go beyond this and are often suicidal in nature. Cases of anxious attachment are seen as patterns in the records of the elderly but are not necessarily accompanied by the other symptoms noted above. Therefore, these individuals are more amenable to reassurance alone, whereas the more complicated patterns (self-destructive) require more careful supervision. Both types of cases can profit from psychotherapy precisely because they are so needful and are consciously suffering emotional pain.

Another type of clinical phenomenon seen in the elderly on the S.A.T. is termed "acting out." They are individuals who express themselves on the test by reduced attachment levels and a combination of high individuation and hostility responses. These are persons who can be described as readily moved to excessive complaints, arrogant comments, evasive tactics, negativism and refusals to cooperate. In some cases of this kind, a constriction is present on the test, and when this occurs, therapeutic efforts are far more difficult. Generally, persons of this nature are handled best through management techniques rather than through attachment relationships. These individuals could not be characterized as emotionally detached because they express considerable hostility.

Detachment disorders are manifested largely by low emotional responsiveness to the test. The individual expresses high levels of individuation, only fair attachment and limited affect, either in hostility or in pain. These persons have often been classified as narcissistic, acting out characters who prefer to go their own way and are little influenced by others. These cases are rare and, in the present study population, represented by only 4% of the cases.

Some elderly, like some adolescents, show a very poor response to both the attachment and individuation reactions, while, at the same time, demonstrating an intense reaction to hostility and pain responses. In my clinical experience, I have found such persons to be narcissistically dependent characters who not only lack adequate attachment capacity but also show limited resourcefulness and are readily influenced by infantile emotional feelings. About 4% of the test group fell into this category.

DISCUSSION

The results of this study point rather strongly to the probability that the S.A.T. increases our insights into ways of studying and handling the elderly, even though the test was originally constructed for use with adolescents. The elderly respond to the test and do not manifest any more or less testing problems on this instrument than adolescents. Therefore, it would be clinically useful to develop an instrument of this type with separation situations more related to the lives of old people.

We might well raise the question why elderly people react in such a way to separation situations meant for adolescents and demonstrate patterns very similar to those seen in youngsters. Further, why do the obtained data from varied life conditions, age groups, marital status and male-female differences present us with material which apparently is quite defensible on known psychological principles? To answer this question, one can first resort to Bowlby's theories of attachment (1969) and separation (1973). The development and retention of attachments, while essentially an early developmental process and one which establishes the making and breaking of significant life relationships, go through further elaboration and sophistication as life proceeds through adolescence, adult life and old age. The nature and intensity of separation experiences throughout the life span may be reacted to by earlier patterned tactics but may, nevertheless, alter these very tactics if they be sufficiently traumatic and of long duration. Horrendous environmental changes and pressures have been known to create personality changes, even in old age. Additionally, internal changes, especially cerebral ones, may well alter long-standing reactive characteristics. At the same time, we can expect that those individuals who are not exposed to serious environmental changes may well retain the patterns which grew out of the second individuation period of adolescence (Blos, 1967). Thus, without an adequate history, it would be difficult to ascribe the test patterns to current life situations or to early life development alone.

The explanation for the separation patterned differences among the elderly living varied lives seems within our grasp. Any situation that confines and isolates and reduces capacity for functioning must, of necessity, produce increasing helplessness, depression, and need for care and attention. This must, apparently, be reflected in a person's attitude toward separation from significant others. Further, it must be reflected in attachment and separation disorders, whether or not the individual has suffered from such disorders in his previous life. Conversely, those life situations that, for various reasons, afford the individual with expanded opportunity to utilize his available powers, must also be reflected in a more positive way toward his handling of necessary life separations. However, as this study has indicated, long-standing personality patterns may show separation disorders, even in more favorable life circumstances. Further, already developed separation disorders may well determine what the life circumstances of an elderly person will be.

Apparently, separation disorders do not differ especially because one is 70, 80 or 90 years old. During the old-age period, separation problems appear to remain constant as long as life-style changes are not enforced. This appears to be a corollary of our preceding remarks that environmental factors are of considerable importance in determining separation reactions. Life experience would suggest that, as one aged from 65 to 90, differences would occur in the reactions to separation from significant persons. This seems to occur mainly because of changes in the life situation, such as loss of contact with jobs, social activities, physical capacities and so on. It is not a function of age unless these occur. If they do not occur or if they occur to a limited extent, our data suggest that reactions to separation will not become more pathological.

It should also be noted that a goodly percentage of the elderly handle separation very well. This is especially true among those who are actively engaged in life activities, including employment, social life and avocational pursuits. Even in the most confining situations, where death is approaching, some elderly do very well on the test. It seems likely that some individuals have such strong personality cores, in terms of attachment capacity and counterbalancing separation acceptance, that they can withstand the encroachment of age disabilities. If one examines the comparative data with youngsters, there is evidence of as much separation pathology as among the elderly, while we do not see much difference in the presence of healthy reactions. Without further investigation, it would be difficult to evaluate the presence of health and pathology in separation reactions in other age groups.

Marital status does appear to be one of those life circumstances which are related to separation reactions. Married persons tend, on the whole, to do somewhat better on the test than widowed and those never married. The widowed appear to be more vulnerable and more sensitive, but it is difficult to say whether this would be the effect of widowhood or the basic personality structure. Those never married show a trend toward lesser affect and more limited personality structures. It seems likely that living in contact with others has a beneficial effect on separation dynamics, whether it is related to job, social life or marital status. Intimate contact with others appears to be salutary to the healthy separation reactions of the elderly.

Our data suggest that women in old age are somewhat more sensitive to separation than men. They appear to be more needful of contact and less able to withstand the inroads of old age separations. Is it possible that this is a cultural artifact because of the years of dependency relationships of women in our society? While it is true that the current generation has shown considerable change in this respect, the present group included individuals who were raised during the time of, and somewhat after, the First World War, a time when the average woman was not as much in the throes of the so-called women's liberation movement. It remains to be seen whether vast cultural changes in the role of women will alter this condition.

CONCLUSIONS

The current study has been a cursory attempt to study the reactions of elderly persons in the age group 65 to 90 to separation situations depicted in pictures originally designed for adolescents. The test was given to approximately 100 persons in five groups, including employed, unemployed living at home and unaffiliated, those attending a senior citizen's club, elderly in a nursing home and a group confined to a hospital for the permanently disabled or terminally ill.

The evidence from the results suggests a number of interesting conclusions:

1.   There are considerable differences in the reactions of elderly persons, depending upon the conditions and style of living to which they have either consigned themselves or are forced to live due to various disabling conditions. These differences strongly suggest that elderly persons, where possible, should be employed in useful work. If not possible, they should be engaged in social and avocational pursuits which provide opportunities for social and emotional contacts with others.

2. Separations for a percentage of the elderly, especially those who are most emotionally vulnerable, should be accomplished under mental health management. Isolation is a great danger for the elderly and should be avoided as a steady diet. The S.A.T. is a useful instrument in detecting vulnerable elderly and should be utilized, especially in nursing homes and hospitals.

3. As long as the elderly are engaged, as suggested in (1), age ranges from 65 to 90 will not significantly affect their reactions to separation. Pathological reactions to separation are less a function of age in the elderly than of life-style or environmental conditions.

4. Married elderly show generally better separation patterns than widowed and unmarried elderly. There is evidence that widowed persons are more vulnerable and, therefore, generally require more mental health care regardless of whether they are involved in useful life endeavors.

5. Although our culture is undergoing continuous change in the role of women, elderly women still appear to be more sensitive and vulnerable to separations. It is therefore likely that they will need more attention, care and mental health management than males. It is also likely that women will seek out mental health services more readily, as they generally appear to be more needful of closer contact with others.

6. From the theoretical viewpoint, the present study seems to confirm the theory that separation problems are of considerable importance in old age as well as in childhood and adolescence. Attachment needs are as intense toward the end of life as in the earlier stages and, perhaps, this was the origin of the expression "second childhood." The ongoing nature of what Bowlby refers to as the elastic band and what I have termed the attachment-individuation balance seems to be verified by the present study.

7. There is an indication that, among the elderly, one may detect separation pathology (or attachment pathology) as readily as one may discern this among

youngsters. I would therefore recommend that a
special test be devised for elderly persons to uncover
particular problems in the attachment and separation
areas, and, thereby, aid in the mental health care of
the elderly.

REFERENCES

Bowlby, J., *Attachment and Loss*, Vol. I, *Attachment*. New York: Basic Books,
1969.
Bowlby, J., *Attachment and Loss*, Vol. II, *Separation: Anxiety and Anger*.
London: Hogarth Press, 1973.
Conte, H. R., Weiner, M., Plutchik, R., and Bennett, R. "Development and
Evaluation of a Death Anxiety Questionnaire." Paper presented at the
83rd Annual Convention of the American Psychiatric Association,
Chicago, September 1975.
Goldfarb, A. I., "Threats of Aging." *N.Y. Journal of Medicine*, Vol. 55, 1955.
Hansburg, H. G., *Adolescent Separation Anxiety: A Method for the Study of
Adolescent Separation Problems*. Springfield, Ill.: C. C. Thomas, 1972.
Reprinted: Melbourne, Fla.: R. E. Krieger, 1980.
Hansburg, H. G., "The Use of the Separation-Anxiety Test in the Detection of
Self-Destructive Tendencies in Early Adolescence," in *Mental Health in
Childhood*, Vol. III. Ed. D. V. Siva Sankar. Westbury, N. Y.: P. J. D.
Publications, 1976.
Hansburg, H. G., *Separation Disorders: A Manual for the Interpretation of
Emotional Disorders Manifested by the Separation Anxiety Test*. (Fall
1976, unpublished.)
Kubler-Ross, C., *On Death and Dying*. New York: Macmillan, 1969.
Parkes, C. M., *Bereavement: Studies of Grief in Adult Life*. New York: In-
ternational University Press, 1972.
Rapaport, D., *Diagnostic Psychological Testing*. Chicago Year Book, 1946.
Schneidman and Farberow, *Cry for Help*. New York: McGraw-Hill, 1961.
Sternschein, I., "The Experience of Separation Individuation in Infancy and
Its Reverberations through the Course of Life: Maturity, Senescence and
Sociological Implications." *Journal of the American Psychoanalytic
Association*, Vol. 21 (3). New York: International University Press, 1973.
Train, G., "The Aged—With Tender Interest and Concern." *Psychosomatics*,
Vol. 16 (Second Quarter), 1975.

19

Extended Family Availability and Maternal Reactions to Separation (1981)

INTRODUCTION

This study of mothers' reactions to personal separation experiences was undertaken as a means of comparison to similar studies of adolescent separation problems (Hansburg, 1972, 1976, 1980). It was intended as a means of acquiring further normative understanding of the value of the S.A.T. when viewing responses of mothers in various studies of special problem areas. The test method had limited use with adults. These include my own study of families (see Chapter 16)—one of which was previously reported in *Adolescent Separation Anxiety* Volume II (Case 7)—a study of the elderly (see Chapter 18); a study of abusive mothers with a control group by DeLozier (1979); a study of 18- and 19-year-olds (college freshmen) by Sherry (1980); and a number of studies in process or close to completion and unavailable to me at this writing. From these studies, normative data for adults have been, and are being, developed and may be compared to those obtained from the earlier studies with adolescents, as well as more recent ones. While the test was developed for use with early and middle adolescents, it has proven to be of considerable value in studying persons in later life.

All women are, of course, not necessarily mothers, and those who are mothers may, for genetic, developmental or experiential reasons, differ to some degree either in personality traits, behavioral reactions and/or internal intrapsychic feelings toward other human beings.

Reactions to separation experiences, whether mild, strong or traumatic, may also differ. While this study is not directed toward studying such differences, it is devoted to a study of the separation reactions of mothers and will be a preliminary evaluation, with the further intention of later correlating such reactions to those of their own children. (This study was never completed.)

Maternal behavior toward children is a highly complicated phenomenon and has been studied very intensively at various stages of the child's life, beginning from infancy. The manner in which children develop close ties to the maternal figure and the significant factors involved have already been well documented by Ainsworth (1978), Bowlby (1958, 1969, 1973) and Mahler (1967, 1968). There is no need here to go into any extensive detail with regard to these works. The effect of maternal behavior on children's behavior, while well known in many respects, still leaves much that is either not known or inadequately understood. Careful researches, especially those by Ainsworth, reveal that mothers may, by their own avoidant or harsh or ambivalent contact reactions to infants, instill very early "unpleasant associations" to physical contact (1978). Maternal behaviors which are more responsive to infant signals of need generally result in happier and less troubled infant behavior. These behaviors, described by Ainsworth (1978), involved responsiveness to infant crying, to close bodily contact, face-to-face interaction, feeding and general emotional reactions.

The mother's inclination to behave in such positive ways toward her children would appear to bear some relationship to similar experiences with her own maternal figure. As Ainsworth pointed out (1978), " . . . maternal behavior and attitudes relevant to close bodily contact in the early months are significantly associated with later quality of attachment. . . ." A comparative study of three groups of mothers confirmed this conclusion. In addition, much recent interest has been shown in the mothers' current experiences with their spouses and with available close relatives.

The fact that mammals instinctively feed, care for and protect their young against natural calamities and predators has been well established, although with some exceptions (Rheingold, 1963). The mutual seeking for each other, the one to protect and the other seeking to be protected, has apparent survival characteristics, whether seen from the point of view of the individual or the tribe or the race or the species. Without such a behavioral phenomenon, survival would become questionable. The disabling of this instinctive pattern by deactivation of attachments runs the danger of destruction. In a certain percentage of cases, mothers abandon their young, especially when, for a variety of reasons, they are unable to care for them or their attachment capacities have been warped, damaged or deactivated. Under some circumstances, mothers may even injure or seriously abuse their children. Finally, mothers may even murder or leave their children to die unattended. While such abandonment, abuse or murder by mothers may occur, the large majority of mothers would condemn such behavior.

The maternal care of the infant has been ascribed both to identification and to what is referred to as object relations. This formulation has evolved from psychoanalysis, and a sample discussion may be obtained in Coleman, Kris and Provence (1953). Maternal fantasies about infants and their relationships to the maternal self have been invoked to explain maternal care. Thus, it is stated, "The earliest variations in maternal attitudes suggest that much of the ability of the mother to handle the small child and much in the difficulty to adjust to its growth depends on the capacity to shift from one type of identification to another." One must assume that these shifts in identification are unconsciously stimulated and not related to conscious choices. There are some plausible elements in these concepts, especially as one studies clinical data.

Aside from the instinctive trend of protectiveness by the mother for the child, and the fantasies the mother may develop with regard to the child, one must consider the elements in the closeness experiences of the mothers with their extended families. The quality and the extent of such closeness represent, for most mothers, the support systems which have been, continue to be, and remain present during the period of parental care for children. This might be illustrated by a study of gorillas by Nadler (Rock, 1979) at the Yerkes Regional Primate Research Center in Atlanta, Georgia. Nadler found that captivity warps the gorilla's normal parental behavior. "When they are caged alone with their babies, abuse by gorilla mothers seems to be the norm." Nadler thought at first that the gorilla mothers abused their infants because they had been separated from their own mothers when they were still infants. He later discovered that it was loneliness and isolation that produced this effect. By grouping the gorilla mothers in the same compound, the abuse of the infants by their mothers ceased. Subsequently, the isolation cage for gorillas at the Yerkes laboratory was abandoned. This more natural habitat produced improved behavior toward their infants.

If we were to interpret this study in terms of the behavior of human mothers, we might conclude that isolation and loneliness may be reacted to by the abuse of their children (DeLozier, 1979). It would seem likely that social support systems for mothers reduce the effect of pathological attachment disorders. A support system for a mother most often consists of her husband, her own parents, brothers, sisters, uncles, aunts, cousins, in-laws and close friends. The degree and nature of this closeness, while of considerable significance, must obviously depend upon how it is utilized and how it is returned by the support system. An active and healthy attachment system within the mother is more likely to stimulate active attachment reactions from the support system, as well as to create reciprocal reactions in her child. Attachment disorders may, on the other hand, be ameliorated to some extent by the presence of adequate support systems in the extended family so that the child may not receive the full impact of the disorder. These are theoretical assumptions for which adequate research data need to be accumulated.

Various concepts are involved here: To what degree did the mother as a child receive adequate support from her own parents for her own instinctive need for protection? To what degree were adequate support systems available from the extended family to reinforce this need? To what degree did these support systems survive the ravages of time until the mother was able to establish her own family system with spouse and children? To what degree are these support systems maintained while the child is young?

The community also affects the nature and quality of support systems by maintaining adequate safeguards against the destruction of the family and extended family. The threat of loss of such safeguards may well introduce problems that, under ordinary circumstances, would be considered pathological. For example, natural and man-made disasters, such as the Managua, Nicaragua, earthquake or the Three Mile Island nuclear accident, may create panics sizeable enough to bring on almost pathological attachment behavior on the part of mothers as well as other individuals. Data on the latter incident (Bromet, et al., NIMH, 1980) pointed up the panic among mothers for the safety of their children. This may be replicated by subjective observations of mothers' behavior in their protection of their children in a recent (February, 1981, Dix Hills, Long Island, N.Y.) event in which the serious disease and death of two children appeared to threaten the health and life of the entire child population. It would not be difficult to document the observation that mothers normally rush to the aid of their infants or children when there appears to be a threat to their existence.

Separation from one's close kin or from familiar surroundings has already been proven to be such a threat (DeLozier, 1979; Hansburg, 1980). It has also been demonstrated that, when separation threats appear with great strength, maternal protection, far from encouraging dependency, improves the chances for the development of the individuation process (Bowlby, 1973; Hansburg, 1972). The problem with which we are concerned in this paper deals to some degree with where the mother derives the capacity to provide closeness for the child. As was mentioned above, the sources appear to come from (1) instinct, (2) the experience of closeness and protection from her own maternal figure and (3) the continued presence of support systems in the extended family, community, etc. The continued activation of the attachment system would appear to be an important characteristic. The presence of an active attachment system does not necessarily guarantee a healthy interaction between the maternal figure and child because there are pathological forms which this system may take which may be damaging to this relationship (*Adolescent Separation Anxiety*, Vol. II). The same is true of the individuation system and other psychological systems.

I should like to say a word here about the variations in the maternal instinctive equipment. It has been demonstrated that variations in the behavioral patterns of twins reared apart (Farber, 1981) show many similarities. It does not seem a far cry to assume that there are varying degrees of capacity to develop attachments based on the degree to which the internal organismic systems are equipped with the genetic patterns. The variations in these genetically determined developmental sequences may well be of significance in determining how the individual will deal with environmental influences.

To return to the major problem of this study, it should be noted that the quality and nature of family closeness need to be considered. Some close families are maintained by a strong, hostile, anxious, attachment which creates considerable ambivalence in many of the family members. In others, there is a severe anxious attachment which is highly pathological, demanding and destructive of individuation. Variations of attachment patterns have been discussed extensively in a previous volume (Hansburg, 1980). In the present study, the character of mothers' reactions to separation is presented as the major concern and family closeness is considered in the mother's personal report.

METHOD OF THIS PRELIMINARY INVESTIGATION

Thirty-one mothers of 5-year-olds were seen during the course of evaluating the children of a kindergarten group. The mothers were interviewed with regard to the closeness of the extended family and were given the S.A.T. The children were attending a parochial school and were being considered for admission into the first grade. Obviously, both the children and the mothers were a select group, culturally, economically and intellectually. Therefore, they could not be considered typical of the general population. There were very few single parent families, either through separation, divorce or death.

While the mothers were present for a few minutes during the initial contact with the child, they were interviewed separately, both for family closeness and for their responses to the S.A.T. The queries with regard to relatives included listing each available relative —maternal grandmother, grandfather, uncles, aunts, brothers, sisters, cousins—and the degree of closeness which the mother felt toward them. Each degree was presented on a scale of 1 to 5, with the mothers rating each relative in this fashion. In addition, the mothers were asked if this closeness was similarly reciprocated. Ratings were listed and a median closeness was obtained. Medians of 4 or 5 were considered high, and the remainder were simply described as less than high. It should be noted that most of the mothers had other children. The median age of the mothers was 31 with a range from 27 to 42 and a mid-50% range of 29 to 35. The median number of children was 2, with a range of 1 to 6 and a mid-50% range of 2 to 2. All of the mothers were of the Hebrew faith and, on the average, were observant of religious customs.

All except two of the mothers were living with their husbands of a first marriage. One mother was living with her husband but contemplating a separation. Another was divorced and living with her second husband for six years. She had a child by her first husband, for whom it had been a second marriage. Further, this mother will be discussed later because of pathological patterns and disturbed history.

ANALYSIS OF DATA

The data were first analyzed by means of a clinical study of the protocols of the S.A.T. to determine the nature of the patterning that each mother presented. These clinical patterns were classified according to the clinical categories described in *Adolescent Separation Anxiety*, Vol. II, as follows: (1) mild anxious attachment, (2) strong anxious attachment, (3) severe anxious attachment, (4) hostile anxious attachment, (5) hostile detachment, (6) dependent detachment, (7) self-sufficiency pattern, (8) excessive self-sufficiency, (9) depressive syndrome, (10) exceptionally healthy pattern.

The extent of the presence of these clinical categories in this maternal population was then recorded and appears in Table 19.1 (p. 284).

Subsequently, all cases in each category were divided into two groups according to whether a high level of family closeness was or was not reported by the mothers. This comparison is presented in Table 19.2 (p. 286).

Following this, an analysis of the data for each of the patterns of the S.A.T. was made, including (1) attachment, (2) individuation, (3) separation hostility, (4) separation pain system, (5) defensive system, (6) the self-evaluative systems—(a) self-love loss, (b) self-esteem preoccupation system, (c) identity stress, (7) attachment-individuation balance, (8) absurd responses, (9) mild-strong response difference, (10) total responsiveness and (11) mental set questions—frequency of separations. This data provided some further adult norms for the various categories and are shown in Table 19.3 (p. 288).

Subsequently, each of the above factors was classified according to the extent of family closeness and is reported in Tables 19.4 and 19.5 (p. 289, 290).

A further analysis of the responses to each picture and the median number and range of responses for each was examined, and the results will be found in Table 19.7 (p. 292).

An analysis of the relationship between family closeness and two further indexes was made—attachment and the separation pain system on the one hand and individuation and separation hostility on the other. These combinations were originally thought to be significant and first offered in a study of children of divorce by Miller (1980). It is presented here again as a suggested way of studying differences between styles of reaction to separation and is detailed in Table 19.6 (p. 291).

SUMMARY OF THE RESULTS

Attachment and Self-Sufficiency Patterns (Table 19.1)

Among this group of mothers, varying degrees and forms of anxious attachment patterns in the face of separation experiences are present in 51½% of the cases, while self-sufficiency patterns are less

Table 19.1

PERCENTAGE OF CLINICAL PATTERNS ON S.A.T. FOR 31 MOTHERS

CLINICAL PATTERN	#	PERCENTAGE
Mild Anxious Attachment	7	22½
Strong Anxious Attachment	5	16
Severe Anxious Attachment	1	3
Hostile Anxious Attachment	3	10
(Total Anxious Attachment)	(16)	(51½%)
Self-Sufficiency Pattern	9	29
Excessive Self-Sufficiency	2	6½
(Total Self-Sufficiency)	(11)	(35½%)
Hostile Detachment	1	3
Generally Excellent Pattern	3	10
Total	31	100

Among the above cases, thirteen (13) included the depressive syndrome, indicating 42% of the group.

common and occur in 35½% of the mothers. Pathological or severe anxious attachment was noted in only one mother, or 3%. Another form but less pathological and probably more common than the latter, hostile anxious attachment, was found in three mothers, or 10%. Of the 51½% of anxious attachment, 38½% were either mild or strong and not considered pathological.

Self-sufficiency patterns of a relatively healthy type were found in nine mothers, or 29%, while two mothers, 6½%, showed excessive self-sufficiency, which is beyond the healthy state and probably indicates some character problems. One mother, 3%, demonstrated a condition of hostile detachment, a definite pathological indicator. Exceptionally healthy patterns were shown in three mothers, or 10%. Further, a careful study of the depressive syndrome in all of the records indicated that this tendency was present in thirteen mothers, 42% of the total group. The latter finding suggests that a large percentage of typical mothers will show depressive reactions to separation experiences, and this is likely evidence of a necessary phase of distress from which the individual later recovers.

Thus, in this group of mothers of Jewish origin and culture, separation stimuli result in forms of anxious attachment ranging from mild to severe in more than half of the cases. On the other hand, self-sufficiency patterns ranging from mild to excessive are less common and are found in slightly more than ⅓ of the cases. On both sides, that is, anxious attachment or self-sufficiency, 13% are somewhat pathological, either in anxious attachment or excessive self-sufficiency. Further, and what appears to be very significant, 42% show a tendency to a depressive syndrome in reaction to separation. There were no cases of dependent detachment and only one case of hostile detachment. While degrees of detachment are present, as shown by the cases of excessive self-sufficiency, they are neither hostile nor dependent in nature. Mild anxious attachment and mild self-sufficiency were the most common patterns and balanced against each other.

As may be seen by the graph (p. 298, Figure 19.1), there is a U-shaped curve if one considers the movement of severe anxious attachment to severe detachment. It is noted that, as one decreases the severity of anxious attachment, the number of cases increase until it falls into the category of excellent forms of attachment. Then, it rises again to mild forms of detachment and gradually drops as it approaches severe detachment.

Family Closeness as Related to Attachment and Self-Sufficiency

In Table 19.2, we see results which help to clarify some aspects of the meaning of the results in Table 19.1. When the 31 mothers are divided into two groups, the first group (17 mothers) representing high family closeness (refer to previous explanation of this term and how it was arrived at) and the second group (14 mothers) representing the mothers who reported lower levels and less qualitative closeness, the presence of both variations of anxious attachment and variations of self-sufficiency patterns show interesting phenomena.

High levels of family closeness show a much stronger trend in the direction of forms of anxious attachment in the 17 mothers, while the 14

Table 19.2

PERCENTAGE OF MOTHERS RATED HIGH IN FAMILY CLOSENESS
IN RELATION TO CLINICAL CATEGORY

CLINICAL CATEGORY	HIGH FAMILY CLOSENESS	NOT HIGH FAMILY CLOSENESS
Mild Anxious Attachment	16	6½
Strong Anxious Attachment	10	6½
Severe Anxious Attachment	3	0
Hostile Anxious Attachment	6½	3
(Total Anxious Attachment)	(35½%)	(16%)
Self-Sufficiency Patterns	10	19½
Excessive Self-Sufficiency	0	6½
(Total Self-Sufficiency)	(10%)	(26%)
Hostile Detachment	3	0
Healthy Patterns	6½	3
Total	55	45

SUMMARY

Anxious Attachment	35%	16%
Self-Sufficiency	10%	26%
Depressive Syndrome	30%	12%

mothers in the not-high family closeness group show a much stronger trend in the direction of self-sufficiency patterns of varying strength. There are no mothers with severe anxious attachment in the not-high family closeness group, and there are no cases of mothers of excessive self-sufficiency in the high family closeness group. The summary table on page 296 (Table 19.2) is quite striking in demonstrating this result.

Family closeness is also related to the separation reaction of depressive syndrome. Thirteen (42%) mothers show a depressive syndrome reaction to separation, but 9 mothers (70%) of these are high in family closeness while only 4 (30%) mothers are in the not-high family closeness group. It appears that separation experiences are more likely to result in a depressive syndrome in mothers with high levels of family closeness. These are mild depressive signals and in only a few cases are these of severe potential.

In the summary, variations of the anxious attachment patterns occur in 35.5% of the mothers rated high in family closeness, while only 16% of variations in anxious attachment show in the not-high family closeness group. At the same time, only 10% of the mothers who showed self-sufficiency patterns fell into the high family closeness group and 26% of the mothers appeared in the not-high family closeness group. The contrast is unmistakable, and its implications will be discussed later.

It is difficult to explain the one mother who showed a clinical picture of hostile detachment and yet fell into the high family closeness group. This woman, a refugee from Roumania, will be discussed later in the section on discussion and indicates how experiences in flight from dangerous situations may affect individuals who are raised in close-knit families.

Trends in Pattern Summaries for Mothers on the Separation-Anxiety Test

This is a small group of mothers for normative trends on the test patterns. Table 19.3 is presented as tentative, awaiting corroboration by further data. (This Table may be compared to Table A.1, *Adolescent Separation Anxiety*, Vol. II, p. 188.) Higher levels in the mothers appear mainly in attachment, hostility, pain and self-love loss, while lower levels appear in defensiveness, identity stress, self-esteem preoccupation, absurd responses and total responses. Mild responses

are definitely less frequent and result in a much higher mild-strong difference percentage median.

Table 19.3

SUMMARY OF PATTERN CHART DATA ON S.A.T.'S OF MOTHERS

PATTERN	MEDIAN	RANGE	MIDDLE 50%
Attachment	26%	0-42%	20-31%
Individuation	21%	4-57%	16-30%
Hostility	16%	1-40%	9-19%
Pain	21%	1-35%	16-25%
Defensiveness	9%	0-27%	6-12%
Concen.-Sublima.	8%	0-23%	5-12%
Self-Love Loss	8%	0-21%	5-11%
Mild-Strong Diff.	32%	-7-62%	16-42%
Identity Stress	4%	0-13%	0-7%
Absurd Responses	1%	0-6%	0-2%
Attach-Indiv Balance	52%	-4-97%	38-78%
Separation "Yeses"	5%	2-12%	4-7%
Total Responses	38%	18-75%	27-50%
Mild Responses	12%	7-32%	10-16%
Strong Responses	26%	10-53%	17-32%

Family Closeness and Pattern Summaries on the Separation Anxiety Test

A comparison of family closeness with the reaction patterns of the
S.A.T. shows some significant trends. A comparison of Tables 19.4 and
19.5 strongly suggests that the degree of family closeness is associated
with strong separation pain reactions (compare 76% to 43%). This is
the major significant trend. Further, the attachment-individuation
balance is far stronger (71% to 43%) in the high closeness mothers,
although the attachment level itself is not differentiating.

Table 19.4

PERCENTAGE OF HIGH FAMILY CLOSENESS MOTHERS (17)
WHO ALSO HAVE HIGH S.A.T. PATTERNS

S.A.T. PATTERN HIGH	% OF HIGH FAMILY CLOSENESS MOTHERS	
High Attachment	70%	(Data obtained by checking
High Separation Pain	76%	the 17 mothers who were
High Attach-Indiv Balance	71%	high in family closeness
High Depressive Syndrome	65%	for highs in the S.A.T.
High Separation Hostility	41%	patterns shown to the left
High Defensiveness	35%	of this Table. The Table
High Individuation	47%	represents an agreement of
High Identity Stress	35%	highs between the S.A.T.
Low Separation Frequency	51%	pattern and family close-
High Mild-Strong Difference	76%	ness.)

Table 19.5

PERCENTAGE OF NON-HIGH FAMILY CLOSENESS MOTHERS (14)
WHO ALSO HAVE HIGH S.A.T. PATTERNS

S.A.T. PATTERN HIGH	% OF NON-HIGH FAMILY CLOSENESS MOTHERS	
High Attachment	64%	(Data obtained by checking
High Separation Pain	43%	14 mothers who were not
High Attach-Indiv Balance	43%	high in family closeness
High Depressive Syndrome	29%	for highs in the S.A.T.
High Separation Hostility	29%	patterns shown to the left
High Defensiveness	29%	of this Table. The Table
High Individuation	50%	represents an agreement of
High Identity Stress	7%	the S.A.T. pattern highs
Low Separation Frequency	42%	and non-family closeness.)
High Mild-Strong Difference	50%	

An examination of the depressive syndrome (higher self-love loss than self-esteem preoccupation) demonstrates that high closeness is associated with far more cases of depressive syndrome (65% to 29%). Identity stress is also a differentiating factor, being very much stronger in the high closeness mothers (35% to 7%). Defensive patterns, individuation and low separation frequency are not especially differentiating. Separation hostility appears to trend more in the direction of high family closeness (41% to 29%) but does not appear as strongly differentiating as separation pain.

The differences between the responses to mild and strong pictures show a trend in the direction of high family closeness (76% to 50%). Generally, there appears to be a trend to rather strong differences between the high closeness mothers and the non-high closeness group. Separation stimuli for the high closeness mothers appears to produce stronger separation pain, higher levels of attachment-individuation balance, stronger separation hostility, greater identity stress, more frequency of mild depressive trends and greater differences between the responses to the mild and strong stimuli. Whether this is peculiar to mothers of the Jewish faith remains to be seen by further study.

Comparison of Attachment-Pain and Individuation-Hostility Patterns with Levels of High Family Closeness

Another way of studying the relationship between high family closeness and the S.A.T. is to compare the patterns of attachment-separation pain combination and the individuation-hostility pattern. These are summations of six factors of the Test dealing with attachment needfulness and the fear-anxiety-pain system as compared to six factors in the individuation and the hostility systems. The closer these two patterns move to each other, the less control attachment has over either hostility or aggression. The theoretical formulation for this lies in the fundamental nature of whether separation produces greater attachment needfulness and emotional pain or whether it stirs up a self-sufficiency and hostile reaction. The greater control the former has over the latter in developmental sequences, the less likelihood of impulsive aggression.

It can be seen from Table 19.6 that high family closeness mothers have far more control over aggression than non-high family closeness mothers (pattern differences of 17% to 1%). These data corroborate

Table 19.6

FAMILY CLOSENESS AND ATTACHMENT-SEPARATION PAIN INDEX
COMPARED TO INDIVIDUATION-HOSTILITY INDEX

INDEX	HIGH F.C. MEDIAN (17 Cases)	NOT-HIGH F.C. MEDIAN (14 Cases)
Attach.-Sep. Pain	52%	41%
Indiv.-Sep. Host.	35%	40%
Difference	17%	1%

Median Difference for Total 31 Mothers: 9.0%

previously presented data that family closeness appears more related to anxious attachment and much less to excessive self-sufficiency. The differences in the data are quite striking.

Mild and Strong Picture Responses and a Comparison of These to Family Closeness

The responses to individual pictures (Table19.7) indicate that the strong pictures still elicit more responses than the mild pictures. Note that the median number of responses to each of the mild pictures is 2 or less, while the median number for each of the strong pictures is 3, 4, 5, or 6. The picture eliciting the most responses is the death of the mother, while the picture of the judge runs a close second. This is similar to the reactions of adolescents to these pictures.

When the responses to the pictures are divided into two groups—a high family closeness group and a not-high family closeness group—Table 19.8 (p. 293) points up the greater responsiveness of the high family closeness group to most of the strong pictures. This is in line with the higher levels of anxious attachment in the high family closeness group and the higher level of self-sufficiency in the not-high family closeness group.

DISCUSSION OF RESULTS

This study corroborates, in some ways, the concepts of attachment theory. The notion that degrees of family closeness and the continuity of such close relationships are of great moment in the adjustment of

Table 19.7

RESPONSES TO EACH PICTURE OF THE S.A.T. BY 31 MOTHERS

PICTURE	MEDIAN RESPONSE NUMBER	RANGE RESPONSE NUMBER	MID-50% RESPONSE NUMBER
I Grandmother	3	1-8	2-5
II Classroom	2	1-6	1-4
III Moving	2	1-5	2-4
IV School	2	1-7	2-3
V Camp	2	1-7	1-3
VI Argument	3	1-9	2-5
VII Sailor	2	0-5	1-3
VIII Judge	5	1-11	3-7
IX Sleep	1	1-7	1-2
X Hospital	4	1-8	2-5
XI Death	6	2-10	4-8
XII Runaway	4	1-10	3-5

persons of all ages is strongly indicated. Nevertheless, there are certain problems which are clearly portrayed here and which require clarification. As with all talents, capacities and positive characteristics, there are conditions under which these very capacities can be temporarily handicapping or incapacitating.

First, let us examine our data from the point of view of attachment theory and the positive outcomes of family closeness. Among the group of 31 mothers, 17 demonstrated, in interview and in the factual background of family closeness, that they were very close to many family members, including parents, uncles, aunts, brothers, sisters, etc., while 14 mothers were not considered as high in closeness. This division into two groups facilitated an interesting study of the relationship between the family closeness of a group of mothers and their performance on the S.A.T.

The analysis of the data indicated that the group showing the highest levels of closeness demonstrated evidence of anxious attachment in varying degrees. This group was quite different in this

Table 19.8

RESPONSES TO EACH PICTURE OF THE S.A.T. BY 31 MOTHERS
DIVIDED ACCORDING TO
HIGH FAMILY CLOSENESS (17) AND NON-HIGH FAMILY CLOSENESS (14)

	PICTURE	MEDIAN RESPONSE NUMBER		RANGE RESPONSE NUMBERS		MID-50% RESPONSE NUMBERS	
		HIGH FC	NON-HIGH	HIGH FC	NON-HIGH	HIGH FC	NON HIGH
I	Grandmother	4	3	1-8	1-7	3-5	2-3
II	Classroom	2	3	1-6	1-4	2-5	2-3
III	Moving	2	2	1-5	1-4	2-3	2-4
IV	School	2	2	1-5	1-7	2-3	2-3
V	Camp	2	2	1-5	1-7	1-3	2-3
VI	Argument	4	3	1-9	1-7	2-4	2-4
VII	Sailor	2	1	1-8	0-5	2-3	1-2
VIII	Judge	4	5	2-9	1-11	4-7	3-6
IX	Sleep	2	1	0-4	0-7	1-2	1-2
X	Hospital	4	3	1-8	1-8	3-5	2-4
XI	Death	6	5	3-10	2-9	4-9	3-7
XII	Runaway	4	3	2-10	1-9	4-5	3-5

respect from the mothers whose reports of family closeness and availability of relatives showed more limited scope. We should not forget that this result was obtained on a test which requests reactions to separation experiences. For this reason, the above result has to be confined to such experiences and not necessarily referable to others. Nevertheless, since separation experiences stimulate the response of closeness needfulness, the test results indicate a heightened painful reaction for such mothers. *Thus, if loss or threats of loss are presented to a group of mothers, those who represent themselves as very close to the threatened loss experience greater emotional stress. At the same time, and conversely, when loss or threats of loss are presented to mothers who represent themselves as less close to the threatened loss, less stress is experienced and more self-sufficiency is registered.*

It has been posited (Bowlby, 1969) that such need for closeness has survival value in our culture. Families which maintain a strong interaction with each other may be less prone to attack by predatory persons. They are afforded warmth, communication, mutual love, financial assistance, vocational and avocational aid and emotional support during crises. The role of the availability of the extended family has been well documented.

On the other hand, there are handicapping problems in closely knit families when separation experiences are threatened either by real events or fantasies. The data indicate that the depressive syndrome on the S.A.T. occurs in 30% of the high family closeness group while only 13% showed the depressive syndrome in the non-high family closeness group. Such deactivation of the self-evaluative system by separation experiences, mild though it be in most of the mothers, would need further corroboration by other in-depth investigations. Data on depression have generally indicated that larger numbers of persons suffer from depression as a result of the early death of a parent—especially before the age of 11 (Brown, et al., 1977).

In this study, mild depressive reactions to separation and loss appear, therefore, to be more frequent in closely knit families than in families that are less close. Yet, severe depressive reactions, such as are found in severe anxious attachment problems, are nearly non-existent in both groups of this study (only one case was found). Severe attachment pathology of any kind was relatively rare in this group of 31 mothers.

The depressive syndrome was distributed among the clinical categories as follows:

Clinical Category		Number of Cases of Depressive Syndrome
Mild Anxious Attachment	5	
Strong Anxious Attachment	3	(2 of 3 would be mild without the D.S.)
Severe Anxious Attachment	1	
Hostile Anxious Attachment	2	
Hostile Detachment	1	
Excellent Healthy Pattern	1	

The one case of severe anxious attachment was a 32-year-old mother (A.G.), who, at the time of the study, was living with her second husband, a song writer who earned his living mainly by driving for a car service. This marriage was also her current husband's second. In her history, she reported that, within the space of one year, her mother and her brother (aged 30) had died, and she had divorced her first husband. Then, later, she was required to undergo a hysterectomy. Both her parents had been very close to her, but the series of events resulted in a depression, an attempt at suicide and hospitalization. She was the mother of two children, one boy aged 13½ by her first marriage and a 5-year-old girl. Although close to her family, her father and a sister live in other states and her mother-in-law is in a nursing home. Thus, in this case, although there was closeness in the family, the support systems were gradually withdrawn by death and by distance. At the time of the study, she was concerned that her 5-year-old would develop fears and anxieties. Her youngster was already demonstrating anxious attachment problems at night and wanted to be close to the mother.

In the case of the mother showing hostile detachment, the history was somewhat different. At the time of the study, she was 33 years old and had been a native of Roumania. From here, she had migrated to Israel and, after a period of time, had moved to the United States. Once in this country, she moved from one home to another. She has a large extended family consisting of parents, uncles, aunts, cousins, brothers, sisters and in-laws. Yet, the patterning suggests a strong depressive tone, with 21% of the responses in the area of self-love loss involving strong feelings of rejection. From the one interview, it was not possible to account for this patterning.

Precisely how does the depressive syndrome in the face of separation threats occur in close-knit families? To be more specific, why do 42% of a group of mothers, who represent a non-clinical population derived from close-knit families and are maternal enough to care about the kind of school their children are educated in, report such frequent feelings of rejection and intrapunitiveness on separation pictures? Our interpretation of the test phenomenon itself has been proven correct by clinical data. When we compared the high closeness mothers to the non-high closeness mothers on this syndrome, the percentages were 30% compared to 12%.

It seemed likely that the presence of this syndrome fell into the normal area in nine out of thirteen cases. There were only two very serious cases, as described above, and two others of hostile anxious attachment, one of which had to be considered within the norm because she showed a strong personality core (high attachment and high individuation), but the affect was strongly dominated by anger. The latter woman, age 32, indicated that she worked in a store to keep her from thinking about a brutal past in Russia where her father died in a prison camp when she was 5 years old. However, one of the cases of hostile anxious attachment showed weaknesses in the individuation area, powerful affect and a depressive syndrome. Although not considered seriously pathological, there were problems. She is married to a man for whom this is a second marriage who has an 8½-year-old child by the first marriage who does not live with them. Both parents work and the 5-year-old is alone a good deal. The mother was quick to point out that the 5-year-old girl "understands" the situation and does not complain. Yet, she admits that this child has been quite babyish since the 1½-year-old was born. A third case of hostile anxious attachment was also considered to be within the normal range and did not show the depressive syndrome.

The depressive syndrome in the face of separation experiences in this population must, therefore, be interpreted as a healthy and acceptable phenomenon. Bowlby (1980, p. 246) states ". . . depression as a mood that most people experience on occasion is an inevitable accompaniment of any state in which behavior becomes disorganized, as it is likely to do after a loss. So long as there is an active interchange between ourselves and the external world, either in thought or action, our subjective experience is not one of depression; hope, fear, anger, dissatisfaction, frustration or any combination of these may be experienced. It is when interchange has ceased that depression occurs (and continues) until such time as new patterns of interchange have become organized toward a new object or goal . . . such disorganization and the mood of depression that goes with it, though painful and perhaps bewildering, is nonetheless potentially adaptive. . . . It is characteristic of the mentally healthy person that he can bear with this phase of depression and disorganization and emerge from it, after not too long a time, with behavior, thought, and feeling beginning to be reorganized for interactions of a new sort."

Further, it would appear that threats of loss or actual loss in many persons produces temporary injury to the self-evaluative system. As noted previously (*Adolescent Separation Anxiety*, Vol. I), a part of the self suffers injury and strong feelings of rejection and intrapunitiveness result. Such feelings may well be associated with feelings of weakness and inadequacy. This reaction seems possibly more associated with persons in close-knit families because the very closeness tends to invest and incorporate the family members as part of the self. Thus, strong attachments may produce more vulnerability to pain and depression when the attachment is threatened or broken. In this connection, it is noteworthy that, during wars, a soldier who loses a close buddy shows a strong inclination to refuse to adopt a new one for fear of the pain of loss should the new buddy also be killed. In view of the significant survival value of attachments and the positive values to be derived from them, the temporary disorder which follows separation and loss must be considered as a necessary phase of distress from which most individuals recover.

Let us now consider the data with regard to the group of 14 mothers classified as being not as high in family closeness as the group of 17 discussed above. Here, various levels of self-sufficiency dominated the scene. This is not to say that the group that was high in closeness did not have mothers with self-sufficiency patterns, but rather that the group of 14 showed many more such mothers—26% to 10%. It would appear that, in this group of Jewish mothers with less family closeness, self-sufficiency patterns are a natural response. Where closeness is not as high, greater self-sufficiency is necessary at separation. This is not to say that self-sufficiency patterns on the S.A.T. are not survival based and are not healthy but, rather, that it is a variation of a life-style adaptation, just as mild and strong anxious attachment is such a variation in response to separation. It is only when the self-sufficiency becomes excessive (as previously described) that the nature of the adjustment becomes maladaptive.

It is noteworthy that the mothers in the not-high family closeness group did not respond as strongly (less frequency) to the strong pictures as the mothers in the high closeness group. Instead, they showed a trend toward lower responsiveness to the strong pictures. If we combine this with the trend toward greater self-sufficiency patterns, we increase the evidence that the non-high closeness group showed a greater tendency to be less distressed by separation experiences. This is further proof that the less closeness, the less distress up to a point. A glance at Figure 19.1 indicates that increasing attachment shows greater disturbance and increasing self-sufficiency shows greater disturbance, with the healthiest patterns lying in the center and the less healthy eventually branching out in both directions. This bi-modal curve suggests that both anxious attachment, on the one hand, and self-sufficiency, on the other, have their limits of health. The separate curves for the two groups of mothers indicate that both groups show a slightly bi-modal arrangement, although, for the high closeness group, the curve shows the high point in the anxious attachment area and the non-high closeness group shows the high point in the self-sufficiency area. (See Figure 19.2)

Figure 19.1

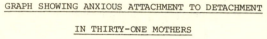

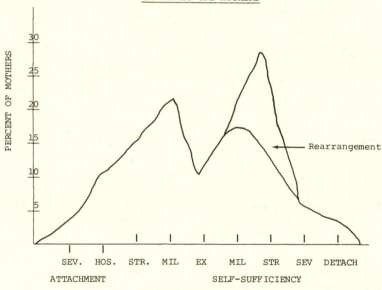

CLINICAL PATTERNS

FOOTNOTE: If cases of self-sufficiency are arranged to
            parallel cases of anxious attachment, i.e., mild,
            strong and severe, the curve shifts somewhat and
            eliminates the upward bulge on the self-sufficiency
            side.

SUMMARY AND CONCLUSIONS

This study has been a preliminary investigation of the relationship between the extent of family closeness and the response to the S.A.T. in 31 mothers of a group of 5-year-old children. The families were all of the Jewish faith, and the children were attending a Hebrew parochial school. The results of the study have been analyzed from the point of view of a set of clinical criteria developed in part around Bowlby's attachment theory and out of the concept of anxious attachment. These clinical criteria have already been presented in Volume II of *Adolescent Separation Anxiety*. Using a continuum of both anxious attachment and self-sufficiency (also detachment), I have attempted to present a picture of a relatively typical population on this scale.

Figure 19.2

GRAPH SHOWING ANXIOUS ATTACHMENT TO DETACHMENT

IN TWO GROUPS OF MOTHERS IN CONTRAST

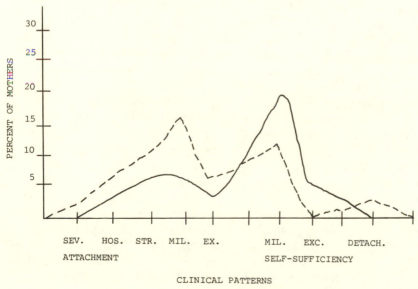

CLINICAL PATTERNS

LEGEND: ------ High Closeness Mothers

           _____ Non-High Closeness Mothers

Instead of using the term "separation anxiety" as an applicable
term for typical reactions, I have adapted Bowlby's term "anxious attachment," which he had originally developed for use in pathological
conditions. The central theme is that separation anxiety can only occur
if there are varying degress of anxious attachment present, that is, from
mild to very severe. Further, that mild degrees of anxious attachment
are a necessary aspect of survival in a family setting and that, without
it, mutual interaction of protection and needing protection between
mother and child becomes more difficult. We then consider separation
anxiety as an aspect of the mutually anxious attachment which normally exists between a mother and her child. At the same time, there
are degrees of self-sufficiency which have to exist so that, eventually,
degrees of autonomy will develop. The interaction and dominance, as
well as balance, between these two phenomena are therefore important issues in this study.

The 31 mothers were faced with separation experiences via a series
of pictures. Not only were their reactions to the pictures studied, but
they were divided into two groups according to the degree of family
closeness reported by them in interviews. The group of 17 mothers,
classified as high in family closeness, and the group of 14 mothers,
designated as not-high in family closeness, were then compared in their
reactions to the S.A.T. From the obtained data, we have drawn certain
tentative conclusions which will require further verification through
replicative studies.

High family closeness among Jewish mothers tends to result in
higher degrees of stress for them under threat of separation than among
those for whom family closeness is less strong or extensive. This stress is
manifested in separation pain, anxious attachment, and depressive syndrome of varying strengths. Those in whom family closeness is less extensive tend, on the other hand, to show greater degrees of self-
sufficiency.

The varying degrees of typical patterns of separation reactions
tend, in the former group, to emphasize anxious attachment and, in
the latter group, self-sufficiency. There appears to be a bi-modal curve
when these characteristics are arranged in a continuum, with the
healthiest patterns in the middle of the scale and fewer in number. The
best patterns of response are obviously not the most frequent, while the
mild distress on both sides of the scale are most frequent. Minor
deficiencies or problems in "separation health" are more frequent in

terms of anxious attachment or self-sufficiency than in excellent separation health. Severe forms of separation disorder are infrequent in this population and are present in small numbers.

Do these results suggest that high family closeness is an evil to be avoided? On the contrary, they indicate that its value lies in the arousal of the necessary forms of pain, depressive feelings and anxious attachment that are part of the survival mechanisms. Strong forms of separation normally produce grief and mourning to which the individual succumbs for a period of time and from which he eventually finds new forms of growth. At the same time, those who show such characteristics also maintain sufficient individuation and other strengths to see them through their separations. On the other hand, those with mild self-sufficiency dominance also maintain sufficient anxious attachment to give them the necessary stress outlet for relief of grief. Mothers in close families appear, on the whole, to manage separations very well, and only a small percentage show separation pathology of any severity.

REFERENCES

Ainsworth, M. D. S. *Patterns of Attachment*. Hillsdale, N. J.: Lawrence Erlbaum Associates, 1978.

Bowlby, J. "The Nature of the Child's Tie to His Mother." *International Journal of Psychoanalysis*, Vol. 39, Part V, 1958.

Bowlby, J. *Attachment and Loss*, Vol. I, *Attachment* (1969). Vol. II, *Separation: Anxiety and Anger*. (1973). Vol. III, *Loss: Sadness and Depression*. (1980). New York: Basic Books.

Health Findings. University of Pittsburgh School of Medicine, Dept. of Psychiatry, October 1980.

Browne, G. W. et al. "Depression and Loss." British Journal of Psychiatry, 1977, *130*, 1-18.

Coleman, R. W., et al. "The Study of Variations of Early Parental Attitudes." *Psychoanalytic Study of the Child*, Vol. 8, pp. 20-47. New York: International Universities Press, 1953.

DeLozier, P. P. "An Application of Attachment Theory to the Study of Child Abuse." Doctoral Dissertation, Calif. School of Professional Psychology, Los Angeles: 1979.

Deutsch, H. *The Psychology of Women*, Vol. II. New York: Grune & Stratton: 1945.

Farber, S. *Identical Twins Reared Apart: A Re-analysis*. New York: Basic Books, 1981.

Hansburg, H. G. *Adolescent Separation Anxiety*, Vol. I, *A Method for the Study of Adolescent Separation Problems*. Springfield, Ill.: C. C. Thomas, 1972. Reprinted: Melbourne, Fla.: R. E. Krieger, 1980.

Hansburg, H. G. *Adolescent Separation Anxiety*, Vol. II, *Separation Disorders*. Melbourne, Fla.: R. E. Krieger, 1980.

Hansburg, H. G. *Separation Anxiety Test Pictures and Scoring Materials*. Melbourne, Fla.: R. E. Krieger, 1980.

Hansburg, H. G. "The Use of the Separation Anxiety Test in the Detection of Self-Destructive Tendencies in Early Adolescence." In *Mental Health in Children*, Vol. III, Ed. D. V. Siva Sankar. Westbury, N.Y.: P.J.D. Publications, 1976, pp. 161-199.

Hellman, I. "Some Observations on Mothers of Children with Intellectual Inhibitions." *Psychoanalytic Study of the Child*, Vol. 9. New York: International Universities Press, 1954, pp. 259-273.

Kinard, E. M. "Emotional Development in Physically Abused Children." American Journal of Orthopsychiatry, Vol. 50 (4), October 1980, pp. 686-695.

Levy, D. "Maternal Overprotection." *Psychiatry*, Vol. I (4), November 1938, p. 570.

Mahler, M. S. *On Human Symbiosis and the Vicissitudes of Individuation*, Vol. I. New York: International Universities Press, 1968.

Rheingold, H. L. *Maternal Behavior in Mammals*. New York: John Wiley, 1963.

Rock, M. A. "Gorilla Mothers Need Some Help from Their Friends." *Smithsonian*, Sept. 1979. Discussion of Research by Ronald Nadler at Yerkes Primate Research Center.

Sherry, M. "Father Absence and Separation Anxiety Reactions in College Freshmen." Doctoral Dissertation, Michigan State University, East Lansing, Michigan, 1980.

Yahraes, H. "A Study of How the Child Separates from the Mother." (Investigator: M. Mahler) Mental Health Program Reports, *NIMH* pp. 113-124.

SECTION FOUR

This section presents the various ways in which the S.A.T. has been adapted or revised for various ages, groups, and problem situations. Since the time the original test was developed for adolescents, it has also been used to study latency-age children, young adults, middle-aged individuals, and the elderly. However, some researchers found it difficult to use the test for other groups as it was originally created, so they proceeded to vary either the directions, the pictures, the associated phrases, the scoring system and/or the statistical procedures.

Obviously, the test could not be used for very young children, and the reader will note that Chapters 20 and 21 are devoted to two efforts to develop more adaptable measures. For latency-age children, one investigator retained the test essentially as it was constructed but changed the method of administration. Eight-year-olds did not have sufficient reading ability to deal with the test. The same was true of children who were older but who could not read; so not only were the directions changed for them but also the manner of responding. Chapter 22 contains a presentation and discussion of these methods. The S.A.T. was used with impunity in many adult studies with the exception of a change in directions. One effort to change the pictures for adults was undertaken in a study of divorce, and this is described in Chapter 23. (Also, since the test would be useless for those who could not understand English, efforts were made to translate the original test into foreign languages. One such effort is in the Appendix.)

Other methods of studying human reactions to separation have been developed and utilized in research. M. D. S. Ainsworth, formerly of Johns Hopkins University and now at the University of Virginia, studied separation problems in infancy and very early childhood. Referring to these studies as "strange situations," she placed the children in a room with the mother, and the child's behavioral reactions were observed. Subsequently the mother left the room and the child was alone with the experimenter, and behavior was observed further. The return of the mother made possible further observations of the child's behavior. Studies of both attachment and exploratory behavior, as well as the accompanying emotional reactions, revealed the degree to which each child was affected by the presence or absence of the mother.

These observational studies included the behavior of the mother as well. Maternal behavior included responsiveness to infant crying, acknowledgment of baby's behavior when entering the room, behavior relevant to bodily contact, behavior relevant to infant obedience, etc.

Infant behavior included crying, response to physical contact, and face-to-face behavior with the mother, such as smiling, vocalizing, bouncing, etc. In children of ages two to four, interactive behaviors were observed, such as proximity seeking, contact maintaining, avoidance, resistance, exploratory behavior, crying, etc. Behavior patterns were classifed in groups (see Ainsworth, et al., 1978).

Bowlby (in a personal discussion with me) has indicated his personal preference for observational methods which have been objectively developed. However, he is not averse to accepting test methods if the purpose is to determine the degree to which the personality has been affected by separation experiences and also to predict separation behavior.

I have heard and read about a number of innovations used to measure the effects of separation on children and adults but have not investigated them.

On research techniques, scoring methods, and statistical ideas in the use of the S.A.T., a few remarks are in order. Revisions in an effort to simplify scoring for research purposes run the risk of over-simplification—with a resultant destruction of the rich clinical material to be derived from it. In any given individual, the impact of separation experiences is highly complicated, and the internal results are in motion, ebbing and flowing within limits and forming differing and shifting patterns. To attempt to represent this process by a simple score becomes very misleading. For this reason any research concerned with the effects of separation experience upon human feelings, thoughts, and behavior should employ a schema which involves clinical patterning rather than simple scoring techniques.

In the Introduction, I discussed the variations in statistical methods used to derive norms and to establish reliability and validity of the method. In the course of working with the S.A.T. method, various researchers have used some of the usual measures of central tendency, reliability of differences, and, more significantly, the differences in variability of the data known as ANOVA, or analysis of variability. Many have used partial correlation techniques in order to eliminate the effects of certain variables on the data. I have strongly advised workers in the field to use clinical analysis of the patterns and make comparisons between groups by X^2 techniques. Our experience has shown that studying populations for the relative presence or absence of disorders in particular psychological systems as a result of separation experiences will be rewarding if we use these methods. Obviously, when populations are small, more refined statistical techniques are necessary, as well as more careful pairing or matching of sample individuals.

A number of investigators have raised the issue of standard scores rather than the percentage ratings which have been in use for the S.A.T. Originally, it was conceived that the reactions to individual patterns should be scored as a percentage of the total responses for each individual. The raw score for each pattern was highly subject to the total responsiveness of the subject, and, therefore, the pattern score would be better represented by its relationship to the total number of responses. Continued studies have shown that these pattern percentages in relation to each other are quite meaningful. Ordinarily, standard score measures are derived from standard deviations. The problem of how to derive standard scores which will provide an adequate relationship to other standard scores within an individual protocol on this test remains open. Until we have such a scoring system, I would suggest that we retain the present method and concentrate on developing meaningful interpretive test patternings—for example, the Separation Test Index used by Varela (see Chapter 7).

The following chapters present the current revisions of the S.A.T.:

- The Klagsbrun-Bowlby Scale for 4- and 5-year-olds
- Varela's revision of the Klagsbrun-Bowlby Scale
- Brody's method of using S.A.T. with 8-year-olds
- Duplak's method of using S.A.T. material for a study of learning-disabled children of latency age
- Burger's revision of the S.A.T. for adult male divorcees

The following examples of revisions and adaptations of the S.A.T. method suggest that others may readily be developed. The method is so flexible as to permit of variations for different cultures, special situations, age groups, etc. The significant question is whether each variation will need to establish comparability to the original and its own validity and reliability.

20

A Clinical Test for Young Children

The earliest effort at adapting the S.A.T. was undertaken by a student, Micheline Klagsbrun, under the direction of John Bowlby at the Tavistock Clinic in London, and published in 1976. Klagsbrun was particularly interested in developing the technique for children 4½ to 5½ years of age and adapting the method in pictures, phrases, psychological terminology, method of scoring, and interpretation closer to Bowlby's attachment theory. She used six realistic photographs of separation experiences (one set for girls and one for boys) to study eighty-two children. A complete description of this revision is given in the following paper, entitled "Responses to Separation from Parents: A Clinical Test for Young Children," by Micheline Klagsbrun and John Bowlby, reprinted with the kind permission of the British Journal of Projective Psychology and Personality Study, 21 (2), December 1976.

SUMMARY

The test described, based on a test developed by Hansburg (1972) for older children, aims to throw light on how a child in the age-range of about 4 to 7 would respond to situations in which he is separated for shorter or longer periods from his parents. The results of a pilot study with five-year-olds during their first term at a London School are regarded as promising with respect both to the validity of an overall score as a measure of health or disturbance and also to the range and relevance for clinical and educational assessments of the responses given.

INTRODUCTION

An increasing number of psychiatrists and psychologists have come to regard the way a person responds to situations of actual or threatened separation from a loved person, either temporary or permanent, as a major indicator of personality development and possible psychopathology. Among those who have drawn attention to the key role of such responses are Freud (1917, 1926), Fairbairn (1952), Winnicott (1965), Jacobson (1965), and Mahler (1968). Currently one of us is attempting to examine the empirical evidence with a view to developing a consistent theoretical model, drawing on concepts from ethology and cognitive psychology as well as from psychoanalysis (Bowlby, 1969, 1973).

Recently, Hansburg (1972) has published particulars of a test intended to help assess an individual's modes of responding to situations entailing a separation from or loss of parents. Hansburg's Separation Anxiety Test, designed to be given to adolescents in the 11 to 17 years age range, consists of a dozen pictures, all but three of which depict a situation in which either a child is leaving his parents or a parent is leaving the child. Some of the situations, such as a child leaving to go to school or a mother leaving her child at bedtime, are of a kind that any child of over six would be expected to take in his stride. Others are of a more disturbing character. They include a picture in which the child's mother is being taken by ambulance to hospital, and another in which the child is going off to live permanently with his grandmother.

Under each picture is written a title making explicit what the picture represents. In presenting each picture the clinician asks the child or adolescent, first, "Did this ever happen to you?" and then, if the answer is no, "Can you imagine how it would feel if it did happen?" Responses to each picture are found to fall into some 17 categories from which various scores, ratios and indices can be derived.

Although Hansburg has as yet published only preliminary evidence for the validation of the test, his results have seemed to us to be of sufficient interest and promise to warrant the construction of a version suitable for younger children. This was done and tried out in a pilot study by one of us (M.K.) The study was undertaken in part requirement for the Diploma in Clinical Psychology awarded by the Tavistock Institute of Human Relations. An account of the test as devised for five-year-olds and of the results of a pilot study follow.

The Test

To suit a younger age group not only was the series of pictures shortened to six, but realistic photographs were substituted for the original ink drawings. Two corresponding sets of pictures were assembled, one for boys and one for girls [see pages 310–317]. The pictures were chosen to combine maximum situational focus with a minimum of facial expression, so that with the help of a caption the situation is made clear but the emotions aroused remain ambiguous. Three of the situations are considered more severe (and unanimously judged to be so by four independent judges) than the other three, in that the milder ones are more everyday and familiar (Hansburg's main criterion). This differentiation into mild and severe types of situation is of much significance in interpreting test responses since different sorts of response are to be expected to each type.

The situations specified, in the sequence in which they are presented to the children and labeled M for mild or S for severe, are as follows:

1. parents go out for the evening, leaving child at home (M)
2. mother (father) goes away for the weekend, leaving little girl (boy) with aunt (uncle) (S)
3. child's first day at school; moment of parting from parent (S)
4. parents are going away for two weeks; prior to their departure they give the child a specially attractive toy: pedal car for boys, party dress for girls (S)
5. park scene; parents tell child to run off and play by himself for a while, they want some time alone together to talk (M)
6. father (mother) tucks little girl (boy) up in bed and leaves room (M)

In these situations, although the child is not always physically alone, he is very much out on his own in that he must cope without having his parents at hand to fall back on.

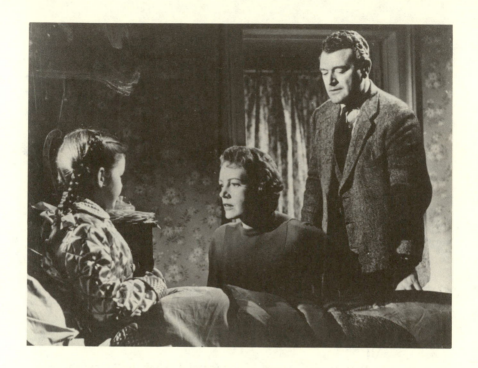

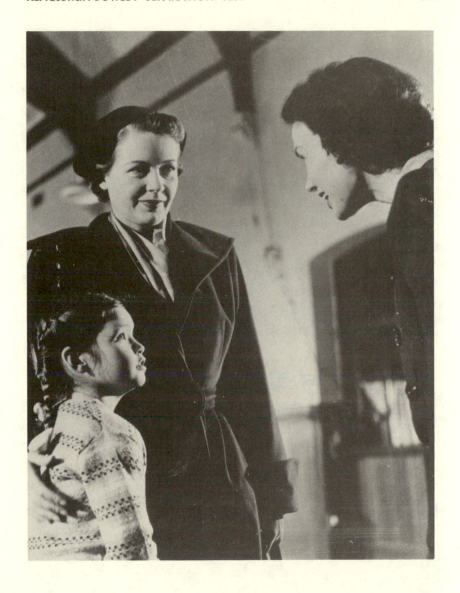

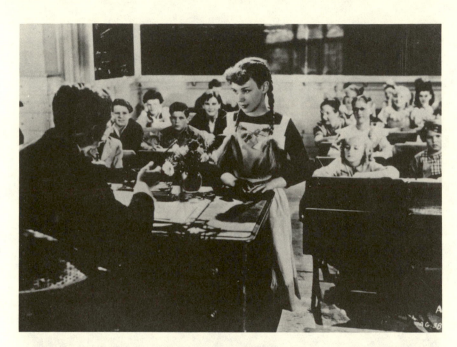

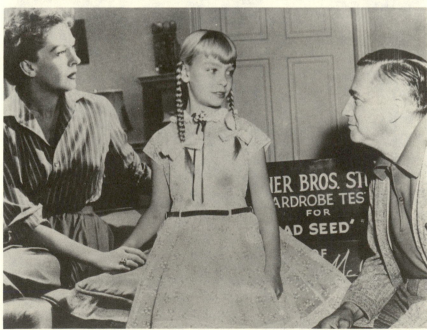

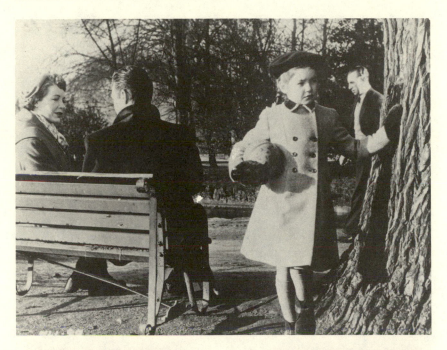

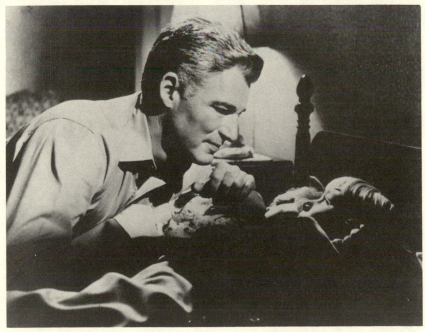

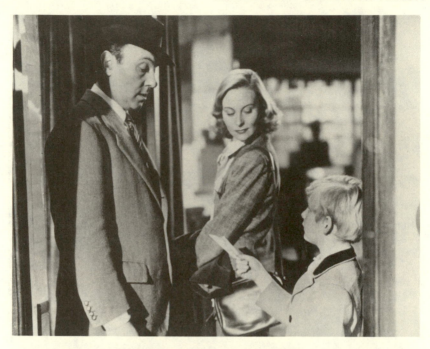

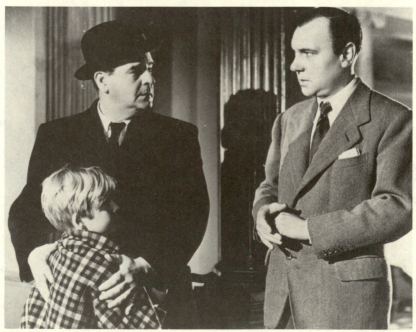

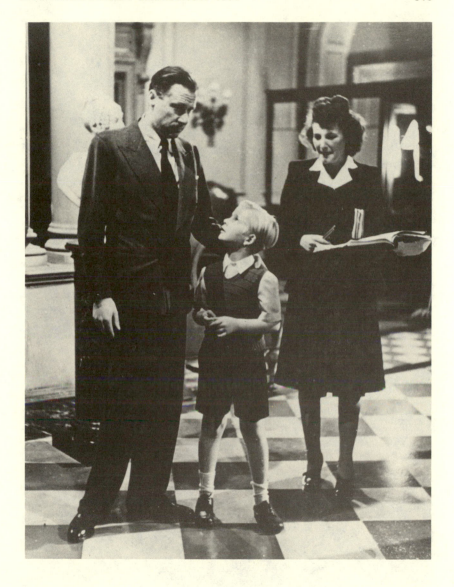

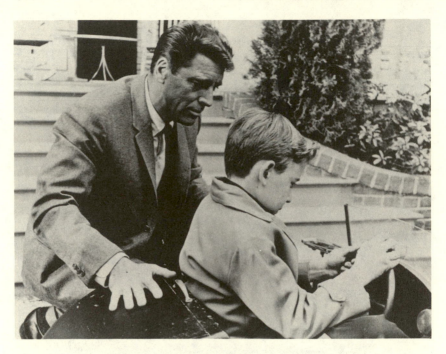

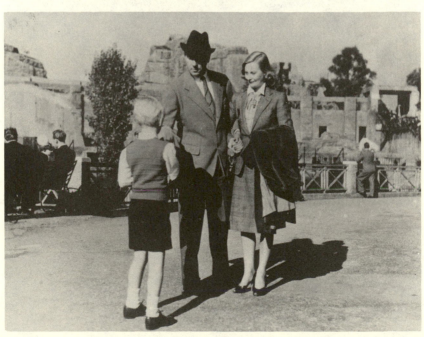

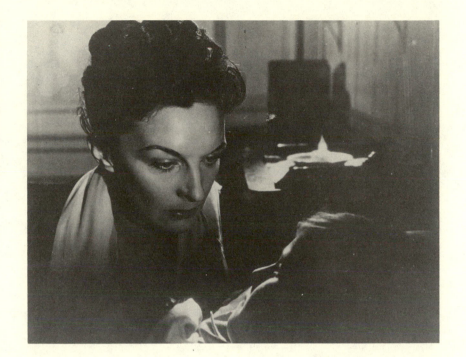

Administration

Children are tested individually. After a few minutes of conversation to establish rapport, the child is shown the pictures, one by one, and told what is happening in each. He/she is asked, "How does the little boy (girl) in the picture feel?" If he has difficulty in responding, a list of possible responses (based on those presented by Hansburg to his subjects, and ordered randomly) is read to him. It is emphasized that he does not have to choose any of them, that they are merely suggestions as to how he might put his feelings into words. The list is as follows:

"Does the little boy feel lonely—or does he feel sad—or does he feel angry—or does he feel that his parents don't love him anymore—or that it's not really happening—or does he feel like hiding away—or does he feel like he just doesn't care—or does he feel that if he'd been a good boy it wouldn't have happened—or that it's someone else's fault—or that something bad is going to happen—or does he feel now he's going to have a good time—or that he's hungry—or getting a tummy ache or a headache."

It was rarely necessary to go through the whole list in this manner. Most children would interrupt when one of the responses seemed suitable to them. (Although it would be possible to continue reading the list to see if a child selected additional responses, this procedure was not followed.)

Not only a child's feelings but the means he considers for coping with the situation also seemed a promising area for investigation. For example, in stressful situations an anxious child is liable to be inhibited, to withdraw or to hide, a depressed child to respond with apathetic resignation or passive withdrawal, a child prone to delinquency to respond with anger and violence or by pilfering or running away. Accordingly, each child was asked, after his response to each picture, "What does the little boy (girl) do?"

Method of Scoring

Hansburg has conducted several studies in which he has tested samples of adolescents from diverse backgrounds. Certain patterns of response appear to be associated with different forms of emotional disturbance and others with healthy development.

Although in our scoring we have adhered closely to Hansburg's ideas and procedures, we have adopted a different terminology. Hansburg employs a number of fairly traditional clinical terms, but these are often ambiguous and laden with theory that we do not necessarily accept. The terms we use are at a simple descriptive level and, when linked to theory, are linked to the ideas developed in Bowlby's *Attachment and Loss* with which Hansburg's findings are highly compatible. A glossary of equivalent terms is in Appendix 2.

Our scoring procedure is as follows. The children's responses are first classified into 14 categories, based on those used by Hansburg but omitting three of his categories as inappropriate for a younger age-group. Again following Hansburg, these categories are next grouped into six main classes of response, a few of which overlap with others (see Table 20.1). Using the number of responses falling into each class, it then becomes possible to calculate a variety of indices.

The first index takes account of the balance between attachment-type responses and self-reliant responses, with special reference to whether the situation being responded to is mild or severe. For a favorable result a child is expected to show more self-reliant responses

Table 20.1

Category of Response	Class of Response
1. Loneliness	Attachment
2. Sadness	Loss of Self-esteem
3. Rejection ("his parents don't love him any more")	
4. Self-reproach ("if he'd been a good boy it wouldn't have happened")	
5. Anger	Hostile
6. Blames others ("it's someone else's fault")	
7. Well-being ("fine," "now he's going to have a good time")	Self-Reliant
8. Disbelief ("it's not really happening")	Avoidant
9. Withdrawal ("he feels like hiding away")	
10. Evasion ("he doesn't care")	
11. Generalized dread/anxiety ("he feels like something bad's going to happen")	Anxious
12. Fear (of ghosts, monsters, burglars etc.)	
13. Somatic reaction ("he's getting a tummy ache")	
14. Hunger	(Classified as both Attachment and Anxious)

in mild situations and more attachment-type responses in severe situations. The resulting index is termed the Attachment-Self Reliance index.

The second and third indices refer to the frequency of Hostile responses compared to those of attachment-type and of anxious responses respectively. For a favorable result the number of hostile responses is expected to be fewer than the number of each of the latter kinds.

The fourth index is the number of Anxious responses as a percentage of total responses. For a child to be scored favorably it is expected that some proportion of his total responses will express anxiety but that the proportion will not be too high.

The fifth index is a simple score of Avoidant responses. The lower the score the more favorable the result.

The sixth index is a simple score of responses indicating Loss of self-esteem. Once again the lower the score the more favorable the result.

The seventh index is a simple score of responses that seem bizarrre or absurd together with responses referring to death.

The eighth index derives from the children's answers to the question, "What then would you do?" Answers are categorized as follows:

> Appropriate activity, including active attempts to master the situation (with or without engaging the help of adults) and diversions (playing, reading, watching television, etc.)
> Unrealistic optimism, including disbelief ("they won't really go"), fantasy solutions ("he'll run away to Africa") and pseudo-mature solutions ("he'll be able to take a car and drive to school")
> Unrealistic pessimism, including catastrophes and total rejection ("they'll never come back")
> Withdrawal or inaction, including sleep (if inappropriate), and being totally overwhelmed ("he just cries")

The index of Appropriate Action derived from these answers is the ratio of the number of appropriate responses to the sum of those judged to indicate unrealistic optimism, unrealistic pessimism or inactive withdrawal.

Finally, by allocating either positive or negative points to scores on each of these indices, it is possible to give each child an overall test score designed to indicate how favorably or unfavorably he seems to be developing. The method of assigning such points is empirical and derived from the results of Hansburg's clinical experience with the test. Particulars of how the indices and the Test Score are arrived at are in Appendix 1.

The Test Score, which represents an ordinal not an interval scale of measurement, is no more than a crude indicator of health and disturbance. For clinical and educational purposes a profile made up of the eight indices is more informative since it gives a picture of the directions in which a given child deviates from the norm. Further information still can be derived from a study of the particular categories into which most of a child's responses fall.

PILOT STUDY

It was decided to administer the test to all the children newly admitted to a local authority day school in inner London during their first term of attendance. This enabled us to obtain a reasonably representative sample of children drawn from every socioeconomic level, and to test them at an age at which our society expects them to be able to adapt to a six-hour day away from home. Class teachers were asked to classify all the children in their care according to the following two-step procedure:

First Step
    Divide all the children into three groups:
    1. adjusting to school well; no difficulties
    2. some short-lived difficulties in adjusting to school; nothing to cause serious concern
    3. definite and persistent problems in adjusting to school

Second Step
    Subdivide children in group (1) into two subgroups (1a) composed of children doing slightly better than those in (1b). Subdivide children in group (3) in a similar way

Children in each of these five groups are assigned a Teacher's Rating ranging from 1 to 5.

By correlating the results of the test with the Teachers' ratings it was hoped to get a first impression of the probable validity of the test.

The sample comprised 49 boys and 33 girls, whose ages ranged from 4 years 6 months to 5 years 6 months, with a mean of 5 years 1 month. All were believed to be "getting along all right" and to have no known history of professional consultation for mental health reasons. The first 21 children to whom the test was administered were used as a preliminary sample for refining the administration of the test, leaving a main sample of 61 children, 37 boys and 24 girls.

The children were extremely interested in the task and only a few had difficulty expressing themselves. Little prompting was needed and what there was proved unrelated to a child's test score. Only two children refused the test; one came from overseas and hardly spoke English.

No difficulties were encountered in classifying the responses. Although no test of reliability was conducted, it is expected to prove satisfactory.

Correlation of Test Scores and Teachers' Ratings

Test scores were well distributed, the extremes ranging from $+6$ to -12, and gave four easily defined and roughly equal groups of children designated groups A, B, C, and D. All but eleven of the children scored between $+4$ and -3. Teachers' Ratings were less evenly distributed, with ratings 2 and 4 little used. Since neither Teachers' Ratings nor Test Scores were correlated either with age or sex, results are pooled. The distribution of the children's Test Scores and Teachers' Ratings is shown in Table 20.2.

Table 20.2

DISTRIBUTION OF CHILDREN BY TEST SCORES
AND TEACHERS' RATINGS

Group	Test Score	Teachers' Rating					Totals
		1	2	3	4	5	
A	+4 and over	9	0	1	1	1	12
B	+1 to +3	8	2	6	0	2	18
C	0 to -2	6	4	3	2	3	18
D	-3 and below	0	0	8	2	3	18
		23	6	18	5	9	61

To test for significance the Spearman Rank Relation Coefficient (Siegel 1956) was used, which gives the following results:

		Value of t or rs	Significance
Girls Only	(n = 24)	rs = 0.05865	$p.$ 01
Boys only	(n = 37)	t = 3.3393	$p.$ 01 with 35 df
All children	(n = 61)	t = 5.5674	$p.$ 001 with 59 df

There is thus a significant degree of correlation between the two measures, not only for all the children but for boys and girls separately. This provides initial evidence that the test has some degree of validity.

Range of Responses

The children's responses to the pictures covered a strikingly wide range of feeling and behavior and brought home to us the strong emotions aroused in children of this age when confronted by situations of the types depicted. In illustration we give a selection of responses to the first two cards, the first of which depicts a mild situation and the second a severe one.

The group in which the overall Test Score places the child who gave each response is indicated.

Responses to Card 1
(Parents going out for evening—mild situation)
1. "Not very well. (Not very well?) She's got a cold and she's got a headache. (What does she do?) Go to sleep." *Group C*
2. "Tired. (Does she feel any of these . . . ?) She's lonely. (Do?) Go to bed and go to sleep." *Group A*
3. "Very well. She feels happy. My friend looks after me when mummy and daddy go out. (Do?) She's going to stay in bed." *Group C*
4. "Upset. (Upset?) Crying upset, she's crying. (Do?) Nothing." *Group B*
5. "He doesn't feel all right because he's alone. He's angry and lonely (makes a face and a roaring noise). (Do?) He's going to play with his toys." *Group A*
6. "He feels O.K. (Do?) I'd hide in a corner. (Why?)

Because there might be a dragon in the house." *Group C*

7. "He feels like something dangerous is going to happen and they don't love him anymore. (What might happen?) A robber. (Do?) He's going to put on his pajamas and get into bed and then play." *Group A*

8. "All right. My sister looks after me. Maybe his sister will stay with him. (What if he's alone?) Horrid. He'd be hungry, and scared. (Do?) He might get lost and he might run away from his house and he might think they don't love him. (Which do you think is most likely?) He'll run away I should think."

9. "He might feel very well, he could feel upset, he could feel something touching, he could feel something with his mouth like kissing. (Which do you think?) He's sad, and he's scared. He's scared of a barking man. He's heartbroken. If I loved my mummy and she ran away I would be heartbroken." *Group C*

10. "Lonely. (Any of these . . . ?) No. (Do?) Watch TV. I never cry you know. I was playing football and my leg broke and I never cried." *Group B*

11. "She starts to cry. (Do?) I'd pinch everything that I could get to eat. (Any of these . . . ?) I'd feel all of them. (Any one in particular?) Hungry." *Group C*

12. "All right. (Any of these?) She feels like hiding away, because she doesn't want to see her mummy and daddy in the morning. (Why?) I don't know. (Do?) Hide." *Group C*

13. "She's not very well. (Any of these?) She's scared and she's got a tummy ache. She's sick and she's hungry. It's only a dream. (Do?) She's going to be very sick. But it's all a dream so then she'll wake up." *Group D*

Responses to Card 2
(Mother (father) goes away for weekend, leaving little girl (boy) with aunt (uncle)—severe situation)

1. "Sicky and sad. (Do?) She's going to stay with her nanny." *Group B*

2. "She feels happy again. (Any of these . . . ?) No, she's

very well. (Do?) She's going to bring her toys to auntie's and play with them." *Group C*

3. "He's sad and angry. He's angry with his daddy. (Do?) He's going to play with his toys." *Group A*

4. "Nasty. The toys are nasty and he doesn't want to play. He wants to drink his milk and go to bed. He's going to hide under the bed. (Why?) Because it's nighttime and the Bad is coming." *Group A*

5. "He hopes that his daddy will come back soon. (Any of these . . . ?) If he'd been a good boy it wouldn't have happened. (Do?) He's going to ask his uncle if he can have some lunch." *Group A*

6. "He's frightened. He doesn't want his daddy to go away. His uncle might get cross. (Do?) Play games with his uncle." *Group A*

7. "She's worried. (What about?) She's worried with her mum gone away, worried about aunty. She wants to go with her mum. (Do?) She hides under the bed away from her nanny." *Group C*

8. "All right. (Any of these . . . ?) He's hungry, and his father might say he hasn't bought any food, there might not be any food in the house for him. (Do?) He's going to play with his toys, get dressed, comb his hair, go to school, comb his own hair and do his own shoelaces up." *Group B*

9. "He's uncomfortable because the bed is cold. (Any of these . . .) It's lonely but it's really only a dream. He feels sorry for himself. (Do?) Don't know." *Group C*

10. "He'll cry because daddy doesn't love him anymore. He's scared, of . . . (Of what?) That he might get killed. (Do?) I don't know." *Group D*

11. "He's crying his eyes out. (Any of these . . .?) Scared. A man might come and take him away. (Do?) Play with him" (pointing to uncle). *Group B*

12. "Terrible bad. I mean, because he's cuddling him. He's scared. (Do?) Hide away in the bath." *Group D*

13. "She feels afraid, of her mummy going and not coming back again. (Do?) Don't know." *Group D*

14. "Sad, and scared that she might get hurt. (How would

she get hurt?) There might be some bombs drop on
her. (Do?) Don't know, just play." *Group C*

Portraits of Individual Children

Turning now to individual children we formed the impression as
we read each child's responses that we were presented with a relatively
consistent and revealing picture. In some cases it was a disturbing one.
There follow the responses given by one boy and one girl from each of
the four groups into which the children are divided by Test Score.

The actual Test Score (T.S.) and Teacher's Rating (T.R.) is given
after each child's name. Cards 1, 5 and 6 depict mild situations; Cards
2, 3 and 4, severe ones.

GROUP A—12 children

Annabel (T.S. +4 T.R. 1)
This little girl gave responses that seem typical of children who are
developing well.

> Card 1   evening out (M)
> > She cries, she's lonely. She feels like maybe it's
> > in a dream. (What's she going to do?) Hide un-
> > der the bedclothes. I do that sometimes when
> > there's a crack in the ceiling. Something dan-
> > gerous might come out of the crack in the ceil-
> > ing. But nothing really comes, it's only made
> > up, in a story.
>
> Card 2   weekend (S)
> > She feels all right (Any of these . . . ?) No,
> > she's all right. (Do?) Drawing and painting.
>
> Card 3   school (S)
> > I felt lonely at school. I was crying because I
> > didn't want mummy to go home. (Do?) Cry.
>
> Card 4   two weeks (S)
> > Who's looking after her? (Who do you think?)
> > I think the lady in the black hat in the second
> > picture is going to come and look after her. So
> > she'll be all right. She would be sad if she was
> > alone.

Card 5   run off and play (M)
         She feels all right. (Does she feel any of these
         . . . ?) No. (Do?) There's a hole in the tree,
         and she's putting her hand in it, she's feeling
         the tree and then she's going to play ball.
Card 6   tuck up (M)
         She feels all right. (Any of these . . . ?) No.
         She's going straight to sleep. It's easy.

Although Annabel shows a tendency to withdraw (Cards 1 and 3) and some disbelief (Card 1), she also shows a capacity to experience and tolerate the pain of separation. Her Attachment-Self-Reliance Balance is good, with more Self-Reliant responses in the milder situations, and more Attachment-type responses in the severe ones. The response to Card 4 seems a particularly good way of coping with the situation. It was very rare for a child to remember the aunt (or uncle) in Card 2, and to use her (him) so aptly and effectively; this was done only by children of this group. Similarly, the expression of mixed feelings was rare, and confined to these children. Examples from the records of other children are:

Card 3   Nice and sad. . . .
Card 5   Happy. And that his mummy and daddy don't
         love him anymore. (Can he be happy if his
         mummy and daddy don't love him anymore?)
         Yes, because he just feels one, just for a
         minute, and then he feels the other. . . .

David (T.S. +4 T.R.1)

Card 1   evening out (M)
         He thinks that he should go to sleep soon. He
         feels hungry. (Do?) He's going to see if he
         could make himself some toast.
Card 2   weekend (S)
         He hopes that his daddy will come back soon.
         (Any of these . . . ?) If he'd been a good boy it
         wouldn't have happened. (Do?) Ask his uncle
         if he can have some lunch.

Card 3 school (S)

I felt like I was going to have a nice time, and I could tell my mummy things when I came back home. (Any of these . . . ?) No. (Do?) Some reading from a reading book.

Card 4 two weeks (S)

He wishes that he had someone to look after him. He feels a bit sad (Do?) He's going to see if he can make himself some lunch, and then play.

Card 5 run off and play (M)

He thinks he'll go and see if there's a playground. (Any of these?) No. He's fine.

Card 6 tuck up (M)

He feels that he wants to go to sleep so morning will come sooner. (Any of these . . .?) No. It's easy for him to sleep.

Throughout the record David is giving responses that show a good balance between attachment-type responses and self-reliance, combined with decisive and appropriate action.

GROUP B—18 children

Yvette (T.S. + 2 T.R. 1)

Card 1 evening out (M)

Upset. (Upset?) Crying upset, she's crying. (Do?) Nothing.

Card 2 weekend (S)

I'd stay with my uncle. (How does she feel?) She feels all right, she wouldn't feel upset then. (Do?) Have some food.

Card 3 school (S)

I didn't like it. First I was in class 10, then in class 7. It was a Friday. I was only 4 then, I'm 5 now. (Does she feel any of these . . . ?) No, but I wouldn't like to be alone. Mummy and daddy wouldn't leave me alone because I didn't like Miss C (teacher). (Do?) She plays in the Wendy House and makes a book.

Card 4 two weeks (S)
> I don't stay on my own. If she's all on her own she's very upset, and she's got a tummy-ache. (Do?) Cry.

Card 5 run off and play (M)
> She's upset, and she's got a headache. (Do?) She runs away, to the park, because she doesn't like her mummy and daddy any more.

Card 6 tuck up (M)
> She feels happy. (Any of these . . . ?) No. (Do?) Go to sleep. I say the ABC and then I go to sleep. (Why the ABC?) Because I like saying it, and because I don't like sleeping, I like to watch T.V. better.

Lionel (T.S. 3 + T.R. 3)

Card 1 evening out (M)
> All right. (Any of these . . . ?) No, he's O.K. (Do?) He's going to wait till his mummy's back and his daddy. He'll wait for them and after they'll go shopping.

Card 2 weekend (S)
> He's crying his eyes out. (Any of these . . . ?) He's scared. A man might come and take him away. (Do?) Play with him (pointing to uncle).

Card 3 school (S)
> Nice. He feels real nice. (Do?) He's going to have some rock.

Card 4 two weeks (S)
> He's sad because they don't love him anymore. And he's scared. Something might come and take him away. (Do?) Play with his car.

Card 5 run off and play (M)
> He's sad, and he's got a tummy ache because he thinks someone will take him away. (Do?) Play hide and seek.

Card 6 tuck up (M)
>   Sleepy. His mummy reads him a story and
>   then he looks at a book and then he's asleep.

Of these two Group B children, Yvette shows a good deal of
distress and a somatic reaction on two cards (4 and 5). On cards 2, 3
and 6, however, she is able to take some appropriate action. Lionel also
shows a somatic reaction on one card (5); and on no less than three
cards he expresses fear that someone will come and take him away.
Nevertheless, to most of the cards he, too, is able to decide on something appropriate to do.

GROUP C—18 children

Mabel (T.S. 0 T.R.2)

Card 1 evening out (M)
>   I wouldn't cry because I never cry. My sister
>   would cry because she's scared that someone
>   might come in the door. (Does the little girl
>   feel scared?) No, because mummy locks the
>   door. (Does the little girl feel any of these
>   . . . ?) No, I can't think. (What does she do?)
>   Go to sleep.

Card 2 weekend (S)
>   She's sad. (Do?) Cry.

Card 3 school (S)
>   I was in class 10, seven years ago. (How does
>   she feel?) Horrible. I felt horrible because I
>   didn't like the teacher. (Do?) Nothing. I've
>   forgotten.

Card 4 two weeks (S)
>   Is she on her own? (Yes, what if she's on her
>   own?) It's nice. She feels like she's going to
>   have a good time. (Do?) Play a game.

Card 5 run off and play (M)
>   Sad (Do?) Cry.

Card 6 tuck up (M)
>   She's upset. (What kind of upset?) Crying and
>   her tummy hurts. (Do?) She'll go to sleep. I go
>   to sleep but my sister doesn't and she keeps
>   waking me up.

The deficiencies in Mabel's development are reflected in the Attachment-Self-Reliance (a higher proportion of Attachment responses
given to the mild situations, and one Self-Reliant response to a severe
one), and an apathetic quality to many of her Action responses. Her
unwillingness to admit to feelings that are often regarded as "babyish"
and her attribution of these to her sister conflict with her manifest
distress at being separated from her parents. Her responses to Card 4,
in which she seems not to notice the severity of the situation, suggests
unrealistic optimism.

Archie (T.S. − 2 T.R.5)

      Card 1 evening out (M)

             Scared because he's on his own. He's scared of
a burglar (Do?) Nothing. Burglars can only go
in one of the bottom flats, can't they?

      Card 2 weekend (S)

             Feels all right. I can think of lots of things
that's happening to him. (How does he feel?)
Sad. (Do?) Stay at home.

      Card 3 school (S)

             I don't remember. It feels very good because I
liked it. I like it at home best of all. (How does
he feel?) Nothing. (Any of these . . . ?) No.
(Do?) Nothing.

      Card 4 two weeks (S)

             He's worried. (About what?) Daddy, because
he hasn't got daddy with him. (Any of these
. . . ?) Lonely, and scared that something bad
might happen. In case a burglar comes. (Do?)
Nothing.

      Card 5 run off and play (M)

             This is a hard one, isn't it? (How does he feel?)
Hungry (Do?) Nothing.

      Card 6 tuck up (M)

             I don't know. All right (plays with pictures).

(Any of these . . . ?) No. I don't know. (Do?)
Go to sleep.

There were several indications in Archie's manner that the situations presented in the pictures were disturbing to him. His voice became progressively more babyish and took on a lisp, and he began to rock himself back and forth. His responses are characterized by fear and persistent inability to take any action.

GROUP D—13 children

All but one of these children had Test Scores in the range − 3 to − 7, the exception being a boy who scored as low as − 12. The responses of each of these children gave the impression of a seriously disturbed child. That, if valid, would give an incidence of psychiatric disorder for the sample of about 20%, which is close to the incidence found by other methods for London children (Rutter and others, 1975).

Claire (T.S. − 4 T.R. 3)

In her responses Claire expressed much anger with her parents and also envious dissatisfaction. Throughout the testing she chewed aggressively on her fingers.

Card 1   evening out (M)
She feels lonely, and angry with her mummy and daddy. (Do?) She's going to get out of bed and hide. She wants to go with them.
Card 2   weekend (S)
She feels as if she wanted to go with mummy. (Do?) She wants to go with them, if they're going to do anything nice. (Anything else?) Sort of lonely and angry.
Card 3   school (S)
I've forgotten. It feels strange. Some children you hadn't seen before and some children you had. Rather long playtimes and things like that. She gets a bit bored. (Do?) Rather do nothing. (Does she feel any of these . . . ?) No.
Card 4   two weeks (S)
She's angry with mummy and daddy. (Do?)

She's going to shout at them when they come back.

Card 5 run off and play (M)

She feels everybody else has got something to play with and she hasn't. She feels angry. (Do?) She's going to find someone to play with.

Card 6 tuck up (M)

She doesn't want to go to sleep, because she's wondering what her mummy and daddy are doing, and she's trying to listen to the telly. That's what I do. I lie down and shut my eyes and pretend to sleep, and if mummy or daddy come in they think I'm asleep, but I keep quiet and listen to the telly.

Amanda (T.S. − 6 T.R. 5)

Card 1 evening out (M)

She's got a tummy ache. (Do?) She's going to run away, to see mummy and daddy. I stay by myself with my brother and *he* wants my mummy and daddy.

Card 2 weekend (S)

She wants mummy. She feels like hiding away by herself, because mummy comes back and doesn't love her.

Card 3 school (S)

Yes, I remember. It's pains in my stomach. (Do?) Go to the medical room.

Card 4 two weeks (S)

She wants her mummy and daddy, she's hungry. (Do?) She's going to cook the dinner and *burn* herself.

Card 5 run off and play (M)

She's going to run away, because it feels as if they don't love her anymore.

Card 6 tuck up (M)

She feels sick. (Do?) Get out of bed and play with her toys.

Amanda was the lowest scoring among the girls. To two cards (2 and 5) she expresses the view that her mother does not love her anymore and also to two (1 and 5) that she will run away. On three cards (1, 3, and 6) she shows a somatic response and on a fourth (4) she expects to damage herself.

Such constant recourse to one or two modes of response proved characteristic of children with low Test Scores. Some made repeated reference to a specific situation feared; others repeatedly withdrew. One such boy, Theo (T.S. − 3 T.R. 4) was preoccupied during the test measuring the pictures, trying to fit them exactly on top of one another, and then arranging them side by side with great precision. He expressed fear of catastrophe (Card 4), of an intruder (Card 6) and of unspecified danger (Card 3), and also a desire to control his parents' movements by controlling their supply of money.

Julian (T.S. − 12 T.R.5)

This boy was the lowest scoring of all the children. In each of the last two cards he expresses a fear that his parents wish to be rid of him.

> Card 1 evening out (M)
> He thinks they're still at home. He forgets that they've gone out. He don't like it. (Feels?) If you're alone, you can get a tummyache by crying. Something's going to happen to him. (What?) He doesn't know, but he'll get a tummyache when he cries. (Do?) He forgets. He only remembers in the morning.
>
> Card 2 weekend (S)
> He feels a bit better because uncle's there. He feels a bit better if uncle takes him somewhere where there's lots of people, because he'll feel better, better if there's hundreds of people. But not if they make a lot of noise and it's a wedding. (Have you been to a wedding, with your uncle?) Yes.
>
> Card 3 school (S)
> I didn't mind very much. But when I first saw the teacher I thought it was going to be Miss M (headmistress). (Any of these . . . ?) (Do?) Don't know, don't remember.

Card 4 two weeks (S)
>He feels all right, but how would he feel if he didn't know how to work the motor car? *This* time he might think his parents *did* like him, because they did buy him a motor car. (Do?) He's going to drive the car, and if he's tired, he might want to eat and he forgot to ask his dad to give him something to eat. (Do you think he's hungry?) Yes.

Card 5 run off and play (M)
>He might find other children, but he'll be worried because of mummy and daddy, that they might want something. (Want something?) Yes, they might want him to die. It might be something for him to be killed there. To get rid of him.

Card 6 tuck up (M)
>He feels as if mummy's going to go to another country and leave him there and never come back, and leave him there for all his life, and not let him know when it's morning. Mother's not nice to him any more. That's the last time.

Others of the children in Group D expressed fear that they might die, e.g.,

>Response of girl (T.S. − 5) to Card 2: "She's scared that something bad's going to happen . . . she's going to die."
>Response of boy (T.S. − 7) to both Cards 2 and 3: "He might get killed."
>Response of boy (T.S. − 4) to Card 6: "Something might kill him if he's in the dark."

or that they might be abandoned, e.g.,

>Response of girl (T.S. − 5) to Card 2: "She feels afraid of her mummy going and not coming back again."
>Response of girl (T.S. − 3) to Card 4: "She's scared that they're never going to come back again."

One of the basic differences between these responses and similar-sounding responses given by children with good test scores is the ability of the latter to do something effective despite fear. This is illustrated by a response to Card 4, from a girl scoring +3:

"She thinks that something bad's going to happen. Something might come and take her away. (What does she do?) She's going to go and stay at her nana's."

Family Relations

There is now strong evidence that the pathway of personality development which a child, adolescent or young adult follows is correlated with the pattern of interaction within his family (see review in Bowlby, 1973, Chapter 21).

In our pilot project we had hoped to be able to test this hypothesis by interviewing the parents of the ten children with the highest test scores and those of the ten with the lowest. Difficulties arose, however, partly from time being limited and partly from difficulty in obtaining cooperation, especially (and probably significantly) from the parents of the low scorers. From what was done, however, including asking parents to predict how they thought their child would respond to the situations depicted on the cards, we formed a strong impression that the parents of the higher scoring children were more likely than parents of low scorers to empathize with and to be responsive to their child's feelings, to be more aware of the value of their being available at critical times (e.g., when the child comes home from school), more flexible about practical arrangements, and more skillful at preparing their child realistically for an upsetting situation without allowing their own anxieties to intrude.

DISCUSSION

In contrast to most projection tests which present a deliberately undefined stimulus situation, the test described presents a series of clearly specified situations which are selected because of their relevance to a particular theory of personality development and psychopathology. We regard the results of our small pilot study as promising on account of the range of responses the test gives, the extent to which Test Scores correlate with Teacher's Ratings, and the relevance that the responses have for understanding how each child construes his family situation and is likely to react to unsought separations from, or to loss of, a parent.

The test proves interesting to children in the age-group concerned, appears not to engender undue anxiety even in disturbed children, is relatively quick and easy to give and is not difficult to score. Responses are readily related on the one hand to clinical problems and on the other to theory. This leads us to believe that the test may prove of use both in routine clinical settings and for research.

Nevertheless much further work is required before the test can be regarded as a valid and reliable instrument. Information is needed regarding the reliability of classifying responses and the degree to which results correlate with other methods of assessing personality. With further experience some simplification of scoring methods may prove possible.

REFERENCES

Bowlby, J. *Attachment and Loss*, Vol. I. London: Hogarth Press. New York: Basic Books, 1969. London: Penguin Books, 1971.

Bowlby, J. *Attachment and Loss*, Vol. II. London: Hogarth Press. New York: Basic Books, 1973. London: Penguin Books, 1973.

Bowlby, J. *Attachment and Loss*, Vol. III. London: Hogarth Press. New York: Basic Books (in preparation).

Fairbairn, W. R. D. *Psychoanalytic Studies of the Personality*. London: Tavistock/Routledge. Published in the USA under the title *Object Relations Theory of Personality*. New York: Basic Books, 1954.

Freud, S. "Mourning and Melancholia." *S.E. 14*, 1917, 243–258.

Freud, S. "Inhibitions, Symptoms, and Anxiety." *S.E. 20*, 1926, 87–172.

Hansburg, H. G. *Adolescent Separation Anxiety: A Method for the Study of Adolescent Separation Problems*, Springfield, Ill.: C. C. Thomas, 1972.

Jacobson, E. "The Return of the Lost Parent," in M. Schur (ed.), *Drives, Affects, Behavior*, Vol. 2. New York: International Universities Press, 1965.

Mahler, M. D. *On Human Symbiosis and the Vicissitudes of Individuation*, Vol. 1: *Infantile Psychosis*. New York: International Universities Press, 1968.

Rutter, M., Cox, A., Tupling, C., Berger, M., and Yule, W. "Attainment and Adjustment in Two Geographical Areas: 1. The Prevalence of Psychiatric Disorder," *British Journal of Psychiatry 126*, 1975, 493–509.

Siegel, S. "Non-parametric Statistics for the Behavioural Sciences." New York: McGraw-Hill, 1956.

Winnicott, D. W. *The Maturational Processes and the Facilitating Environment*. New York: International Universities Press, 1965.

APPENDIX I: Method of Calculating Indices and Test Score

As described in the text, responses are first classified into 14 categories and the categories then grouped into six main classes of response (see Table 20.1). Using the number of responses falling into each class it is then possible to calculate the following eight indices. Finally, positive and negative points can be assigned to scores on each of these indices, and an overall Test Score reached by summing these points.

Index 1: Attachment-Self-Reliance Balance

This index is reached by taking account of each of three comparisons, the results of which are expressed as positive or negative marks. When these marks are summed the total received by each child can be used for assigning him positive or negative points towards his overall Test Score.

For a child to be scored favorably his responses should be as follows:

1. In mild situations more self-reliant responses are expected than attachment responses; therefore, for this comparison two positive marks are awarded for each self-reliant response given to a mild situation and two negative marks to each attachment type response.
2. In severe situations more attachment type responses are expected than self-reliant; therefore, for this comparison the scoring is reversed.
3. In all six situations together more attachment type responses are expected than self-reliant; therefore, for this comparison each attachment type response is awarded one positive mark and each self-reliant response one negative.

In assigning points for calculating a child's overall Test Score the following method is used:

> children with + 6 marks and above receive 2 positive points.
> children with between + 5 and − 1 mark receive 1 positive points
> children with − 2 marks and below receive 1 negative point.

Index 2: Hostility-Attachment Ratio

For a child to be scored favorably the number of attachment type responses is expected to exceed the number of hostile responses. When that is so a child receives one positive point towards his Test Score; otherwise zero.

Index 3: Hostility-Anxiety Ratio

In a similar way, for a child to be scored favorably the number of anxiety responses is expected to exceed the number of hostile responses. When that is so, he receives one positive point towards his Test Score; otherwise zero.

Index 4: Anxiety Ratio

For the sample of children tested, the median percentage of anxiety responses to total responses falls between 20 and 25%. In assigning points towards a child's Test Score, the following formula is used. When anxiety responses as a percentage of total responses are

> over 50% a child receives one negative point.
> between 35 and 50% a child receives one positive point.
> between 10 and 35% a child receives two positive points.
> less than 10% a child receives one negative point.

Index 5: Avoidant Responses

Hansburg has found that avoidant responses are characteristic of severely disturbed children. In the sample tested, it was rare for a child to give more than one such response and none gave more than three. In assigning points the following formula is used. A child who gives

> 2 avoidant responses receives one negative point.
> 3 avoidant responses receives two negative points.

Index 6: Responses Showing Loss of Self-Esteem

Hansburg has found that responses showing loss of self-esteem are characteristic of depressed children and that, if numerous, they indicate suicidal tendencies in early adolescence. In the sample tested nine children gave one such response, three gave two, and one gave three. In assigning points it was decided to give one negative point for each such response.

Index 7: Idiosyncratic Disturbed Responses

Hansburg has found that responses that appear bizarre or absurd or that refer to death are rare but characteristic of severe disturbance. In the present sample they were shown by only 13 children. It was decided to assign one negative point for each such response.

Index 8: Ratio of Appropriate Actions to Those Showing Unrealistic Optimism or Pessimism or Withdrawal

For a child to score favorably it is expected that the number of appropriate actions described in response to the six situations will exceed the sum of all the other types of action. Expressed as a ratio the range runs from 6:0 to 0:6. When the ratio is below unity one negative point is assigned.

APPENDIX II: Terms Used by Hansburg and Equivalent Terms Used Here

Hansburg's term	Our term
intrapunitive	self-reproach
projection	blames others
denial	disbelief
phobic feelings	fear
symbiosis	attachment
individuation	self-reliance
reality avoidance	avoidance
painful tension	anxiety

21

Modification of a Clinical Test for Young Children

In 1980, Lynn M. Varela, a graduate student at the California School of Professional Psychology, revised the Klagsbrun-Bowlby Scale to suit the needs of her study of hospitalized young children and their mothers. Preferring to use drawings rather than photographs, she devised a different scale in which she read all of the thirteen possible responses to the children—a change of procedure from that of Klagsbrun. The system of scoring resembled that of the S.A.T. This revision is discussed and presented in its entirety in the following paper, entitled "Revisions in Responses to Separation from Parents: A Clinical Test for Young Children," by Lynn Millikin Varela.*

The author made a number of changes in the set of pictures used in the pilot study (Klagsbrun and Bowlby, 1976). These modifications are discussed in the following sections:

1. the original set of photographs
2. development of a new set of drawings
3. assessment of content and subsequent changes
4 similarities between the photographs and the drawings
5. modifications in test administration.

---

*This is a complete copy of Appendix C from the unpublished doctoral dissertation entitled *The Relationship between the Hospitalized Child's Separation Anxiety and Maternal Separation Anxiety*, California School of Professional Psychology, Los Angeles, 1982.

THE ORIGINAL SET OF PHOTOGRAPHS

The two sets of six pictures, one set for females and one set for males, which were utilized in the pilot study (Klagsbrun and Bowlby, 1976) were black and white photographs which appeared to be stills from a number of motion pictures. The author felt that the primary strength of the photographs was their realistic quality. However, she felt that the appearance of the individuals pictured, in terms of their mode of dress and hair styles, as well as the settings, lacked a feeling of contemporaneousness. Although the photographs may have accurately reflected life in the United States a number of years ago, they did not mirror life in the early 1980s.

The author felt that the dated quality of the photographs would tend to decrease their usefulness with the children in the present study. The aim was that each child in the study would be able to identify to some degree with the child pictured and attribute to that child his/her own feelings regarding the separation depicted. However, there was concern about the extent to which the children would identify with children whose modes of dress, postures, and hair styles appeared very different from their own. Therefore, the decision was made to develop a new set of pictures for use in the present study.

DEVELOPMENT OF THE NEW SET OF DRAWINGS

The possibility of a new set of photographs, which would resemble the Klagsbrun-Bowlby set, was considered. However, the author felt that the black and white drawings developed by Hansburg for the Separation Anxiety Test had been utilized quite effectively with adolescents and adults (Hansburg, 1972; 1980). Therefore, she decided to work with an artist to develop a set of drawings that could be used with the Klagsbrun-Bowlby scale for young children.

The artist, James Allen, was contacted, and the study was described to him. The author requested that the artist follow three guidelines in the drawings for the study: (1) keep facial expression to a minimum; (2) provide focus upon the separation taking place; and (3) depict the children in the drawings as within the age group of the present study (4- through 7-year-olds).

ASSESSMENT OF THE CONTENT AND SUBSEQUENT CHANGES

Once the decision had been made to substitute a set of drawings for the original photographs, it became clear that there was an opportunity to evaluate the content and captions of the photographs in order to see if improvements could be incorporated in the new drawings. The process of evaluation and the subsequent changes in content are discussed in the following sections: (1) consistency within the test; (2) one picture: a change in content and caption; and (3) replacement of one picture.

Consistency within the test

In three of the original photographs, both parents are involved in separations from their child. However, in three other photographs, the separations involve only one parent. In the three photographs administered to the females in the pilot study, the separation is between mother and daughter. In the corresponding photographs administered to the males, father and son are separating. The author felt that the parent pictured in the one-parent pictures should be the same in the set for females as in the set for males. That is, the attachment figure should be either father *or* mother in all the one-parent pictures. Whether mother or father is depicted should not be varied as a function of the subject's gender. Clearly, it was essential that the identical test be administered to both the females and males in the present study. Otherwise, if results were obtained that indicated significant differences in test response patterns between females and males, there would be a real question as to the degree to which the differences in the test rather than differences in subject attributes contributed to the differences in test results. It was decided that in the three one-parent drawings, the parent depicted would be the mother.

Certainly, research into how young females and males feel about separation from father—when father is the only attachment figure pictured—is warranted. The author hopes that future studies with the scale will address precisely this issue.

One picture: A change in content and caption

Two changes were made in one of the original Klagsbrun and Bowlby photographs. The caption of the photograph is as follows: "Parents are going away for two weeks; prior to their departure they give the child a specially attractive toy: pedal car for boys, party dress for girls" (pages 8 and 9). The author of the present study aimed to have the drawing focus on the child's separation from mother and father rather than on both the separation and the toy the child received prior to the separation. Otherwise, response to separation could be confounded with response to the presentation of the toy. It was decided that in the new drawing the presentation of a gift prior to departure would be eliminated.

An addition was also made to the new drawing. The drawing for the present study depicted the child with his/her aunt, who was going to care for the child in the parents' absence. The new caption is as follows: "The mother and father are going away for two weeks. They are leaving their little girl (boy) with her (his) aunt." In retrospect, the author feels that the addition of the aunt to the drawing may not have been a helpful change. The subject's feelings about his/her own aunt may have colored how he/she responds to the drawing. Thus, a drawing with mother and father leaving their child, with the figure of the aunt excluded, might have been more effective.

Replacement of one picture

The theme of one of the original photographs, considered to be strong in intensity, was eliminated entirely from the set of six pictures. The caption of the photograph is as follows: "Mother (father) goes away for the weekend, leaving little girl (boy) with aunt (uncle)" (pages 8 and 9). Because there already was a picture depicting a two-week separation (a picture considered to be strong in intensity) and also a picture depicting an evening's separation (a mild picture), it was felt that the use of the picture showing a separation for a weekend might not be the most useful. As a replacement, the author decided upon the addition of a picture almost identical to one of the black-and-white drawings in the S.A.T. (Hansburg, 1972, 1980). The picture, strong in intensity, depicted the father leaving after an argument with the mother, and provided a grouping of mother, child, and father that was quite different from the other two-parent pictures which showed both parents as a unit. (In one picture, the parents are leaving together; in the other, the child is leaving both parents.) It was thought that a picture closely resembling the Hansburg drawing would tap the child's response to a stressful separation from father in a situation in which mother and father were not acting as a unit. A picture was drawn by the artist and captioned with the Hansburg title: "After an argument with the mother, the father is leaving."

SIMILARITIES BETWEEN FOUR PHOTOGRAPHS AND THE CORRESPONDING DRAWINGS

In four of the new drawings, the themes and the captions are very similar to those utilized in four of the photographs (Klagsbrun and Bowlby, 1976). The captions of the photographs and the drawings are presented in Table 21.1.

Table 21.1

SIMILARITIES BETWEEN THEMES AND CAPTIONS:
FOUR PHOTOGRAPHS AND THE CORRESPONDING
NEW DRAWINGS

Caption of Photographs	Caption of New Drawing
1. Parents go out for the evening, leaving child at home.	1. The mother and father are going out for the evening, leaving their child at home.
2. Father tucks little girl up in bed and leaves room.	2. The mother has just put her child to bed.
3. Park scene: parents tell child to run off and play by himself for a while, they want some time alone together to talk.	3. The mother and father are telling their little girl to run off and play by herself for a while. They want some time alone together to talk.
4. Child's first day at school; moment of parting from parent.	4. The child is leaving her mother to go to school. It is her first day of school.

MODIFICATION IN TEST ADMINISTRATION

Test administration in the pilot study

In the Klagsbrun and Bowlby study, each child was shown the pictures, one by one, and was told what was happening. The child was then asked, "How does the little boy/girl in the picture feel?" The authors state:

If he has difficulty in responding, a list of possible responses (based on those presented by Hansburg to his subjects, and ordered randomly) is read to him. It is emphasized that he does not have to choose any of them, that they are merely suggestions as to how he might put his feelings into words.

The list of 13 possible responses used in the pilot study is as follows:

Does the little boy feel lonely—or does he feel sad—or does he feel angry—or does he feel that his parents don't love him anymore—or that it's *not* really happening—or does he feel like hiding away—or does he feel like he just doesn't care—or does he feel that if he'd been a good boy it wouldn't have happened—or that it's someone else's fault—or that something bad is going to happen—or does he feel now he's going to have a good time—or that he's hungry—or getting a tummy ache or a headache.

The authors state: "It was rarely necessary to go through the whole list in this manner. Most children would interrupt when one of the responses seemed suitable to them."

Klagsbrun and Bowlby include a selection of children's responses to the first two cards. A number of the responses seemed to indicate that if the child responded spontaneously to the examiner's initial question ("How does the little boy/girl in the picture feel?"), the examiner did not begin reading the list of thirteen possible responses to the child. Two of the children's responses to card 1 (parents going out for the evening) are as follows:

Not very well. (Not very well?) She's got a cold and she's got a headache. (What does she do?) Go to sleep.

Very well. She feels happy. My friend looks after me when mummy and daddy go out. (Do?) She's going to stay in bed.

Other children's responses, however, seem to indicate that if the examiner considered the child's response too brief, the examiner began to read the list of possible responses. Examples of children's responses which illustrate this approach are as follows:

Tired. (Does she feel any of these . . . ?) She's lonely. (Do?) Go to bed and go to sleep.

All right. (Any of these . . . ?) She feels like hiding away, because she doesn't want to see her mummy and daddy in the morning. (Why?) I don't know. (Do?) Hide.

In conclusion, it appeared to the author that whether or not the examiner began to read the list of responses to the child was contingent upon the completeness of the child's response to the first question. In addition, it appeared that if the list was begun, how soon the list was terminated was dependent upon how soon the child selected a response.

Test administration in the present study

In the author's view, use of the test administration method of the pilot study in the present study presented two problems. First, if the child selected one of the response possibilities presented early in the list, and the reading of the list was terminated at that time, the child would not be selecting from the total group of possible responses. Secondly, depending on at what point each child selected a response from the list, the total number of possible responses read by the examiner would vary from child to child. Thus, an alternative administration procedure was sought.

The approach utilized in the administration of Hansburg's S.A.T. was considered. As discussed previously, for each of the twelve S.A.T. pictures, there is a set of seventeen responses describing how the child in the picture feels (e.g., "The child feels very angry at somebody."). The subject is asked to select as many of the seventeen statements as desired. Similarly, there is a set of thirteen responses describing how the child in the picture feels in the Klagsbrun and Bowlby scale. It was decided that this approach would be used in the present study and that the children would be asked to select as many of the thirteen statements as desired (see the complete procedure for test administration on pages 352–363).

Prior to beginning the study, the author's only hesitation in using this approach was that it might make the test too long an undertaking for the 4-year-olds in the study, as well as the 5- and 6-year olds who had quite short atttention spans. In practice, however, the technique worked quite well when in the hands of an experienced examiner.

An important oversight occurred in the present study that can be easily avoided in future studies utilizing the scale. The list of thirteen possible responses used in the pilot study and in the present study as well does not include a response relating to fear (see page 353). However, Klagsbrun and Bowlby do include fear as a Category of Response. The problem can be easily remedied by the addition of a question relating to fear ("Does the little boy/girl feel afraid?") to the present thirteen possible responses.

[Only the girl's scale is provided in the following. A boy's scale, of course, is also available—H.G.H.]

Table 21.2

CLASS OF RESPONSE SUMMARY CHART

Response	Number of Responses			Percent of Total Protocol
	Mild (1, 2, 6)	Strong (3, 4, 5)	Total	
1. Attachment (Sum of loneliness, sadness, rejection, hunger)				
2. Self-Reliant (Well-being)				
3. Hostile (Sum of anger, blames others, self-reproach)				
4. Anxious (Sum of generalized dread/anxiety, fear, somatic reaction, hunger)				
5. Avoidant (Sum of withdrawal, evasion, disbelief)				
6. Loss of Self-Esteem (Sum of rejection and self-reproach)				

What would you do?   Appropriate Activity
                      Unrealistic Optimism
                      Unrealistic Pessimism
                      Withdrawal or Inaction

Mild		
1	2	6

Strong		
3	4	5

Picture 1

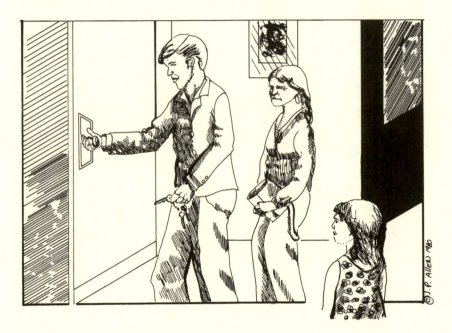

Figure 21.1. The mother and father are going out for the evening, leaving their child at home.

A. Show the picture and read the caption:

"The mother and father are going out for the evening, leaving their child at home with the babysitter."

B. Ask, "How does the girl in the picture feel?"

C. Does the girl feel any of these?

1. Does the girl feel lonely?

2. Does she feel sad?

3. Does she feel angry?

4. Does the girl feel that her parents don't love her anymore?

5. Does she feel that it's not really happening?

6. Does she feel like hiding away?

7. Does the girl feel like she just doesn't care?

8. Does she feel that if she'd been a good girl it wouldn't have happened?

9. Does she feel that it's someone else's fault?

10. Does the girl feel that something bad is going to happen?

11. Does she feel that now she's going to have a good time?

12. Does she feel that she's hungry?

13. Does the girl feel that she's getting a tummy ache or a headache?

D. Ask, "What does the girl do?"

Picture 2

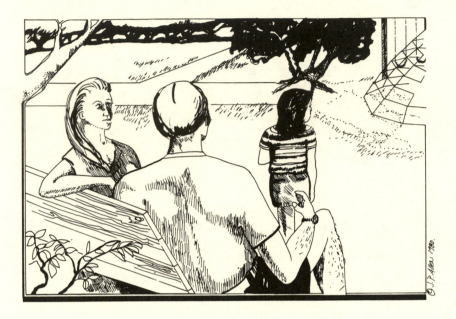

Figure 21.2. The mother and father are telling their little girl to run off and play by herself for a while. They want some time alone together to talk.

A. Show the picture and read the caption:

   "The mother and father are telling their girl to run off and play by herself for a while. They want some time alone together to talk."

B. Ask, "How does the girl in the picture feel?"

C. Ask, "Does the girl feel any of these?"

   1. Does the girl feel that she's getting a tummy ache or a headache?

   2. Does she feel that she's hungry?

   3. Does she feel that now she's going to have a good time?

   4. Does the girl feel that something bad is going to happen?

   5. Does she feel that it's someone else's fault?

   6. Does she feel that if she'd been a good girl it wouldn't have happened?

   7. Does the girl feel like she just doesn't care?

   8. Does she feel like hiding away?

   9. Does she feel that it's not really happening?

   10. Does the girl feel that her parents don't love her anymore?

   11. Does she feel angry?

   12. Does she feel sad?

   13. Does the girl feel lonely?

D. Ask, "What does the girl do?"

Picture 3

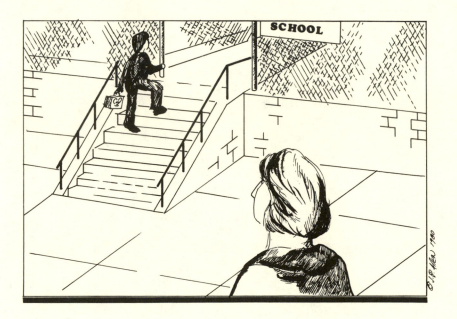

Figure 21.3. The child is leaving her mother to go to school. It is her first day of school.

A. Show the picture and read the caption:

"The child is leaving her mother to go to school. It is her first day of school."

B. Ask, "How does the girl in the picture feel?"

C. Ask, "Does the girl feel any of these?"

1. Does the girl feel like hiding away?

2. Does she feel that her parents don't love her anymore?

3. Does she feel sad?

4. Does the girl feel that it's not really happening?

5. Does she feel angry?

6. Does she feel lonely?

7. Does the girl feel that if she'd been a good girl it wouldn't have happened?

8. Does she feel that she's getting a tummy ache or a headache?

9. Does she feel that something bad is going to happen?

10. Does the girl feel that she's hungry?

11. Does she feel that it's someone else's fault?

12. Does she feel that now she's going to have a good time?

13. Does the girl feel like she just doesn't care?

D. Ask, "What does the girl do?"

Picture 4

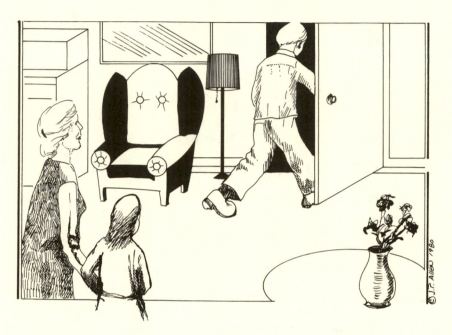

Figure 21.4. After an argument with the mother, the father is leaving.

A. Show the picture and read the caption:

"After an argument with the mother, the father is leaving."

B. Ask, "How does the girl in the picture feel?"

C. Ask, "Does the girl feel any of these?"

  1. Does she feel that something bad is going to happen?

  2. Does she feel that if she'd been a good girl it wouldn't have happened?

  3. Does she feel that she's hungry?

  4. Does the girl feel angry?

  5. Does she feel like hiding away?

  6. Does she feel sad?

  7. Does the girl feel that now she's going to have a good time?

  8. Does she feel that her parents don't love her anymore?

  9. Does she feel that she's getting a tummy ache or a headache?

  10. Does the girl feel lonely?

  11. Does she feel that it's not really happening?

  12. Does she feel that it's someone else's fault?

  13. Does the girl feel like she just doesn't care?

D. Ask, "What does the girl do?"

Picture 5

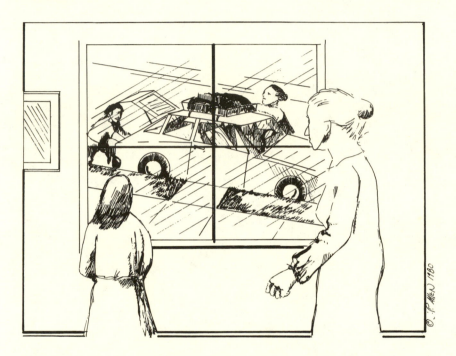

Figure 21.5. The mother and father are going away for two weeks. They are leaving their little girl with her aunt.

A. Show the picture and read the caption:

"The mother and father are going away for two weeks. They are leaving their girl with her aunt."

B. Ask, "How does the girl in the picture feel?"

C. "Does the girl feel any of these?"

    1. Does she feel that now she's going to have a good time?

    2. Does she feel that it's not really happening?

    3. Does the girl feel that it's someone else's fault?

    4. Does she feel sad?

    5. Does she feel that she's getting a tummy ache or a headache?

    6. Does the girl feel that she's hungry?

    7. Does she feel lonely?

    8. Does she feel that something bad is going to happen?

    9 Does the girl feel angry?

    10. Does she feel that if she'd been a good girl it wouldn't have happened?

    11. Does she feel like hiding away?

    12. Does the girl feel that her parents don't love her anymore?

    13. Does she feel like she just doesn't care?

D. Ask, "What does the girl do?"

Picture 6

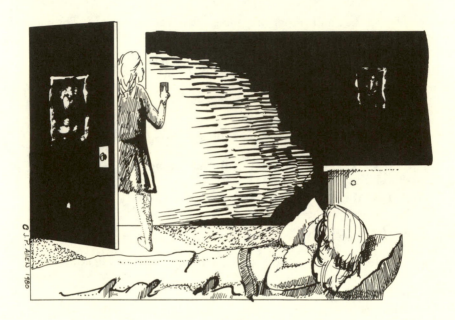

Figure 21.6. The mother has just put her child to bed.

A. Show the picture and read the caption:

"The mother has just put her child to bed."

B. Ask, "How does the girl in the picture feel?"

C. "Does the girl feel any of these?"

    1. Does she feel that it's not really happening?

    2. Does she feel like she just doesn't care?

    3. Does the girl feel sad?

    4. Does she feel that it's someone else's fault?

    5. Does she feel lonely?

    6. Does the girl feel that if she'd been a good girl it wouldn't have happened?

    7. Does she feel angry?

    8. Does she feel that now she's going to have a good time?

    9. Does the girl feel that her parents don't love her anymore?

    10. Does she feel that she's getting a tummy ache or a headache?

    11. Does she feel like hiding away?

    12. Does the girl feel that she's hungry?

    13. Does she feel that something bad is going to happen?

D. Ask, "What does the girl do?"

Table 21.3

CATEGORY OF RESPONSE CHART

	Totals			Mild Separation Intensity			Strong Separation Intensity		
	Mild	Strong	Total	1	2	6	3	4	5
1. Attachment									
Loneliness				1	13	5	6	10	7
Sadness				2	12	3	3	6	4
Rejection				4	10	9	2	8	12
Hunger				12	2	12	10	3	6
2. Self-reliant									
Well-being				11	3	8	12	7	1
3. Hostile									
Anger				3	11	7	5	4	9
Blames others				9	5	4	11	12	3
Self-reproach				8	6	6	7	2	10
4. Anxious									
Generalized dread/ anxiety				10	4	13	9	1	8
Somatic Reaction				13	1	10	8	9	5
Hunger #				12 #	2 #	12 #	10 #	3 #	6 #
5. Avoidant									
Withdrawal				6	8	11	1	5	11
Evasion				7	7	2	13	13	13
Disbelief				5	9	1	4	11	2
6. Loss of self-esteem									
Rejection #				4 #	10 #	9 #	2 #	8 #	12 #
Self-reproach #				8 #	6 #	6 #	7 #	2 #	10 #
Total Responses									

\# Repeated measure—do not include in total response.

The numbers immediately under Mild and Strong Separation Intensity refer to the picture numbers in the test.

22

Tests for Third-Grade Children
and Learning-Disabled Children

Another revision was that developed by Nancy Brody for a study of third-grade children of divorced parents in the Catholic Elementary Schools of Phoenix, Arizona (see Chapter 5). While she used the S.A.T. pictures, she tape-recorded the seventeen statements following each picture, enabling these 8-year-olds to hear the statements while they were reading them silently. The tapes were used because the level of reading of these children was below that required to read and comprehend the statements. A discussion of this method is presented here.

Furthermore, Christine Duplak, a former psychologist in the psychiatric clinic of the JCCA and a former assistant of mine in the original work on the S.A.T. (see acknowledgments in Adolescent Separation Anxiety, *Vol. 1, p. xii), in a study of learning-disabled children at New York University in 1982, revised the method of response. Instead of providing individual phrases for each picture, she substituted cartoon heads with varied facial expressions, which the children were asked to select. After a pilot study using this method to demonstrate that the pictures were indeed a good measure of separation anxiety, she then used the test pictures without the phrases to study the reactions of latency-age children to separation situations (see Chapter 9). A presentation of her method, and that of Brody, appears below.*

Dr. Brody tape-recorded the seventeen statements following each picture, enabling the child to hear the statements while he or she was reading them silently. The tapes were made in order to lessen the effects of the child's reading ability on the test results. Each child was told to select as many of the seventeen statements as he or she believed represented how the child in the picture felt. The child indicated his or her choice of a statement as soon as it was heard by saying "yes," "that one," or the number of the statement. When all seventeen statements had been read, the child was asked if he or she had anything to add about how the child in the picture felt. The child's responses were recorded on a recording chart.

Before giving this test to the children in the sample, Brody practiced its administration with two other third-grade classes. At that time it was learned that some children needed help understanding the vocabulary of the test. The tape recorder was easily stopped, in order to explain those words that needed explanation. Two words, *institution* and *suicide* were routinely defined for all the children. Others needed help with such words as *permanently*, *transferred*, and *coffin*.

A much more radical adaptation of the Separation Anxiety Test was developed by Dr. Christine Duplak. The technique was adopted in the course of determining whether or not the twelve pictures of the test actually aroused separation anxiety with particular reference to children with learning disability.

The twelve separation pictures were prepared as slides and the following group procedure was performed by the examiner:

Now we are going to do something a little bit different. Do you all know what slides are? (If not, explain that they are pictures that we can project—put—onto the wall with a machine.) I'm sure you've all seen these before. We are going to show you some slides of children in different places, doing different things. At the same time that I show you the slide up on that screen, I will tell you what is supposed to be happening in the picture. Now I am going to give you each a piece of paper. Look at it carefully and you will see that it has twelve numbers down this side (illustrate). Does everybody see them? Next to each number, there are four faces and under each face it tells with a word how the face looks (illustrate). Can you all read the words under the pictures and see that the word matches how the face looks? Okay, now as you look at each slide, I will call out the number of the picture that we are looking at and you put your finger on that number as I am telling you what is happening in the slide. When I am finished talking, I want you to put a big X over the face that shows what you think the boy in the picture is feeling. Run your finger across the line like this until you come to the face that you want to mark with an X. For example, (holding up a large copy of the answer sheet) after I show you slide Number 1, I want you to think about whether the child in the slide feels happy, sad, etc. If you think he feels happy, put an X over the face like this. If you think he feels sad, put an X over this face. Okay, any questions? Now I will show you the slides one by one. I will go slowly and tell you what is happening in the slide and call out each number so that you can put an X over one of the faces in that line. Mark only one face in each line. If you have any questions, stop me as we go along. Okay, let's see the first slide. This is Number 1, put your finger on line one. Now listen. Here is a slide showing a boy who will live permanently with his grandparents and without his parents.

If a child aks why, he is told that the reason is not important and that he is to make his decision of how the boy feels based only on the fact that the boy will be living without his parents. The investigators monitored the children to see that they understood the task and that they were marking the answer sheets correctly (Duplak 1982, pp. 69–71).

Some of the captions on the pictures were changed in order to accommodate to the specific situation of the experiment. Following are the changed captions as they appear in Duplak's study.

1. The child will live permanently with the grandmother and without his parents.
2. A child is being transferred to a new class.
3. The family is moving to a new neighborhood.
4. The child is leaving the mother to go to school.
5. The child is leaving the parents to go to camp.
6. After an argument with the mother the father is leaving.
7. The child's older brother is a sailor leaving on a trip.
8. The judge is telling the child he/she has to live away from his parents for a long time.
9. The mother has just put this child to bed.
10. The child's mother is being taken to hospital.
11. The child and the father are at a funeral.
12. The child is running away from home.

The answer sheet used for this separation arousal method is shown below. These forms were used in the pilot study for Duplak's dissertation, but were not considered as data for her report since there were measures of attachment that she utilized for her results (see Chapter 9).

The subjects were ages 10 to 13. An instrument consisting of 30 cartoons portraying two interpersonal styles was used to determine attachment style. Each of these 30 cartoons illustrates either a movement away from or a movement toward a figure. The movement away is referred to by Duplak as "detachment" and the movement toward as "attachment." The test was given without stimuli two weeks prior and then repeated two weeks later immediately after being shown the S.A.T. pictures. The cartoons follow.

ATTACHMENT PATTERN SORT

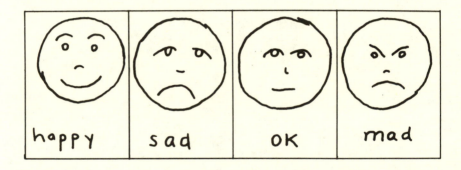

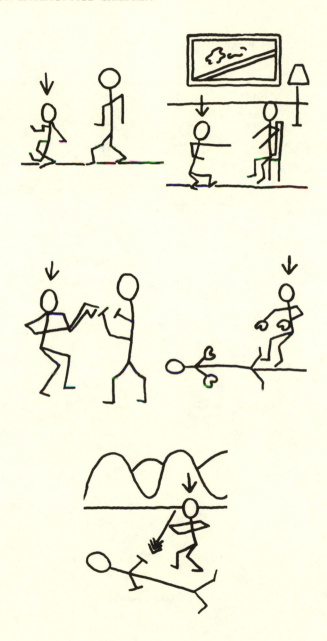

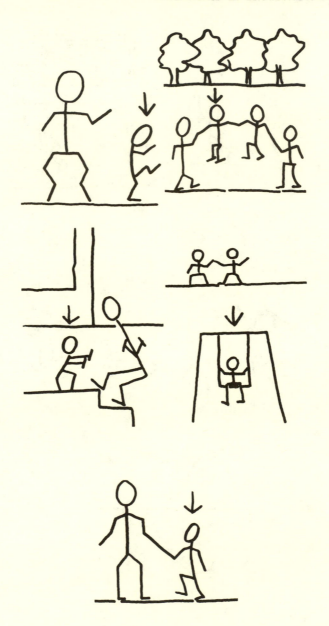

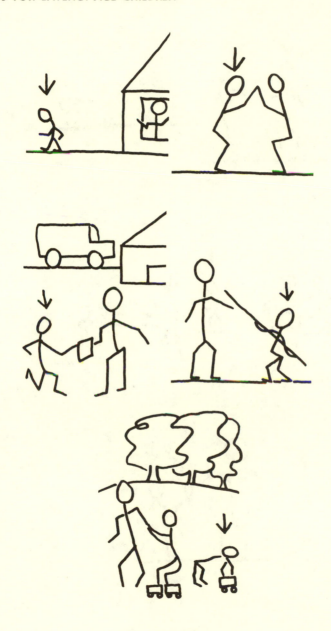

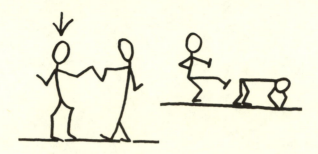

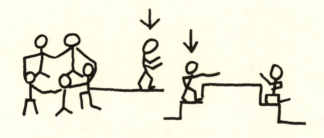

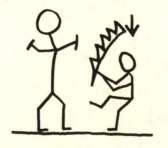

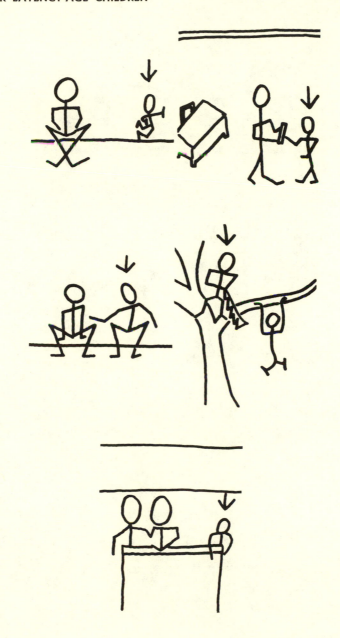

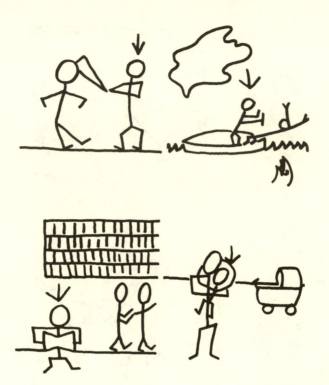

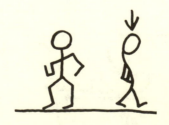

23

A Test for Young Divorced Males

In regard to the use of the S.A.T. with adults, it was obviously found necessary to revise the instructions. This revision may be found in the test itself as published by R. E. Krieger in 1980. However, it has also long been obvious that the test could readily be adapted to a group method of administration with older adolescents and adults, and this has been done by a number of investigators, including Michael Slutsky at the California School of Professional Psychology in San Diego and Rick Schiller at Case Western Reserve University. I have been informed by these researchers that it was accomplished with minimal difficulty and that the results seemed quite comparable to those obtained in individual administration.

Other researchers suggested that it would be worthwhile to revise the pictures for adults so that the situations would be more comparable to adult life. The only such attempt known to me was that of Donald Burger, presented in 1981 at the San Diego branch of the California School of Professional Psychology. In this study Burger was concerned with understanding the reactions of young male divorcees. The twelve pictures of the S.A.T. were redrawn to show the adult divorced males experiencing separation. The response phrases were adapted for these situations and were made similar to those of the original test. This test is presented in this section, while the original study is summarized in Chapter 6.

In the revised pictures, the central figure is a young adult male who has been divorced. It may be noted that the mental set questions with regard to whether or not the event had ever occurred in the man's life have been omitted. The reason for this was not explained by Burger. However, all other instructions were similar to those used with adolescents. Phrases were neces-

sarily altered to accommodate to the alteration in the age level and the some-
what varied situations in the pictures.

The following material is an excerpt from the original dissertation (see
Chapter 6).

Hansburg (1972) made specific assumptions when he developed the
Separation Anxiety Test that were also used in extrapolating this test
for use with adults. These were as follows: that pictures of separation
experiences will stimulate adults sufficiently to be able to project their
reactions; that they can select and report reactions which reflect how
they feel; that these reactions will show patterns; and that the test will
reveal cognitive and affective responses to separation anxiety.

This test consists of twelve pictures, each depicting a separation
situation for an adult male. The situations in this test were designed to
duplicate as closely as possible the ones used by Hansburg in his test.
They vary from low-stress adult experiences with separation to
traumatic experiences. The selection of the situations was achieved
through discussion with a professional committee (psychologists). The
following situations were agreed upon:

1. The man's divorce is final and he is going back to live
    with his parents.
2. The man is being transferred to a new department and
    has a new boss.
3. The man and his family are moving to a new neigh-
    borhood.
4. The man is leaving his wife to go to work.
5. The man is leaving his wife to go to a convention.
6. After an argument between the husband and wife, the
    wife is leaving.
7. The man's best friend's wife has died and he is leaving
    on a voyage.
8. The officer is sending the man overseas without his
    wife.
9. The man's wife is going to visit her parents and the
    man is going to bed alone.
10. The man's wife is sick and is being taken to the
    hospital.
11. The man is standing at his wife's coffin.
12. The man is secretly leaving his wife.

In keeping with Hansburg's test, an effort was made to avoid facial expression in drawing the figures; colors of the spectrum were avoided in order to remove the influence color exercises on affect; the drawings were done in black ink with white backgrounds. Shading followed the scheme used by Hansburg; that is, the more stimulating the picture, the heavier the shading.

In accordance with Hansburg's description, the drawings were made so that the figure with which the subject could identify would be in the foreground of the picture. The pictures were of the same size in order to avoid problems in perception, corresponding to the size of the Murray Thematic Apperception Test. There were captions at the bottom of the drawings defining the twelve separation situations. The deliberate effort to focus on the separation situation made misinterpretation by the subject practically impossible.

The order of presentation of the pictures corresponds to that of Hansburg, which was decided by considering the intensity of the stimulation. The pictures are mixed so that the influence of the effect of one picture on another is reduced, with the exception that four of the least stimulating pictures appear near the beginning and three of the most stimulating appear at the end.

The construction of the S.A.T. was based on the assumption that the selection of specific responses on the pictures represents a tendency to respond with particular cognitive and affective patterns. This reflects the dominant modes or patterns of cognitive and affective responses in adult males. The following cognitive and affective response patterns are dominant in separation literature and were used: separation denial, attachment need, separation hostility, separation pain, separation identity stress, self-love loss, individuation, and self-esteem preoccupation.

Descriptive phrases were patterned after Hansburg and constructed by the author. . . . To portray the cognitive and affective responses that make up the above-mentioned patterns, subjects chose from these appropriate phrases to complete the stem sentences. For example, "The man feels . . . (that he will be much happier now, that his wife doesn't love him anymore, a terrible pain in his chest, etc.)." The phrases were presented in varying order from picture to picture.

The patterns were comprised of phrases describing the following cognitive and affective responses:

Patterns	Responses
Separation denial	Evasive denial
	Withdrawal
	Fantasy denial
Attachment need	Grief or loneliness
	Empathy
	Rejection
Separation hostility	Anger
	Projection
	Intrapunitiveness
Separation pain	Phobic reactions
	Generalized anxiety
	Somatization
Separation identity stress	Identity Stress
Self-love loss	Rejection
	Intrapunitiveness
Individuation	Well-being
	Adaptive reaction
	Sublimation
Self-esteem preoccupation	Concentration
	Sublimation

A chart was used for both recording and scoring the responses. To facilitate recording, a number for each phrase of each picture was utilized. During the testing the subject circled the numbers of the phrases he selected. The test was administered individually.

Quantitative scores on the test consisted of the number of responses for each of the seventeen items; the total number of responses for all twelve pictures; the total number of responses for each of the eight patterns.

The validity of the instrument was tested by submitting it to three clinical psychologists, all of whom had an educational background and interest in projective instruments. The three psychologists were given the seventeen response items and asked to match them with the 204 possible responses to the pictures. Two out of the three psychologists agreed upon the categories that each phrase represented. Reliability was assessed by the split-half method. Coefficients of reliability for each of the seventeen response categories varied because of intentional card pull. The reliability coefficients are reported in the following table; as can be seen, they were comparable to those reported by Hansburg (1972).

The revision of the test itself follows.

Table 23.1

SPLIT-HALF RELIABILITY COEFFICIENTS FOR EACH OF THE
SEVENTEEN RESPONSE CATEGORIES

Response Category	Correlations	
	Burger	Hansburg
Rejection	.58	.57
Impaired Concentration	.71	.68
Phobic Reaction	.62	.63
Generalized anxiety	.67	.64
Loneliness	.72	.57
Withdrawal	.60	.64
Somatization	.79	.74
Adaptive reaction	.71	—
Anger	.47	.41
Projection	.49	.34
Empathy	.57	.59
Evasive denial	.71	.63
Fantasy denial	.69	.55
Well-being	.54	.50
Sublimation	.60	.48
Intrapunitiveness	.51	.50
Identity stress	.68	—

Note: Responses to pictures 1, 3, 5, 7, 9, and 11 were correlated with responses to pictures 2, 4, 6, 8, 10, and 12.

Picture 1

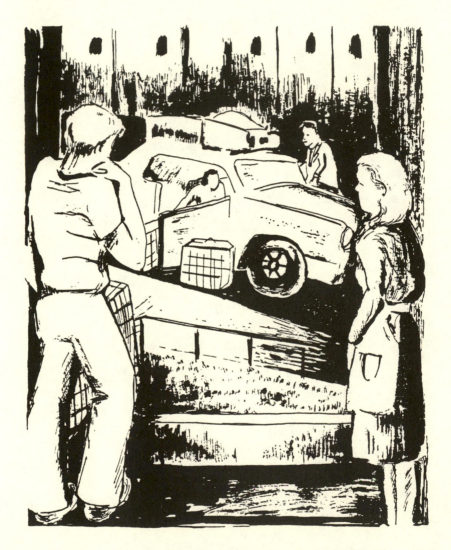

Figure 23.1. The man's divorce is final and he is going back to live with his parents.

Check as many of the statements below which you think would tell how this man feels.

The man feels:

1. that he will be much happier now.

2. that his wife doesn't love him anymore.

3. like curling up in a corner by himself.

4. a terrible pain in his chest.

5. alone and miserable.

6. that he doesn't care what happens.

7. that he will do his best to get along.

8. that his parents' house will be a frightening place to live in.

9. that something bad is going to happen to him now.

10. that it's all the fault of their neighbors.

11. angry at somebody.

12. that he won't be the same person anymore.

13. that if he had been a good husband, this wouldn't have happened.

14. that it's only a dream—it isn't really happening.

15. like reading a book, watching TV, or playing games.

16. sorry for his wife.

17. that he won't be able to concentrate on his job anymore.

Picture 2

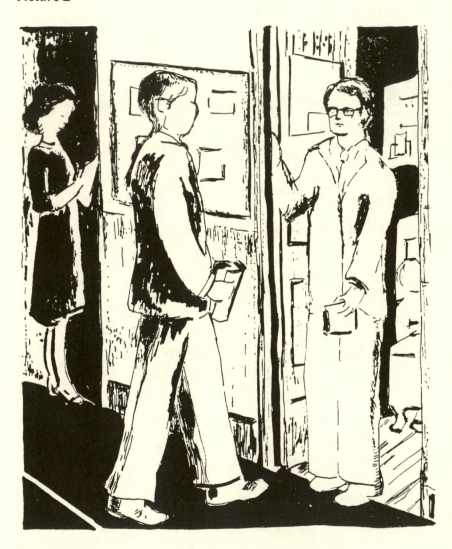

Figure 23.2. The man is being transferred to a new department and has a new boss.

Check as many of the statements below which you think would tell how this man feels.

The man feels:

1. that he doesn't care what happens.

2. that the new department is a frightening place to be.

3. sorry for his past boss.

4. that if he had been a good worker, this wouldn't have happened.

5. like playing cards with his friends.

6. that something is happening to change him.

7. that he will make the best of the situation.

8. that nobody really likes him.

9. that now he is going to have a good time.

10. that it's not really happening—it's only a dream.

11. that he won't be able to concentrate on his job.

12. like sitting alone in the corner of the room.

13. very angry at somebody.

14. like he's getting a stomachache.

15. alone and miserable.

16. that something terrible is going to happen.

17. that somebody who wishes him harm is responsible for doing this to him.

Picture 3

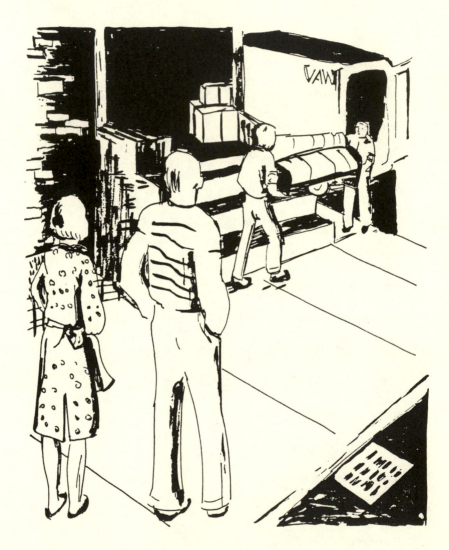

Figure 23.3. The man and his family are moving to a new neighborhood.

Check as many of the statements below which you think would tell how this man feels.

The man feels:

1. afraid to leave.

2. a pain in his stomach.

3. that the neighbors made them move.

4. glad to get away from this bad neighborhood.

5. alone and miserable.

6. that he doesn't care what happens.

7. that it's only a dream.

8. like hiding somewhere.

9. that the new house will be a frightening place to live in.

10. that now he will be a different person.

11. that he won't be able to concentrate on his job.

12. sorry for his family.

13. that he will make the best of the situation.

14. like punching somebody in the face.

15. that nobody likes him anymore.

16. that now he can make some new friends.

17. that if he had been a better neighbor, he wouldn't have had to move.

Picture 4

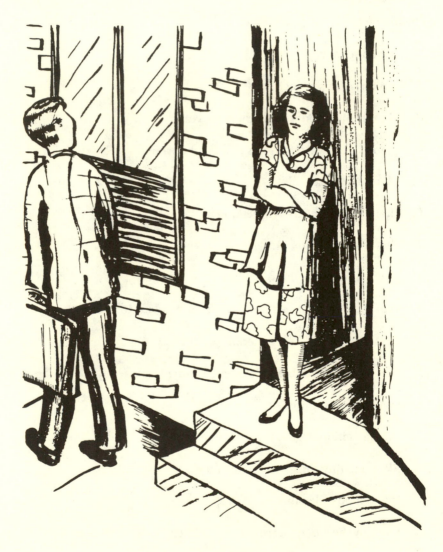

Figure 23.4. The man is leaving his wife to go to work.

Check as many of the statements below which you think would tell how this man feels.

The man feels:

1. that he won't be able to concentrate on his job.

2. afraid to leave.

3. that work is a frightening and unpleasant place to be.

4. that his wife doesn't care about him.

5. that he doesn't care what happens.

6. angry at having to go to work.

7. like joining his friends and going to work.

8. glad to get away from the house.

9. sorry for his wife.

10. like he's going to be sick.

11. that something is happening to change him.

12. that if he had been a better husband, his wife would let him stay home.

13. like staying home in bed.

14. that he will do his best to get along.

15. that it's not really happening—it's only a dream.

16. alone and miserable.

17. that somebody else is causing all this trouble.

Picture 5

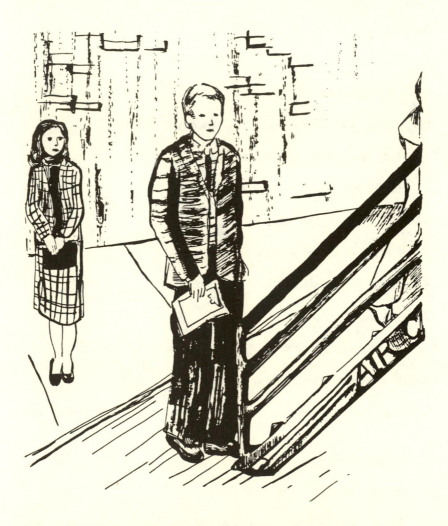

Figure 23.5. The man is leaving his wife to go to a convention.

Check as many of the statements below which you think would tell how this man feels.

The man feels:

1.   sorry for his wife.

2.   angry about going.

3.   that this is a threatening place to be.

4.   that now he will be a different person.

5.   that it's not really happening—it's only a dream.

6.   that his mind can't think straight.

7.   like sitting alone in the back of the plane.

8.   that someone else made this happen to him.

9.   like reading a book and playing cards.

10. that he doesn't care what happens.

11. that something terrible is going to happen to him.

12. that a bad headache is coming on.

13. that nobody really loves him.

14. that he will make the best of the situation.

15. that if he had been a better husband, his wife wouldn't let him go.

16. that now he is really free to enjoy himself.

17. alone and miserable.

Picture 6

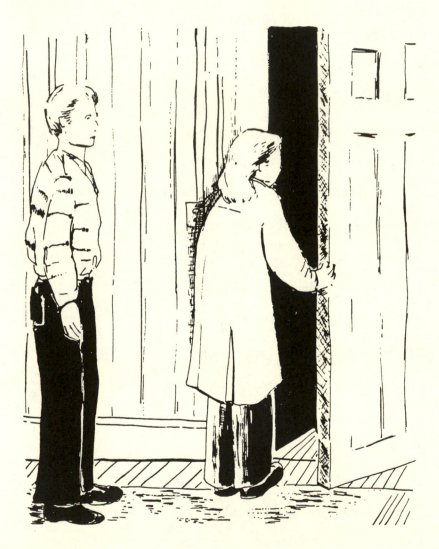

Figure 23.6. After an argument between the husband and wife, the wife is
leaving.

Check as many of the statements below which you think would tell how this man feels.

The man feels:

1. very angry at the wife.

2. that now he is free to do anything he wants to.

3. that his home will now be a scary place.

4. that he won't be able to concentrate on his job.

5. that something terrible is going to happen to him now.

6. that someone else has been causing all of this trouble.

7. like reading a book, fixing something, or watching TV.

8. that something is happening to change him.

9. lonely and unhappy.

10. that nobody really likes him.

11. that he is going to be very sick.

12. like being alone in their bedroom.

13. sorry for his wife.

14. that he doesn't care what happens.

15. that he will try hard to work things out.

16. that he himself caused her to leave.

17. that it's only a dream—it really isn't happening.

Picture 7

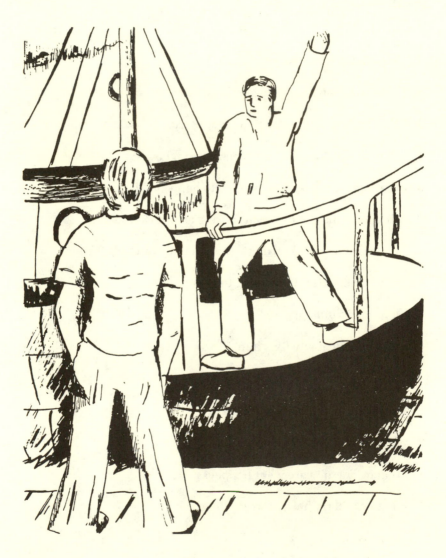

Figure 23.7. The man's best friend's wife has died and he is leaving on a voyage.

Check as many of the statements below which you think would tell how this man feels.

The man feels:

1. sorry for his best friend.

2. that if he had been a better pal, his friend would not have to leave.

3. that it's not really happening—it's only a dream.

4. that this is a very scary thing.

5. very angry.

6. lonely and miserable.

7. that he will not be the same person anymore.

8. like being alone at home.

9. that someone else caused all this trouble.

10. like playing cards with another friend.

11. that he won't be able to concentrate on his job.

12. that he will try hard to work things out.

13. that something terrible is going to happen to him.

14. that nobody really likes him.

15. that a bad stomachache is coming on.

16. that he doesn't care what happens.

17. that now he is free to enjoy himself in any way he likes.

Picture 8

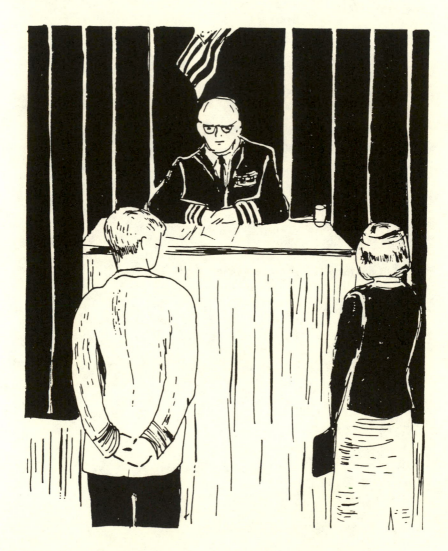

Figure 23.8. The officer is sending the man overseas without his wife.

Check as many of the statements below which you think would tell how this man feels.

The man feels:

1. that the world is full of corrupt people who did this to him.

2. that it's only a dream and he will wake up soon.

3. like committing suicide.

4. that he will go and make the best of it.

5. sorry for his wife.

6. that this is a frightening place.

7. like curling up in a corner.

8. dizzy and faint.

9. that he doesn't care what happens.

10. happy to get overseas as soon as possible.

11. that he is not very well liked.

12. terrified at what will happen to him.

13. like reading a book or watching TV.

14. angry at the officer.

15. that now he won't be able to concentrate.

16. all alone and unhappy.

17. that now he will be a different person.

Picture 9

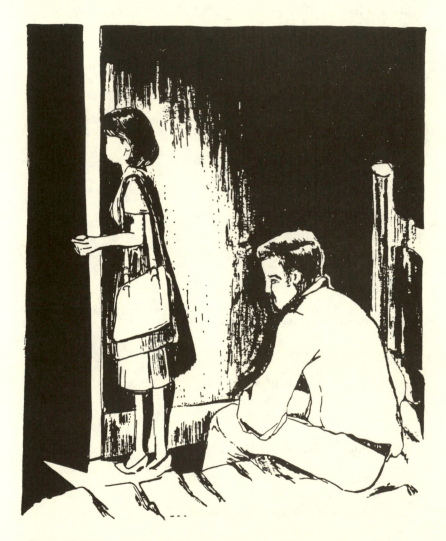

Figure 23.9. The man's wife is going to visit her parents and the man is going to bed alone.

Check as many of the statements below which you think would tell how this man feels.

The man feels:

1. angry at his wife.

2. that it's frightening to be alone here.

3. like pulling the covers over his head.

4. like he doesn't care what happens.

5. that something is happening to change him.

6. that someone else made the wife leave.

7. that now he's free to enjoy himself any way he likes.

8. that his wife doesn't stay with him because he's a bad husband.

9. it's not really happening—it's only a dream.

10. that he will make the best of the situation.

11. like reading a book or watching TV.

12. that something bad is going to happen to him.

13. sorry for his wife.

14. that he is getting sick.

15. that his wife doesn't really care about him.

16. that he won't be able to concentrate at work tomorrow.

17. very lonely.

Picture 10

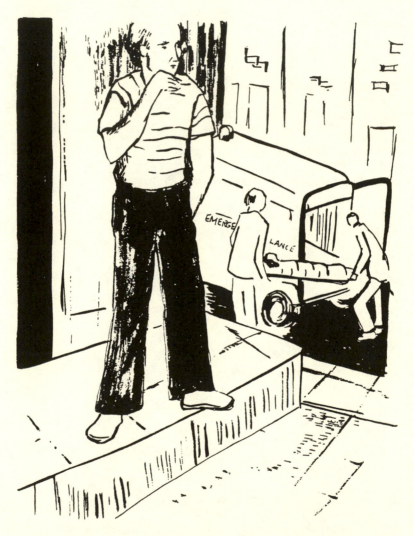

Figure 23.10. The man's wife is sick and is being taken to the hospital.

Check as many of the statements below which you think would tell how this man feels.

The man feels:

1. very angry at somebody.

2. that he will not be the same person anymore.

3. glad that his wife is leaving.

4. like being alone at home.

5. that he doesn't care what happens.

6. that it's not really happening—it's only a dream.

7. that he's going to have a bad headache.

8. that he will do his best to get along.

9. scared about what is going to happen to him.

10. sorry for his wife.

11. that nobody likes him anymore.

12. like watching TV.

13. that his wife became sick because of what he had done.

14. that somebody else caused all this trouble.

15. that this home is going to be a scary place to stay in now.

16. alone and miserable.

17. that he won't be able to concentrate on his job.

Picture 11

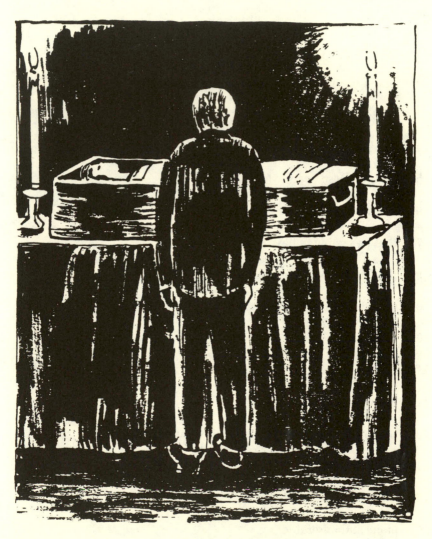

Figure 23.11. The man is standing at his wife's coffin.

Check as many of the statements below which you think would tell how this man feels.

The man feels:

1. that he won't be the same person anymore.

2. frightened about what will happen to him.

3. that if he had been a good husband, it wouldn't have happened.

4. that now he is free to do what he wants.

5. angry about what happened.

6. that nobody will love him anymore.

7. that he doesn't care what happens.

8. that his home will now be a scary place to live in.

9. like sitting in a corner by himself.

10. that other people are to blame for this.

11. that he will make the best of the situation.

12. that it is only a dream.

13. a bad pain in his head.

14. sorry for his wife's mother and father.

15. alone and miserable.

16. that now he won't be able to concentrate on work anymore.

17. like reading a book or watching TV.

Picture 12

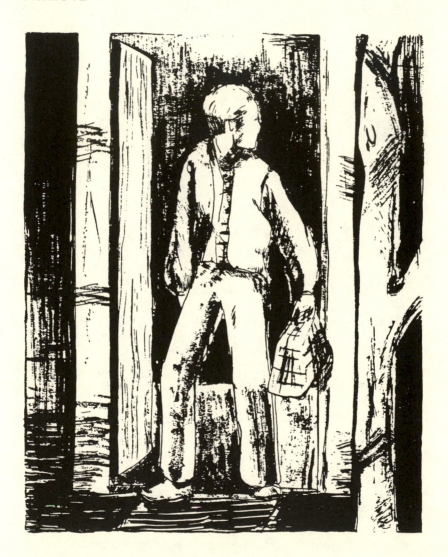

Figure 23.12. The man is secretly leaving his wife.

Check as many of the statements below which you think would tell how this man feels.

The man feels:

1.   that he is just going away to have some fun.

2.   angry at his wife.

3.   afraid that his wife will be angry for something he did.

4.   that he doesn't care what happens.

5.   that his wife doesn't want him around anymore.

6.   that the neighbors have been stirring up his wife against him.

7.   terrible stomach cramps coming on.

8.   that he will do his best to get along.

9.   that he is only dreaming about this and it's not happening.

10.   that something very bad is going to happen to him.

11.   that it is frightening to be leaving.

12.   sorry for his wife.

13.   like watching TV or reading a book.

14.   like being alone somewhere.

15.   that he won't be able to concentrate on work anymore.

16.   that now he will be a different person.

17.   lonely and miserable.

SUMMARY

The title of my last chapter in *Adolescent Separation Anxiety*, Volume I, asked, "Where Has This Study Led Us?" We might well ask the same question with regard to the present volume. We have accumulated considerable information about the S.A.T. through the medium of research, and we have learned to understand the instrument far better than we did when we had first experimented with it. In the foreword to that volume, a statement from John Bowlby indicated, "Were your test to be used in future research, as I much hope it will, there is good prospect that many gaps in our knowledge will be filled." How prophetic those words were!

Examining the data, we realize that we have now learned how truly complicated the problems of attachment, individuation, and separation are. It will be noted how often the researchers have variously referred to these areas of study. Some have used the term "attachment-separation"; others, "separation-individuation," "attachment-individuation balance," etc. All seem to be referring to a balance between the internal growth of capacity for object relations and the capacity for separation as an individual with one's own resources. Various forms of attachment are referred to, such as "secure attachment," "anxious attachment," "detachment," "attachment disorders," "major attachment disorders," "major detachment disorders," "intimacy," "high intimacy," "merger status (enmeshment)," etc. The language that refers to the nature of attachment varies considerably depending on the theoretical orientation and the source in other research. With regard to individuation, Bowlby's term "self-reliance" is often utilized, while excesses in this area may carry the tag "self-sufficiency." Further, the term "autonomy" has been used with the same connotation, while in the early 1960s Bowlby coined a term "autonomous relatedness" to refer to an individuated person's capacity for attachment. The term "separation" has a number of meanings, at one time referring to internal development of separateness from the idealized maternal image and at another to the geographical distancing from parental figures or the sudden departure of close persons.

We have learned that the terms "attachment," "individuation," and "separation" must be constantly characterized by adjectives which describe the nature of these terms.

Interesting research findings on child abuse have been unearthed by the use of the S.A.T. The studies by DeLozier (1979) and by Mitchell (1980) have shown that severe forms of anxious attachment and detachment are characteristic of abusive mothers. DeLozier found that abusive mothers demonstrate an overall sensitivity to separation and feelings of helplessness, anxiety, and anger in response to significant separation experiences. Mitchell's major contribution in using the S.A.T. was to demonstrate that the level of individuation in abusive mothers was markedly decreased and that this was related to familial experience rather than indigence as seen in the Mexican-American community. Her findings agreed with DeLozier with regard to attachment disorders in abusive mothers. On the other hand, it appeared, according to Kaleita (1980), that abused adolescents expressed an excessive self-sufficiency which appeared to be largely related to those who were institutionalized rather than those who were living in intact families. Kaleita also did not find ethnic differences in the S.A.T. reactions to abuse in adolescents.

Excessive self-sufficiency seemed also to be a characteristic of children of divorce, as demonstrated in the S.A.T. This was shown by Miller (1980) in 9- to 12-year-olds and by Brody (1981) in 8-year-olds. The same finding appeared in the research of Burger (1981) on divorced adult males. In addition, he found evidence that in divorced males, during a two-year period there was a mild drop in the individuation level, and subsequently in the second year an almost precipitous rise in the individuation level. Further, attachment need showed a definite rise in the period from 2 to 12 months after the divorce, which he referred to in Bowlby's terminology as "despair." Hostility showed its strongest level in the first two months and then subsided, while the pain of separation seemed to be strongest in the second phase. Thus, divorce as a separation phenomenon appeared in the long run to affect mostly the individuation level, causing an increasing reliance on the self. While this does not affect every individual, child or adult, it rather appears to be generally widespread. It may well explain some of the wariness and detachment behavior of children of divorce, as well as the difficulty in many adults of forming new and more secure attachments of a marital nature.

The studies of college students have provided further evidence of the efficacy of the S.A.T. with adults. Sherry (1980), in a study of college freshmen who came from homes where the father was absent because of death or divorce, found evidence that at this stage of life individuals with such backgrounds are greater prey to separation anxiety and anxious attachment. Those who tended to be in need of more intense attachment were more prone to be avoidant or defensive, as demonstrated by their reaction to the reality avoidance items of the test. Levitz (1982), approaching the problem from a different perspective, was more concerned with the kind and nature of attachments that developed between college women and the opposite sex, which she referred to as "intimacy." Using Mahler's formulation and Erikson's ideas on identity, she probed the capacity of the S.A.T. to differentiate between individuals who showed various intimacy commitment levels in Orlofsky's scale, devised in part out of Erikson's conceptions. More disorders of the separation-individuation process were discovered among low-intimacy and merger groups than among high-intimacy groups, while the higher-intimacy groups demonstrated greater capacity for self-reliance, less depression, and less need to feel defensive about separation experiences.

Schwartz (1980), using the categories described in Volume II of *Adolescent Separation Anxiety*, found that the fear of death among college students was more evident in individuals who showed an ambivalent condition on the S.A.T., that is, hostile-anxious attachment. There seemed to be some indication that it was the uncertainty and ambivalence surrounding the attachment figure that eventually intensified the fear of death. It appeared that those persons with the most secure attachment had the lowest level of death anxiety on a scale constructed to measure this fear.

Similarly, Noble (1984) discovered that the S.A.T. was able to differentiate those who joined cults such as the Moonies and Krishnas from those who did not join after visiting or those who never were involved at all. The former were shown to have more major attachment and detachment disorders. Further, depressive reactions were far more common among the cultists than among the comparison group of college students.

In addition to the studies of mothers by DeLozier and Mitchell and by Hansburg (1981), Varela's (1982) interesting research into the relationship between maternal and child separation anxiety made several contributions to the use of the S.A.T. First, of singular importance was her development of a scale for very young children which had originally been devised by Klagsbrun and Bowlby in 1976 (see Chapter 20). Second, she developed an S.A.T. Index Score which proved to be extremely helpful for research purposes. Third, she discovered that mothers with high attachment scores on the Hansburg S.A.T. tend to report more child separation difficulties in the hospital, but there was no evidence that the child's separation response, as reported by the mother, was related to the child's attachment need. The use of one S.A.T. for the child and another one for the mother made possible some interesting discoveries, especially when descriptions of the child's actual hospital behavior were made available.

The effort to relate mothers' attachment and separation reactions on the S.A.T. to their children's behavior was attempted further by Kelly (1981). By evaluating these reactions of three groups of mothers, Kelly learned that mothers of hyperactive children tended to show rather severe defensive reactions that differentiated them from mothers of nonhyperactive children. No other factors of the test showed any differences. Not only were the defensive reactions checked statistically and found to be reliable, but also inquiries into their child-rearing behavior proved to be corroborative. This study may have helped to prove the possibility that much hyperactivity is basically genetic in origin and that the maternal behavior may have been shaped by the childhood disorder to begin with.

A different use of the S.A.T. by Duplak (1982) showed that the method by which the child may respond to the test could be altered in such a way as to produce a meaningful result, although with some loss. By using cartoon figures selected by the child as a selective method of attachment or avoidance, Duplak was able to demonstrate that the S.A.T. pictures could be used with learning-disabled boys and that these subjects would show increasing detachment behavior in the presence of separation.

Several papers have dealt with the use of the S.A.T. with mothers, a use which was a departure from its origination with children and adolescents. Attention should be drawn to the fact that supportive systems in extended families played some role in the reactions to the test. High levels of mother closeness to relatives placed the mothers in the mild anxious attachment category, while less closeness resulted in mild detachment patterns. Very secure patterns were small in number, and the conclusion was that it is likely that a large section of the population shows minor attachment and detachment disorders which must be considered common or normal. A theory is presented indicating a U-curve stretching from severe anxious attachment to severe detachment, with the greatest security area at a low point in the center. Another paper demonstrates that whole families may be profitably studied with the test.

Another extension of the S.A.T. was made with the elderly. The study, written by me in 1979, was the first effort in this direction. This study clearly demonstrated that those elderly who were most involved in life activities, such as employment or social pursuits, showed generally far better profiles on the S.A.T. than those who for a variety of reasons became relatively more isolated. The greatest sensitivity to separation pictures was shown by those who lost a spouse or who were confined by serious debilitating illness. This accorded well with Bowlby's attachment theory, in which he made similar claims with regard to separation experiences. Because Fisk (1979) studied only a more handicapped group of the elderly, he found a large percentage of depression reactions, which correlated highly with the loss of meaning in life. The S.A.T. demonstrated an increase in absurdity, depression, attachment need, and separation pain in a three-month period after nursing home placement. These results agreed closely with mine in that group of elderly who were similarly confined.

Black's study of the reliability of the S.A.T. was strongly indicative of the usefulness of the instrument. The statistical calculations which he made on the test, using both adolescents and their mothers over a six-month period, verified many of the original data published in 1972. While he found that one or two of the patterns could benefit from some revision, he was surprised at the extent of the reliability of the instrument, especially because of its semiprojective nature. However, he was somewhat puzzled by the absence of reliability for all the categories with the exception of the depressive syndrome. He suggested that further work needs to be done to clarify these categories.

I would like to say some final words about revisions which I believe to have made some contribution to the field. They provide a base for further work in the field of attachment, separation, and loss. Revision of methods of study is a never-ending process because there are so many perspectives from which the problems of these psychological areas may be fruitfully examined. I would urge students, as well as professors and clinical workers, to consider revisions of their own which will increase the armamentaria available. We do need these tests, as well as observational methods which can be utilized at stages of development much beyond those studies of Ainsworth and Main in early childhood.

Lastly, I would like to call attention to a number of other studies not presented in this volume that have been completed. The following list is provided here for those who might be interested in perusing them; these ten studies are available either through me or through University Microfilms International, Dissertation Copies, P.O. Box 1764, Ann Arbor, Michigan 48106. Numerous other studies known to me are in progress at various universities and professional schools throughout the country, and the results will be forthcoming in the ensuing years. (Professor Karl E. Pottharst, who has been one of the pioneers in developing the S.A.T., has accumulated considerable data on the test. These will no doubt become the basis for a new set of test norms which may be especially useful for work with adults. At this writing these data are not available to me but may be published in the near future in a book which Dr. Pottharst is completing.)

REFERENCES

Bennett, M. H. *Father-Daughter Incest: A Psychological Study of the Mother from an Attachment Theory Perspective.* Unpublished doctoral dissertation, California School of Professional Psychology, Los Angeles, 1980.

Bergenstal, K. W. *The Relationship of Father Support and Father Availability to Adolescent Sons' Experience of Loneliness and Separation Anxiety.* Unpublished doctoral dissertation, California School of Professional Psychology, Los Angeles, 1981.

Currie, P. S. *Current Attachment Patterns, Attachment History, and Religiosity as Predictors of Ego-Identity Status in Fundamentalist Christian Adolescents.* Unpublished doctoral dissertation, California School of Professional Psychology, Los Angeles, 1983.

Kroger, J. *Separation-Individuation and Ego Identity Status in New Zealand University Students.* Research supported by grant from Internal Research Committee, Victoria University of Wellington, New Zealand, 1984; submitted for publication.

Lesser, B. *An Application of Attachment Theory to a Follow-up Study of Battered Women.* Unpublished doctoral dissertation, California School of Professional Psychology, Los Angeles, 1981.

Marquart, M. E. *Separation-Individuation and Communication Variables in Families with a Schizophrenic Adolescent Compared to Families with a Non-Schizophrenic Adolescent.* Unpublished doctoral dissertation, California School of Professional Psychology, Los Angeles, 1978.

Miller, L. W. *Individual Differences in Rehabilitation as a Function of Attachment Behavior.* Unpublished doctoral dissertation, California School of Professional Psychology, Los Angeles, 1981.

Rubinstein, R. B. *Female Prostitution: Relationship to Early Separation and Sexual Experiences.* Unpublished doctoral dissertation, California Professional School of Psychology, Los Angeles, 1980.

Schiller, R. *Separation Anxiety and Abuse in Adolescence.* Unpublished doctoral dissertation, Case Western Reserve University, Cleveland, 1984.

Slutsky, M. *Adolescent Separation Anxiety as a Function of Perceived Parental Nurturance and Control.* Unpublished doctoral dissertation, California School of Professional Psychology, San Diego, 1983.

APPENDIX

A Spanish Version of the Separation Anxiety Test, *Marjorie J. Mitchell, translator*

In the course of time the Hebrew translation of the S.A.T. has unfortunately been misplaced and is no longer available to me. The Spanish translation, which was introduced by Marjorie Mitchell in her study of the Mexican-American community (see Chapter 2), is available, and the phrases for each picture are being reproduced here with her permission.

LA NIÑA VIVIRÁ PERMANENTEMENTE CON SU ABUELA Y SIN SUS PADRES

¿Alguna vez le ha pasado a usted esto? Sí ____ No ____
Si nunca le ha pasado a usted, ¿puede imaginarse como se sentiría esta niña(o)? Sí ____ No ____
Marque abajo todas las declaraciones que usted piensa que siente la niña(o).
La niña siente:

1. que ella estará mas feliz ahora.

2. que sus padres no la quieren más.

3. deseos de acurrucarse en un rincón solita.

4. un dolor terrible en su pecho.

5. que a ella no le importa lo que pase.

6. que está sola y miserable.

7. que ella va a hacer lo mejor para salir adelante.

8. que esta casa es un lugar espantoso para vivir.

9. que algo malo le va a pasar a ella ahora.

10. que es toda la culpa de sus vecinos.

11. que está enojada con alguién.

12. que ella jamás será la misma persona.

13. que si ella hubiera sido buena esto nunca hubiera pasado.

14. que es solo un sueño que realmente no está pasando.

15. como que está leyendo un libro, viendo T.V. o jugando.

16. lástima por sus padres.

17. que ella no podrá concentrarse en sus trabajos escolares.
    Si hay cualquier otra cosa que usted piensa que esta niña siente, escríbaloa abajo.

    _____
    _____
    _____

LA NIÑA ES TRASLADADA A UN SALON NUEVO

¿Puede usted recordar la última vez que le pasó esto? Sí ____ No____
¿ Puede usted imaginarse como se siente esta niña(o)? Sí ____ No ____
Marque abajo todas las declaraciones que usted piensa que siente la niña(o).

La niña siente:

1. que a ella no le importa lo que pase.

2. que este salón nuevo es un lugar espantoso.

3. lástima por su maestro anterior.

4. que si ella hubiera sido buena esto nunca hubiera pasado.

5. que es como jugar juegos con otros ninos.

6. que algo está pasando para cambiarla.

7. que ella hará lo mejor de la situación.

8. que realmente nadie la quiere.

9. que ella ahora va a pasarlo bien.

10. que es solo un sueño que realmente no esta pasando.

11. que ella no podrá concentrarse en sus trabajos escolares.

12. deseos de sentarse sola en un rincón del cuarto.

13. coraje con alguien.

14. que ella va a tener un dolor de estómago.

15. que está sola y miserable.

16. que algo terrible va a pasar.

17. que alguien es responsable de hacerle esto a ella.
Si tiene algo más que decir de como se siente esta niña(o) escríbalo abajo.

_____
_____
_____

LA FAMILIA SE ESTÁ TRASLADANDO A UN VECINDARIO NUEVO

¿Nunca le ha pasado esto a usted? Sí ____ No ____
Si no le ha pasado, ¿ se puede imaginar como se sentiria al pasarle esto?
Sí ____ No ____
Ahora trate de imaginar como este nino(a) se sentiria en esta escena.
Marque abajo todas las declaraciones que usted piensa que siente la
niña(o).

La niña siente:

1. miedo de irse.
2. un dolor en el estómago.
3. que los vecinos los forzaron a irse.
4. contenta de irse de este mal vecindario.
5. que está sola y miserable.
6. que a ella no le importa lo que pase.
7. que es solamente un sueño.
8. deseos de esconderse en cualquier lugar.
9. que vivir en la nueva casa será espantoso.
10. que ahora será una persona diferente.
11. que ella no podrá concentrarse en sus trabajos escolares.
12. lástima por sus padres.
13. que ella hará lo mejor de la situación.
14. deseos de pegarle a alguién en la cara.
15. que nadie la quiere más.
16. que ahora ella puede hacer nuevos amigos.
17. que si ella se hubiera portado bien en el vecindario no hubiera
    tenido que mudarse.
    Si hay algo más que usted quiera decir de la manera que esta
    niña(o) se siente, escríbalo abajo.

    _____
    _____
    _____
    _____

LA NIÑA DEJA A SU MADRE PARA IR A LA ESCUELA

Usted ha hecho lo que esta niña está haciendo muchas veces.
Sin duda usted tiene una idea de lo que ella siente, verdad? Si ____
No ____
Marque abajo todas las declaraciones que usted piensa que siente la
niña.

La niña siente:

1. que ella no podrá concentrarse en sus trabajos escolares.

2. miedo de irse.

3. que la escuela es un lugar espantoso.

4. que su madre no la quiere.

5. que a ella no le importa lo que pase.

6. coraje de etener que ir a la escuela.

7. deseos de reunirse con sus amigos e ir a la escuela.

8. que está contenta de alejarse de su casa.

9. lástima por su mamá.

10. que se va a enfermar.

11. que algo está pasando para cambiarla.

12. que si ella hubiera sido buena su mamá la hubiera dejado quedarse en la casa.

13. deseos de quedarse en casa en la cama.

14. que ella tratará lo mejor para llevarse bien con los demás.

15. que es solo un sueño que realmente no esta pasando.

16. que está sola y miserable.

17. que alguien está causando estos problemas.
Si hay cualquier otra cosa que usted piensa que esta niña siente,
escríbalo abajo.

_____

_____

418 RESEARCHES IN SEPARATION ANXIETY

LA NIÑA SE ALEJA DE SUS PADRES PARA IR A ACAMPAR

¿Puede usted recordar si le ha pasado esto a usted? Sí ____ No ____
¿Puede imaginarse como se sintió cuando le ocurrió? Sí ____ No____
Si no le ha pasado a usted, ¿puede imaginarse como se sentiria al pasarle esto? Sí ____ No ____
Marque abajo todas las declaraciones que usted piensa que siente la niña.

La niña siente:

1. lástima por sus padres.
2. coraje por tener que irse.
3. que estar en este lugar es espantoso.
4. que ahora será una persona diferente.
5. que es solo un sueño que realmente no está pasando.
6. que su mente no le ayuda a pensar lógicamente.
7. deseos de sentarse sola en el asiento de atrás del autobús.
8. que alguien hizo que le pasara esto.
9. deseos de leer un libro y de jugar.
10. que a ella no le importa lo que pase.
11. que algo terrible va a pasarle.
12. que va a tener un fuerte dolor de cabeza.
13. que realmente nadie la quiere.
14. que ella hará lo mejor de la situación.
15. que si ella hubiera sido una niña buena sus padres no la hubieran alejado de ellos.
16. que ahora realmente es libre para divertirse.
17. que está sola y miserable.
    Si tiene algo más que decir de como se siente esta niña(o), escríbalo abajo.

_____
_____
_____
_____

EL PADRE SE VA DESPUÉS DE UN PLEITO CON LA MADRE

¿Le ha pasado esto a usted? Sí _____ No _____
Si no le ha pasado, ¿se puede imaginar como se sentiría al pasarle esto?
Sí _____ No _____
Marque abajo todas las declaraciones que usted piensa que siente la niña(o).

La niña siente:

1. coraje con el padre.

2. que ahora es libre de hacer lo que quiera.

3. que su casa ahora será un lugar espantoso.

4. que no podrá concentrarse en sus trabajos escolares.

5. que algo terrible va a pasarle.

6. que alguien más es responsable de hacerle esto a ella.

7. deseos de leer un libro, arreglar algo o ver televisión.

8. que algo está pasando para cambiarla.

9. que está sola e infeliz.

10. que realmente nadie la quiere.

11. que ella va a estar muy enferma.

12. que quiere esconderse en la recámara de sus padres.

13. lástima por su madre.

14. que a ella no le importa lo que pase.

15. que ella tratará duro de resolver sus problemas.

16. que ella fue la causa de que su padre se fuera.

17. que es solo un sueño que realmente no está pasando.
    Si hay cualquier otra cosa que usted piensa que esta niña(o) siente, escríbalo abajo.

_____

_____

EL HERMANO MAYOR DE LA NINA ES UN MARINERO QUE SE VA EN UN VIAJE POR MAR

¿Nunca le ha pasado esto a usted? Sí ____ No ____
¿Puede imaginarse como se sentiría si le pasara esto a usted? Sí ____ No ____
Ahora trate de imaginar como este niño(a) se sentiría en esta escena.
Marque abajo todas las declaraciones que usted piensa que siente la niña(o).
La nina siente:

1. lástima por su hermano.
2. que si ella se hubiera portado bien su hermano no la hubiera dejado.
3. que es solo un sueño que realmente no está pasando.
4. que esto es algo espantoso.
5. que está muy enojada.
6. que ella jamás será la misma persona.
7. que está sola y miserable.
8. que le gustaría sentarse sola en su cuarto.
9. que alguien ha causado estos problemas.
10. deseos de jugar con sus amigas.
11. que ella no podrá concentrarse en sus trabajos escolares.
12. que ella hará lo mejor de la situación.
13. que algo terrible le va a pasar a ella.
14. que realmente nadie la quiere.
15. que ella va a tener un dolor de estómago.
16. que a ella no le importa lo que pase.
17. que ahora es libre de divertirse a su gusto.
    Si hay alguna otra cosa que usted piensa que esta niña siente, escríbalo abajo.

_____
_____
_____

UN JUEZ COLOCA A LA NIÑA EN UNA INSTITUCIÓN

¿Puede usted recordar la última vez que le pasó esto a usted? Sí ____
No ____

Si nunca le ha sucedido, ¿puede imaginarse como se sentiría si esto le ocurriera?

Marque abajo todas las declaraciones que usted piensa que siente la niña(o).

La niña siente:

1. que el mundo está lleno de personas malas que le hicieron esto a ella.
2. que es solo un sueño y despertará pronto.
3. deseos de suicidarse. Que le gustaria suicidarse.
4. que ella irá y tratará de hacer lo mejor posible.
5. lástima por sus padres.
6. que la sala de juicio es un lugar espantoso.
7. deseos de acurrucarse en una esquina.
8. que está débil y mareada.
9. que a ella no le importa lo que pase.
10. que estará feliz de llegar a la institución lo más pronto posible.
11. que a ella no la quieren mucho.
12. terror de lo que le pasará.
13. deseos de leer un libro o ver televisión.
14. coraje con el juez.
15. que ahora ella no aprenderá sus trabajos escolares.
16. que está sola e infeliz.
17. que ahora será una persona diferente.
    Si hay alguna otra cosa que usted piensa que esta niña(o) siente, escríbalo abajo.

_____
_____
_____

LA MADRE ACABA DE ACOSTAR A ESTA NIÑA

Esto probablemente la ha pasado a usted muchas veces.
¿Se puede imaginar que está pasando ahora mismo?
Marque abajo todas las declaraciones que usted piensa que siente la niña(o).

La nina siente:

1. que está enojada con su mamá.

2. que es espantoso estar sola.

3. que le gustaría esconderse debajo de las cobijas.

4. que a ella no le importa lo que pase.

5. que algo está pasando para cambiarla.

6. que alguien en la familia ha causado el alejamiento de su madre.

7. que ahora es libre para divertirse de la manera que a ella le guste.

8. que su madre no está con ella porque es una nina mala.

9. que es solo un sueno que realmente no está pasando.

10. que ella hará lo mejor de la situación.

11. deseos de leer un libro, ver T.V. o hacer modelos de plástico.

12. que algo malo le va a pasar.

13. lástima por su madre.

14. que se está enfermando.

15. que su madre realmente no la quiere.

16. que no podrá estudiar en la escuela mañana.

17. que está muy solitaria.
    Si hay cualquier otra cosa que usted piensa que esta niña siente, escríbalo abajo.

_____
_____
_____

SE LLEVAN LA MADRE DE LA NIÑA AL HOSPITAL

¿Ha pasado algo así en su familia?. Sí ____ No ____

Si no le ha pasado, ¿puede imaginarse usted como se sentiría? Sí ____
No ____

Marque abajo todas las declaraciones que usted piensa que siente la niña.

La niña siente:

1. coraje con alguién.

2. que ella jamás será la misma persona.

3. que está contenta porque su madre se va.

4. deseos de esconderse en su recámara.

5. que a ella no le importa lo que pase.

6. que realmente no está pasando, que solo es un sueño.

7. que a ella le vá a dar un dolor de cabeza.

8. que ella va a hacer lo mejor para seguir adelante.

9. temor de lo que le pueda ocurrir a ella.

10. lástima por su madre.

11. que nadie la quiere.

12. deseos de ver T.V.

13. que su madre se enfermó porque ella es mala.

14. que alguien más está causando estos problemas.

15. que ahora estar en su recámara será espantoso.

16. que está sola y miserable.

17. que ahora no podrá concentrarse en su trabajo escolar.
    Si hay otra cosa que usted piensa que esta niña siente, escríbalo abajo.

    _____

    _____

    _____

LA NIÑA Y SU PADRE ESTÁN DE PIE AL LADO DEL ATAÚD DE LA MADRE

¿Nunca le ha pasado esto a usted? Sí ____ No ____

Si no la ha pasado, ¿se puede imaginar como se sentiría al pasarle esto?
Sí ____ No ____

Ahora trate de imaginar como este niño(a) se sentiría en esta escena.
Marque abajo todas las declaraciones que usted piensa que siente la
niña(o).

La niña siente:

1. que ahora será una persona diferente.

2. temor de lo que le pueda suceder.

3. que si ella hubiera sido buena esto nunca hubiera pasado.

4. que ahora es libre de divertirse como le guste.

5. coraje por lo que le ha sucedido.

6. que nadie más la va a querer.

7. que no le importa lo que pase.

8. que su casa es un lugar espantoso para vivir.

9. deseos de sentarse sola en un rincón.

10. que otras personas son culpables de esto.

11. que ella hará lo mejor de la situación.

12. que es solo un sueño.

13. un fuerte dolor de cabeza.

14. lástima por su padre.

15. que está sola y miserable.

16. que ella no podrá concentrarse en sus trabajos escolares.

17. como que está leyendo un libro, o viendo televisión.
    Si hay cualquier otra cosa que usted piensa que esta niña siente,
    escribalo abajo.

LA NIÑA HUYE DE SU CASA

¿Usted hizo algo parecido? Sí _____ No _____

Si usted no lo ha hecho, ¿ha pensado hacer algo parecido a esto? Sí _____ No _____

¿Puede usted comprender porque esta niña(o) haría algo así? Sí _____ No _____

Marque abajo todas las declaraciones que usted piensa que siente la niña.

La niña siente:

1. que ella se va nada más para divertirse.
2. que está enojada con sus padres.
3. temor de ser castigada por algo que hizo.
4. que a ella no le importa lo que pase.
5. que sus padres no la quieren más.
6. que sus vecinos han incitado a sus padres en contra de ella.
7. que le van a dar unos calambres terribles en el estómago.
8. que ella va a hacer lo mejor para seguir adelante.
9. que es solo un sueño que realmente no está pasando.
10. que algo muy malo le va a pasar a ella.
11. que afuera es terriblemente espantoso.
12. lástima por sus padres.
13. como que está viendo televisión o leyendo un libro.
14. deseos de irse a su escondite.
15. que ella no podrá seguir estudiando.
16. que ahora ella será una persona diferente.
17. que está sola y miserable.
    Si hay cualquier otra cosa que usted piensa que esta niña siente, escríbalo abajo.

    _____

    _____

    _____

AUTHOR INDEX

SUBJECT INDEX

A

Abusive behavior, 4
  and poverty, 14
  predicting with S.A.T., 20
Abusive mothers. *See* Mothers,
  abusive
"Acting out," 271
Adolescents
  comparison of separation prob-
    lems with elderly, 269–270
  in marginal religious cults and
    separation reaction, 151–166
  self-destructiveness in, 226–229,
    248–249, 251–252
  separation anxiety in, 27–34
Aged. *See* Elderly
Aging, theories of, 171–172
Alarming events, 4
ANOVA, 193, 305
Attachment, 15
  and child abuse, 5, 16
  in children of divorce, 61
  in divorced males, 68, 71, 72, 75
  in divorced mothers, 43, 50
  in elderly, 172, 173, 258, 259
  and hospitalized children, 81
  in learning-disabled children,
    105–113

in mothers of hyperactive boys,
  98
in mothers separated from extended family, 281–286
pathological, S.A.T. protocols of,
  6
in religious cultists, 158, 161
and self-destruction, 230, 246
types of, 112
Attachment, anxious, 6, 14
  in abusive mothers, 18, 19
  in children from separated/di-
    vorced families, 41, 43, 49, 53
  in college freshmen, 117, 120
  in elderly, 271
  and fear of death, 146
  in mothers separated from ex-
    tended family, 287, 292, 295,
    298–301
  in mothers of hyperactive boys,
    99
  and separation-individuation in
    college women, 133, 134
  t-test analysis, 19
  x^2 analysis, 7
Attachment and Loss (Bowlby), 183
Attachment anxiety
  in abused and neglected
    adolescents, 27–34

432

F

Family, the
  and closeness, 287–293
  mothers' reaction to separation
    from, 277–301
studies of with S.A.T., 213–223
Family Story Test, 185
Fathers
  absence of, and separation reac-
    tions in college freshmen,
    116–120
  and religious cultists, 155
Fear-anxiety-pain syndrome
  and divorced males, 68–71

G

Glass rank biserial correlation, 6
Gorilla mothers, 279
Guilt
  and mothers of hyperactive chil-
    dren, 103

H

Hare Krishna. *See* International Society for Krishna Consciousness.
Hopkins Symptom Checklist, 172,
  176
Hospitalization
  and effects on children, 81
  revision of S.A.T. for hospitalized
    children and their mothers,
    343–364
  and separation anxiety in mothers
    and children, 79–93
Hostile Anxious Attachment
  and fear of death, 145–147
Hostility
  and children from separated/-
    divorced families, 52
  in divorced males, 71
  and fear of death, 143, 144

Hostility reactions
  in abusive mothers, 7
  in children of divorce, 62
  in college freshmen, 119
  in divorced males, 73
  and fear of death, 143
  hostile anxious attachment,
    145–147
Hyperactivity in boys, 95–103

I

Identity stress responses, 21
  in divorced males, 69, 72
  and fear of death, 145
  and self-destruction, 247
In the Shadow of Man (Goodall),
  229
Individuation, 15
  and children from separated/
    divorced families, 46, 61, 62
  in divorced males, 71, 75
  and fear of death, 142
  and intimacy in college women,
    125–136
  in youths belonging to marginal
    religious cults, 151, 152
Individuation-Hostility Index, 32,
  44
  and separated/divorced children,
    44, 49
  and family closeness, 291
Individuation index, 69
Individuation response pattern, 30,
  31
International Society for Krishna
  Consciousness, 156, 157
Intimacy
  See Orlofsky Intimacy Scale and
    college women, 125–136

J

Jewish Child Care Association, 227